Healing

COMPACT EDITION
Guide to
NATURAL
Healing

First printed in this edition 2004 by Geddes & Grosset,
David Dale House, New Lanark, ML11 9DJ
Reprinted 2004

ISBN 1 84205 307 8

Printed and bound in Poland, OZGraf S.A.

COMPACT EDITION
Guide to
NATURAL
Healing

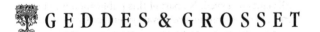

GEDDES & GROSSET

Contents

Natural Healing Through Alternative Medicine

'Alternative medicine' is a commonly used general term to describe all the methods of healing other than those practised by conventional doctors working in general practice or in hospitals. Most people become very familiar with the methods of conventional or orthodox medicine but are less informed about alternative therapies. This may be due partly to the fact that a bewildering variety of alternative therapies exists. However, a more significant factor is almost certainly that, until very recently, methods of alternative medicine were regarded with complete scepticism by much of the medical and scientific establishment. Attitudes have gradually become more enlightened (although doubts still exist in some quarters), and there has been a growing realization that alternative therapies have much to offer in the common aim of helping and healing patients.

Many forms of alternative medicine exist, some being complete methods in themselves, involving both diagnosis and treatment, while others are complementary to conventional practice. An example of the former is homeopathy while massage and aromatherapy fall into the latter category. Some methods of alternative therapy require a period of training at a recognized establishment, which may last for some years and is often undertaken by those with existing medical or nursing qualifications. For other methods, a relatively short training course is needed and the practitioner is not expected to possess medical knowledge to any great extent.

Some alternative therapies have been practised for centuries and date back to the earliest known human civilizations. This is hardly surprising when it is considered that it is orthodox medicine that is, in fact, relatively new, especially in the form in which it is known today. That which is now regarded as 'alternative' may have been the only form of treatment available to people in the past.

In this book, the most well-known and widely practised forms of alternative medicine are described in some detail and other methods are also mentioned. The book does not claim to cover the subject in full detail and some methods have been omitted. It is recommended that a person seeking alternative therapy in any form should obtain advice and as much information as possible, and first consult their own general practitioner.

Acupuncture

Origins

Acupuncture is an ancient Chinese therapy that involves inserting needles into the skin at specific points of the body. The word 'acupuncture' originated from a Dutch physician, William Ten Rhyne, who had been living in Japan during the latter part of the 17th century and it was he who introduced it to Europe. The term means literally 'prick with a needle'. The earliest textbook on acupuncture, dating from approximately 400 BC, was called *Nei Ching Su Wen*, which means 'Yellow Emperor's Classic of Internal Medicine'. Also recorded at about the same time was the successful saving of a patient's life by acupuncture, the person having been expected to die whilst in a coma. Legend has it that acupuncture was developed when it was realized that soldiers who recovered from arrow wounds were sometimes also healed of other diseases from which they were suffering. Acupuncture was very popular with British doctors in the early 1800s for pain relief and to treat fever. There was also a specific article on the successful treatment of rheumatism that appeared in *The Lancet*. Until the end of the Ching dynasty in China in 1911, acupuncture was slowly developed and improved, but then medicine from the west increased in popularity. However, more recently there has been a revival of interest and it is again widely practised throughout China. Also, nowadays the use of laser beams and electrical currents are found to give an increased stimulative effect when using acupuncture needles.

The specific points of the body into which acupuncture needles are inserted are located along 'meridians'. These are the pathways

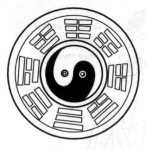

yin and yang

or energy channels and are believed to be related to the internal organs of the body. This energy is known as *qi* and the needles are used to decrease or increase the flow of energy, or to unblock it if it is impeded. Traditional Chinese medicine sees the body as being comprised of two natural forces known as the *yin* and *yang*. These two forces are complementary to each other but also opposing, the yin being the female force and calm and passive and also representing the dark, cold, swelling and moisture. The yang force is the male and is stimulating and aggressive, representing the heat and light, contraction and dryness. It is believed that the cause of ailments and diseases is due to an imbalance of these forces in the body, e.g. if a person is suffering from a headache or hypertension then this is because of an excess of yang. If, however, there is an excess of yin, this might result in tiredness, feeling cold and fluid retention.

The aim of acupuncture is to establish whether there is an imbalance of yin and yang and to rectify it by using the needles at certain points on the body. Traditionally there were 365 points but more have been found in the intervening period and nowadays there can be as many as 2,000. There are 14 meridians (12 of which are illustrated on page 13), called after the organs they represent, e.g. the lung, kidney, heart and stomach as well as two organs unknown in orthodox medicine – the triple heater or warmer, which relates to the activity of the endocrine glands and the control of temperature. In addition, the pericardium is concerned with seasonal activity and also regulates the circulation of the blood. Of the 14 meridians, there are two, known as the *du*, or governor, and the *ren*, or conception, which both run straight up the body's midline, although the du is much shorter, extending

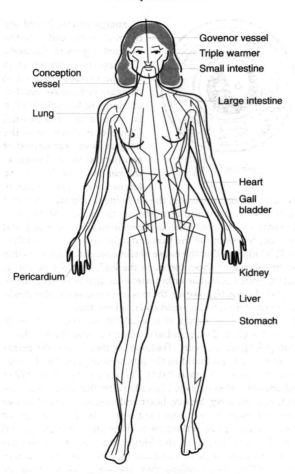

Govenor vessel

Triple warmer

Small intestine

Conception vessel

Large intestine

Lung

Heart

Gall bladder

Pericardium

Kidney

Liver

Stomach

the meridians

13

from the head down to the mouth, while the ren starts at the chin and extends to the base of the trunk.

There are several factors that can change the flow of qi (also known as shi or ch'i), and they can be of an emotional, physical or environmental nature. The flow may be changed to become too slow or fast, or it can be diverted or blocked so that the incorrect organ is involved and the acupuncturist has to ensure that the flow returns to normal. There are many painful afflictions for which acupuncture can be used. In the west, it has been used primarily for rheumatism, back pain and arthritis, but it has also been used to alleviate other disorders such as stress, allergy, colitis, digestive troubles, insomnia, asthma, etc. It has been claimed that withdrawal symptoms (experienced by people stopping smoking and ceasing other forms of addiction) have been helped as well.

Qualified acupuncturists complete a training course of three years duration and also need qualifications in the related disciplines of anatomy, pathology, physiology and diagnosis before they can belong to a professional association. It is very important that a fully qualified acupuncturist, who is a member of the relevant professional body, is consulted because at the present time, any unqualified person can use the title 'acupuncturist'.

The treatment

At a consultation, the traditional acupuncturist uses a set method of ancient rules to determine the acupuncture points. The texture and colouring of the skin, type of skin, posture and movement and the tongue will all be examined and noted, as will the patient's voice. These different factors are all needed for the Chinese diagnosis. A number of questions will be asked concerning the diet, amount of exercise taken, lifestyle, fears and phobias, sleeping patterns and reactions to stress. Each wrist has six pulses, and each of these stand for a main organ and its function. The pulses are felt (known as palpating), and by this means acupuncturists are able to diagnose any problems relating to the flow of qi and if there is any disease present in the internal organs. The first consultation may last an hour, especially if detailed questioning is necessary along with the palpation.

The needles used in acupuncture are disposable and made of a fine stainless steel and come already sealed in a sterile pack. They can be sterilized by the acupuncturist in a machine known as an autoclave but using boiling water is not adequate for this purpose. (Diseases such as HIV and hepatitis can be passed on by using unsterilized needles.) Once the needle is inserted into the skin it is twisted between the acupuncturist's thumb and forefinger to spread or draw the energy from a point. The depth to which the needle is inserted can vary from just below the skin to up to 12 mm (half an inch) and different sensations may be felt, such as a tingling around the area of insertion or a loss of sensation at that point. Up to 15 needles can be used but around five is generally sufficient. The length of time that they are left in varies from a few minutes to half an hour and this is dependent on a number of factors such as how the patient has reacted to previous treatment and the ailment from which he or she is suffering.

Patients can generally expect to feel an improvement after four to six sessions of therapy, the beneficial effects occurring gradually, particularly if the ailment has obvious and long-standing symptoms. Other diseases such as asthma will probably take longer before any definite improvement is felt. It is possible that some patients may not feel any improvement at all, or even feel worse after the first session and this is probably due to the energies in the body being over-stimulated. To correct this, the acupuncturist will gradually use fewer needles and for a shorter period of time. If no improvement is felt after about six to eight treatments, then it is doubtful whether acupuncture will be of any help. For general body maintenance and health, most traditional acupuncturists suggest that sessions be arranged at the time of seasonal changes.

How does it work?

There has been a great deal of research, particularly by the Chinese, who have produced many books detailing a high success rate for acupuncture in treating a variety of disorders. These results are, however, viewed cautiously in the west as methods of conducting clinical trials vary from east to west. Nevertheless trials have been carried out in the west and it has been discovered that a pain message can be stopped from reaching the brain using acupuncture. The signal would normally travel along a nerve but it is possible to 'close a gate' on the nerve, thereby preventing the message from reaching the brain, hence preventing the perception of pain. Acupuncture is believed to work by blocking the pain signal. However, doctors stress that pain can be a warning that something is wrong or of the occurrence of a particular disease, such as cancer, that requires an orthodox remedy or method of treatment.

It has also been discovered that there are substances produced by the body that are connected with pain relief. These substances are called endorphins and encephalins, and they are natural opiates. Studies from all over the world show that acupuncture stimulates the release of these opiates into the central nervous system, thereby giving pain relief. The amount of opiates released has a direct bearing on the degree of pain relief. Acupuncture is a widely used form of anaesthesia in China where, for suitable patients, it is said to be extremely effective (90 per cent). It is used successfully during childbirth, dentistry and for operations. Orthodox doctors in the west now accept that heat treatment, massage and needles used on a sensitive part of the skin afford relief from pain caused by disease elsewhere. These areas are known as trigger points, and they are not always situated close to the organ that is affected by disease. It has been found that approximately three-quarters of these trigger points are the same as the points used in Chinese acupuncture. Recent research has also shown that it is possible to find the acupuncture points by the use of electronic instruments as they register less electrical resistance than other areas of skin. As yet, no evidence has been found to substantiate the existence of meridians.

Auricular therapy
Auricular therapy is a method of healing using stimulation of different acupuncture points on the surface of the ear. Auricular

therapists claim that there are over 200 points on the ear that are connected to a particular organ, tissue or part of the body. If a disorder is present, its corresponding point on the ear may be sensitive or tender to touch and pressure, or there may even be some kind of physical sign such as a mark, spot or lump. Stimulation of the ear is carried out by means of acupuncture needles, or minute electric currents or a laser beam may be used.

It is claimed that auricular therapy is helpful in the treatment of various chronic conditions such as rheumatism and arthritis and also problems of addiction. During a first consultation, the auricular therapist obtains a detailed picture of the patient's state of health, lifestyle and family background. A physical examination of the ears is carried out and any distinguishing features are recorded. The therapist passes a probe over the surface of the ear to find any sensitive points that indicate the areas requiring treatment.

The practice of manipulating needles in the ear to cure diseases in other parts of the body is a very ancient one. It has been used for many hundreds of years in some eastern and Mediterranean countries and in China. Although the method of action is not understood, auricular therapy is becoming increasingly popular in several countries of the world including Great Britain.

The Alexander Technique

Breaking the habit of bad posture

The Alexander Technique is a practical and simple method of learning to focus attention on how we use ourselves during daily activities. Frederick Mathias Alexander (1869–1955), an Australian therapist, demonstrated that the difficulties many people experience in learning, in control of performance, and in physical functioning are caused by unconscious habits. These habits interfere with your natural poise and your capacity to learn. When you stop interfering with the innate coordination of the body, you can take on more complex activities with greater self-confidence and presence of mind. It is about learning to bring into our conscious awareness the choices we make, as we make them. Gentle hands-on and verbal instruction reveal the underlying principles of human coordination, allow the student to experience and observe their own habitual patterns, and give the means for release and change.

Armouring

Most of us are unconsciously armouring ourselves in relation to our environment. This is hard work and often leaves us feeling anxious, alienated, depressed and unlovable. Armouring is a deeply unconscious behaviour that has probably gone on since early childhood, maybe even since infancy. Yet it is a habit we can unlearn in the present through careful self-observation. We can unlearn our use of excess tension in our thoughts, movements, and relationships.

Correct posture

The Alexander technique is based on correct posture so that the body is able to function naturally and with the minimum amount of muscular effort. F. M. Alexander was also an actor and found that he was losing his voice when performing but after rest his condition temporarily improved. Although he received medical help, the condition was not cured and it occurred to him that whilst acting he might be doing something that caused the problem.

To see what this might be he performed his act in front of a mirror and saw what happened when he was about to speak. He experienced difficulty in breathing and lowered his head, thus making himself shorter. He realized that the strain of remembering his lines and having to project his voice, so that people furthest away in the audience would be able to hear, was causing him a great deal of stress and the way he reacted was a quite natural reflex action.

In fact, even thinking about having to project his voice made the symptoms recur and from this he concluded that there must be a close connection between body and mind. He was determined to try and improve the situation and gradually, by watching and altering his stance and posture and his mental attitude to his performance on stage, matters improved. He was able to act and speak on stage and use his body in a more relaxed and natural fashion.

In 1904 Alexander travelled to London where he had decided to let others know about his method of retraining the body. He soon became very popular with other actors who appreciated the benefits of using his technique. Other public figures, such as the author Aldous Huxley, also benefited.

Later he went to America, achieving considerable success and international recognition for his technique. At the age of 78 he suffered a stroke but by using his method he managed to regain

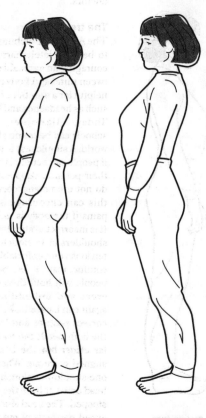

slouching   *too unbending*

the use of all his faculties – an achievement that amazed his doctors.

The treatment

The Alexander technique is said to be completely harmless, encouraging an agreeable state between mind and body and is also helpful for a number of disorders such as headaches and back pain. Today, Alexander training schools can be found all over the world. A simple test to determine if people can benefit is to observe their posture. People frequently do not even stand correctly and this can encourage aches and pains if the body is unbalanced. It is incorrect to stand with round shoulders or to slouch. This often looks uncomfortable and discomfort may be felt. Sometimes people will hold themselves too erect and unbending, which again can have a bad effect. The correct posture and balance for the body needs the least muscular effort but the body will be aligned correctly. When walking one should not slouch, hold the head down or have the shoulders stooped. The head should be balanced correctly above the spine with the shoulders relaxed. It is suggested that the weight of the

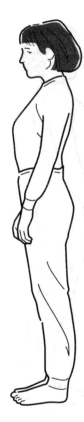

correct posture

body should be felt being transferred from one foot to the other whilst walking.

Once a teacher has been consulted, all movements and how the body is used will be observed. Many muscles are used in everyday activities, and over the years bad habits can develop unconsciously, with stress also affecting the use of muscles. This can be demonstrated in people gripping a pen with too much force or holding the steering wheel of a car too tightly whilst driving. Muscular tension can be a serious problem affecting some people and the head, neck and back are forced out of line, which in turn leads to rounded shoulders with the head held forward and the back curved. If this situation is not altered and the body is not re-aligned correctly, the spine will become curved with a hump possibly developing. This leads to back pain and puts a strain on internal organs such as the chest and lungs.

An Alexander teacher guides a person, as he or she moves, to use less tension. The instructor works by monitoring the student's posture and reminding him or her to implement tiny changes in movement to eradicate the habit of excess tension. Students learn to stop bracing themselves up, or to stop collapsing into themselves. As awareness grows, it becomes easier to recognize and relinquish the habit of armouring and dissolve the artificial barriers we put between ourselves and others.

An analogy of this process can be seen in the now familiar three-dimensional Magic Eye Art. With our ordinary way of looking we see only a mass of dots. When we shift to the 'Magic Eye' way of seeing, a three-dimensional object appears. Through the Alexander technique a similar type of experience is available. But the three-dimensional object we experience is ourselves.

No force is used by the teacher other than some gentle manipulation to start pupils off correctly. Some teachers use light pushing methods on the back and hips, etc, while others might first ensure that the pupil is relaxed and then pull gently on the neck, which stretches the body. Any bad postures will be corrected by the teacher and the pupil will be shown how best to alter this so that muscles will be used most effectively and with the least effort. Any manipulation that is used will be to ease the body into a more relaxed and natural position. It is helpful to be completely aware of using the technique not only on the body but also with the mind. With frequent use of the Alexander technique for posture and the release of tension, the muscles and the body should be used correctly with a consequent improvement in, for example, the manner of walking and sitting.

The length of time for each lesson can vary from about half an hour to three quarters of an hour and the number of lessons is usually between 10 and 30, by which time pupils should have gained sufficient knowledge to continue practising the technique by themselves. Once a person has learned how to improve posture, it will be found that he or she is taller and carrying the body in a more upright manner. The technique has been found to be of benefit to dancers, athletes and those having to speak in public. Other disorders claimed to have been treated successfully are depressive states, headaches caused by tension, anxiety, asthma, hypertension, respiratory problems, colitis, osteoarthritis and rheumatoid arthritis, sciatica and peptic ulcer.

The Alexander technique is recommended for all ages and types of people as their overall quality of life, both mental and physical, can be improved. People can learn how to resist stress and one eminent professor experienced a great improvement in a variety of ways: in quality of sleep; lessening of high blood pressure and improved mental awareness. He even found that his ability to play a musical instrument had improved.

The Alexander technique can be applied to two positions adopted every day, namely sitting in a chair and sitting at a desk. To be seated in the correct manner the head should be comfortably balanced, with no tension in the shoulders, and a small gap between the knees (if legs are crossed the spine and pelvis become out of line or twisted) and the soles of the feet should be flat on the floor. It is incorrect to sit with the head lowered and the shoulders slumped forward because the stomach becomes restricted and breathing may also be affected. On the other hand, it is also incorrect to hold the body in a stiff and erect position.

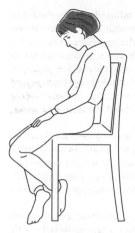

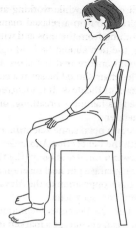

slumped posture   *comfortably balanced posture*

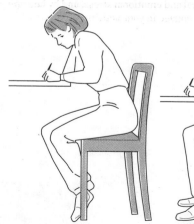

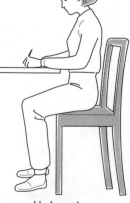

bad posture   *good balanced posture*

To sit correctly while working at a table, the body should be held upright but in a relaxed manner with any bending movement coming from the hips and with the seat flat on the chair. If writing, the pen should be held lightly and if using a computer one should ensure that the arms are relaxed and feel comfortable. The chair should be set at a comfortable height with regard to the level of the desk. It is incorrect to lean forward over a desk because this hampers breathing, or to hold the arms in a tense, tight manner .

There has been some scientific research carried out that concurs with the beliefs that Alexander formed, such as the relationship between mind and body (the thought of doing an action actually triggering a physical reaction or tension). Today, doctors do not have any opposition to the Alexander technique and may recommend it on occasions.

Although the Alexander technique does not treat specific symptoms, you can encourage a marked improvement in overall health, alertness, and performance by consciously eliminating harmful habits that cause physical and emotional stress, and by becoming more aware of how you engage in your activities.

Chiropractic

Origins
Daniel Palmer

The word chiropractic originates from two Greek words *kheir*, which means 'hand', and *praktikos*, which means 'practical'. A school of chiropractic was established in about 1895 by a healer called Daniel Palmer (1845–1913). He was able to cure a man's deafness that had occurred when he bent down and felt a bone click. Upon examination Palmer discovered that some bones of the man's spine had become displaced. After successful manipulation the man regained his hearing. Palmer formed the opinion that if there was any displacement in the skeleton this could affect the function of nerves, either increasing or decreasing their action and thereby resulting in a malfunction i.e. a disease.

Pain relief by manipulation

Chiropractic is used to relieve pain by manipulation and to correct any problems that are present in joints and muscles but especially the spine. Like osteopathy, no use is made of surgery or drugs. If there are any spinal disorders they can cause widespread problems elsewhere in the body such as the hip, leg or arm and can also initiate lumbago, sciatica, a slipped disc or other back problems. It is even possible that spinal problems can result in seemingly unrelated problems such as catarrh, migraine, asthma, constipation, stress, etc. However, the majority of a chiropractor's patients suffer mainly from neck and back pain. People suffering from whiplash injuries sustained in car accidents commonly seek the help of a chiropractor. The whiplash effect is caused when the head is violently wrenched either forwards or backwards at the time of impact.

Another common problem that chiropractors treat is headaches, and it is often the case that tension is the underlying cause as it makes the neck muscles contract. Athletes can also obtain relief from injuries such as tennis elbow, pulled muscles, injured ligaments and sprains, etc. As well as the normal methods of manipulating joints, the chiropractor may decide it is necessary to use applications of ice or heat to relieve the injury.

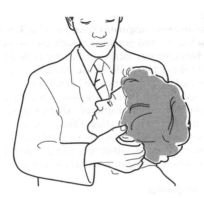

chiropractic treatment of the neck

Children can also benefit from treatment by a chiropractor, as there may be some slight accident that occurs in their early years that can reappear in adult life in the form of back pain. It can easily happen, for example, when a child learns to walk and bumps into furniture, or when a baby falls out of a cot. This could result in some damage to the spine that will show only in adult life when a person experiences back pain. At birth, a baby's neck may be injured or the spine may be strained if the use of forceps is necessary, and this can result in headaches and neck problems as he or she grows to maturity. This early type of injury could also account for what is known as 'growing pains', when the real problem is actually damage that has been done to the bones or muscles. If a parent has any worries it is best to consult a doctor and it is possible that the child will be recommended to see a qualified chiropractor. To avoid any problems in adult life, chiropractors recommend that children have occasional examinations to detect any damage or displacement in bones and muscles.

As well as babies and children, adults of all ages can benefit from chiropractic. There are some people who regularly take painkillers for painful joints or back pain, but this does not deal with the root cause of the pain, only the symptoms that are produced. It is claimed that chiropractic could be of considerable help in giving treatment to these people. Many pregnant women experience backache at some stage during their pregnancy because of the extra weight that is placed on the spine, and they also may find it difficult keeping their balance. At the time of giving birth, changes take place in the pelvis and joints at the bottom of the spine and this can be a cause of back pain. Lifting and carrying babies, if not done correctly, can also damage the spine and thereby make the back painful.

It is essential that any chiropractor is fully qualified and registered with the relevant professional association. At the initial visit, a patient will be asked for details of his or her case history, including the present problem, and during the examination painful and tender areas will be noted and joints will be checked to see whether they are functioning correctly or not. X-rays are frequently used by chiropractors since they can show signs of bone disease, fractures or arthritis as well as the spine's condition. After the initial visit, any treatment will normally begin as soon as the patient has been informed of the chiropractor's diagnosis. If it has been decided that chiropractic therapy will not be of any benefit, the patient will be advised accordingly.

For treatment, underwear and/or a robe will be worn, and the patient will either lie, sit or stand on a specially designed couch. Chiropractors use their hands in a skilful way to effect the different manipulative techniques. If it is decided that manipulation is necessary to treat a painful lumbar joint, the patient will need to lie on his or her side. The upper and lower spine will then be rotated manually but in opposite ways. This manipulation will have the effect of partially locking the joint that is being treated, and the upper leg is usually flexed to aid the procedure. The vertebra that is immediately below or above the joint will then be felt by the chiropractor, and the combination of how the patient is lying, coupled with gentle pressure applied by the chiropractor's hand, will move the joint to its furthest extent of normal movement. There will then be a very quick push applied on the vertebra, which results in its movement being extended further than normal, ensuring that full use of the joint is regained. This is due to the muscles that surround the joint being suddenly stretched, which has the effect of relaxing the muscles of the spine that work upon the joint. This alteration should cause the joint to be able to be used more naturally and should not be a painful procedure.

There can be a variety of effects felt after treatment – some patients may feel sore or stiff, or may ache some time after the treatment, while others will experience the lifting of pain at once. In some cases there may be a need for multiple treatments, perhaps four or more, before improvement is felt. On the whole, problems that have been troubling a patient for a considerable time (chronic) will need more therapy than anything that occurs quickly and is very painful (acute).

Although there is only quite a small number of chiropractors in the UK – yet this numbers is increasing – there is a degree of contact and liaison between them and doctors. It is generally accepted that chiropractic is an effective remedy for bone and muscular problems, and the majority of doctors would be happy to accept a chiropractor's diagnosis and treatment, although the treatment of any general diseases, such as diabetes or asthma, would not be viewed in the same manner.

Hydrotherapy

The healing quality of water

Hydrotherapy is the use of water to heal and ease a variety of ailments, and the water may be used in a number of different ways. The healing properties of water have been recognized since ancient times, notably by the Greek, Roman and Turkish civilizations but also by people in Europe and China. Most people know the benefits of a hot bath in relaxing the body, relieving muscular aches and stiffness, and helping to bring about restful sleep. Hot water or steam causes blood vessels to dilate, opens skin pores and stimulates perspiration, and relaxes limbs and muscles. A cold bath or shower acts in the opposite way and is refreshing and invigorating. The cold causes blood vessels in the skin to constrict and blood is diverted to internal tissues and organs to maintain the core temperature of the body. Applications of cold water or ice reduce swelling and bruising and cause skin pores to close.

Physiotherapy

In orthodox medicine, hydrotherapy is used as a technique of physiotherapy for people recovering from serious injuries with problems of muscle wastage. Also, it is used for people with joint problems and those with severe physical disabilities. Many hospitals also offer the choice of a water birth to expectant mothers, and this has become an increasingly popular method of childbirth. Hydrotherapy may be offered as a form of treatment for other medical conditions in *naturopathy,* using the techniques listed above. It is wise to obtain medical advice before proceeding with hydrotherapy, and this is especially important for elderly persons, children and those with serious conditions or illnesses.

Treatment techniques in hydrotherapy
Hot baths
Hot baths are used to ease muscle and joint pains and inflammation. Also, warm or hot baths, with the addition of various substances such as seaweed extract to the water, may be used to help the healing of some skin conditions or minor wounds. After childbirth, frequent bathing in warm water to which a mild antiseptic has been added is recommended to heal skin tears.

Most people know the relaxing benefits of a hot bath. A bath with the temperature between 36.5°C and 40°C (98°F and 104°F) is very useful as a means of muscle relaxation. To begin with, five minutes immersion in a bath of this temperature is enough. This can be stepped up to ten minutes a day, as long as no feelings of weakness or dizziness arise. It is important to realize that a brief hot bath has quite a different effect from a long one.

There is nothing to be gained by prolonging a hot bath in the hope of increasing the benefit. Immersion in hot water acts not only on the surface nerves but also on the autonomic nervous system (which is normally outside our control), as well as the hormone-producing glands, particularly the adrenals, which become less active. A hot bath is sedative, but a hot bath that is prolonged into a long soak has quite the opposite effect.

Cold baths
Cold baths are used to improve blood flow to internal tissues and organs and to reduce swellings. The person may sit for a moment in shallow cold water with additional water being splashed onto exposed skin. An inflamed, painful part may be immersed in cold water to reduce swelling. The person is not allowed to become chilled, and this form of treatment is best suited for those able to dry themselves rapidly with a warm towel. It is not advisable for people with serious conditions or for the elderly or very young.

Neutral bath

There are many nerve endings on the skin surface and these deal with the reception of stimuli. More of these are cold receptors than heat receptors. If water of a different temperature to that of the skin is applied, it will either conduct heat to it or absorb heat from it. These stimuli have an influence on the sympathetic nervous system and can affect the hormonal system. The greater the difference between the temperature of the skin and the water applied, the greater will be the potential for physiological reaction. Conversely, water that is the same temperature as the body has a marked relaxing and sedative effect on the nervous system. This is of value in states of stress, and has led to the development of the so-called 'neutral bath'.

Before the development of tranquillizers, the most dependable and effective method of calming an agitated patient was the use of a neutral bath. The patient was placed in a tub of water, the temperature of which was maintained at between 33.5°C and 35.6°C (92°F to 96°F), often for over three hours, and sometimes for as long as twenty-four hours. Obviously, this is not a practical proposition for the average tense person.

As a self-help measure, the neutral bath does, however, offer a means of sedating the nervous system if used for relatively short periods. It is important to maintain the water temperature at the above level, and for this a bath thermometer should be used. The bathroom itself should be kept warm to prevent any chill in the air.

Half an hour of immersion in a bath like this will have a sedative, or even soporific, effect. It places no strain on the heart, circulation or nervous system, and achieves muscular relaxation as well as a relaxation and expansion of the blood vessels: all of these effects promote relaxation. This bath can be used in conjunction with other methods of relaxation, such as breathing techniques and meditation, to make it an even more efficient way of wiping out stress. It can be used daily if necessary.

Steam baths

Steam baths, along with saunas and Turkish baths, are used to encourage sweating and the opening of skin pores and have a cleansing and refreshing effect. The body may be able to eliminate harmful substances in this way and treatment finishes with a cool bath.

Sitz baths

Sitz baths are usually given as a treatment for painful conditions with broken skin, such as piles or anal fissure, and also for ailments affecting the urinary and genital organs. The person sits in a specially designed bath that has two compartments, one with warm water, the other with cold. First, the person sits in the warm water, which covers the lower abdomen and hips, with the feet in the cold water compartment. After three minutes, the patient changes round and sits in the cold water with the feet in the warm compartment.

Hot and cold sprays

Hot and cold sprays of water may be given for a number of different disorders but are not recommended for those with serious illnesses, elderly people or young children.

Wrapping

Wrapping is used for feverish conditions, backache and bronchitis. A cold wet sheet that has been squeezed out is wrapped around the person, followed by a dry sheet and warm blanket. These are left in place until the inner sheet has dried and the coverings are then removed. The body is sponged with tepid water (at blood heat) before being dried with a towel. Sometimes the wrap is applied to a smaller area of the body, such as the lower abdomen, to ease a particular problem, usually constipation.

Cold packs

Cold packs were described by the famous 19th-century Bavarian pastor, Sebastian Kniepp, in his famous treatise *My Water Cure*, in which he explained the advantages of hydrotherapy. A cold pack is really a warm pack – the name comes from the cold nature of the initial application.

For a cold pack you need:
A large piece of cotton material; a large piece of flannel or woollen (blanket) material; a rubber sheet to protect the bed; a hot water bottle; safety pins.

First, soak the cotton material in very cold water, wring it out well and place it on the flannel material that is spread out on the rubber sheet on the bed. Lay the person who is having the treatment on top of the damp material, fold it round his trunk and cover him up at once with the flannel material. Safety-pin it all firmly in place.

Now pull up the top bed covers and provide a hot water bottle. The initial cold application produces a reaction that draws fresh blood to the surface of the body; this warmth, being well insulated, is retained by the damp material. The cold pack turns into a warm pack, which gradually, over a period of six to eight hours, bakes itself dry. Usually lots of sweat will be produced, so it is necessary to wash the materials well before using again.

The pack can be slept in – in fact it should encourage deeper, more refreshing sleep. Larger, whole body packs can be used, which cover not only the trunk but extend from the armpits to the feet, encasing the recipient in a cocoon of warmth.

If a feeling of damp coldness is felt, the wet material may be inadequately wrung out, or the insulation materials too loose or too few.

Flotation

A form of sensory deprivation, flotation involves lying face up in an enclosed, dark tank of warm, heavily salted water. There is no sound, except perhaps some natural music to bring the client into a dream-like state. It is exceptionally refreshing and induces a deep, relaxing sleep.

Kinesiology

The function of kinesiology

Kinesiology is a method of maintaining health by ensuring that all muscles are functioning correctly. It is believed that each muscle is connected with a specific part of the body such as the digestive system, circulation of the blood and specific organs, and if a muscle is not functioning correctly this will cause a problem in its related part of the body. The word is derived from *kinesis*, which is Greek for 'motion'. Kinesiology originated in 1964 and was developed by an American chiropractor named George Goodheart who realized that while he was treating a patient for severe pain in the leg, by massaging a particular muscle in the upper leg, the pain experienced by the patient eased and the muscle was strengthened. Although he used the same method on different muscles, the results were not the same. Previous research done by an osteopath named Dr Chapman, in the 1900s, indicated that there were certain 'pressure points' in the body that were connected with particular muscles and, if these were massaged, lymph would be able to flow more freely through the body. Using these pressure points, Chapman found which point was connected to each particular muscle and realized why, when he had massaged a patient's upper leg muscle, the pain had lessened. The pressure point for that leg muscle was the only one that was situated above the actual muscle – all the other points were not close to the part of the body with which they were connected.

The use of pressure points

In the 1930s it was claimed that there were similar pressure points located on the skull and, by exerting a light pressure on these, the flow of blood to their related organs could be assisted. Goodheart tested this claim, which originated from an osteopath called Terence Bennett, and discovered that after only fingertip pressure for a matter of seconds, it improved the strength of a particular muscle. After some time he was able to locate sixteen points on the head, the back of the knee and by the breastbone that were all allied to groups of important muscles. Goodheart was surprised that so little force applied on the pressure point could have such an effect on the muscle, so to further his studies he then applied himself to acupuncture. This is a form of healing that also makes use of certain points located over the body but that run along specific paths known as meridians. After further study, Goodheart came to the conclusion that the meridians could be used for both muscles and organs. The invisible paths used in kinesiology are exactly the same as the ones for acupuncture.

Energy and lymph

A kinesiologist will examine a patient and try to discover whether there is any lack of energy, physical disorders or inadequate nutrition that is causing problems. Once any troublesome areas have been located, the practitioner will use only a light massage on the relevant pressure points (which, as mentioned, are generally not close to their associated muscle). For example, the edge of the rib cage is where the pressure points for the muscles of the upper leg are situated. In kinesiology it is maintained that the use of pressure points is effective because the flow of blood to muscles is stimulated and therefore a good supply of lymph is generated too. Lymph is a watery fluid that takes toxins from the tissues and if muscles receive a good supply of both lymph and blood they should function efficiently. As in acupuncture, it is maintained that there is an unseen flow of energy that runs through the body and if this is disrupted for any reason, such as a person being ill or suffering from stress, then the body will weaken due to insufficient energy being produced. The way in which a kinesiologist assesses the general health of a patient is by testing the strength

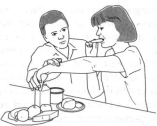

*A – determining sensitivity or
allergy to foods*

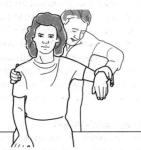

*C – determining whether there are
weak muscles in the stomach*

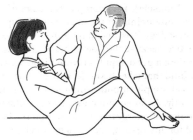

*B – determining whether there is
weakness in the shoulder muscle*

of the muscles as this will provide information on the flow of energy. It is claimed that by finding any inbalance and correcting it, kinesiology can be used as a preventive therapy. If there is a lack of minerals and vitamins in the body or trouble with the digestive system, it is claimed that these are able to be diagnosed by the use of kinesiology. If a person is feeling 'below par' and constantly feels tired, it is believed that these conditions are aggravated by a sluggish flow of the internal body fluids such as the circulation of blood. Kinesiologists can treat the disorder by stimulating the flow of lymph and blood by massaging the pressure points.

Although it is claimed that kinesiology can be of help to all people, it is widely known for the treatment of people suffering from food allergies or those who are sensitive to some foods. It is believed that the chemicals and nutrients contained in food cause various reactions in the body, and if a particular food has the effect of making muscles weak, then it would be concluded that a person has an allergy to it. Allergic reactions can cause other problems such as headaches, tension, colds, tiredness and a general susceptibility to acquiring any passing infections.

There are two simple tests that can easily be tried at home to determine if there is any sensitivity or allergy to certain foods. This is done by testing the strength of a strong muscle in the chest, and to carry this out the person being tested will need the help of a partner. There is no need to exert real force at any time, just use the minimum amount needed to be firm but gentle. To test the chest muscle, sit erect, holding the left arm straight out at right angles to the body. The elbow should be facing outwards and the fingers and thumb drooping towards the table. The partner will then place his or her right hand on the person's nearest shoulder (the right) and the two fingers only on the area around the left wrist. A gentle downward pressure will then be exerted by the partner on the person's wrist who will try to maintain the level of the arm, whilst breathing in a normal fashion. This downward pressure should be exerted for approximately five seconds. If the person was able to resist the downwards pressure and the muscle felt quite firm, then the allergy test can be tried. However, if this was not the case and the person was unable to keep the arm level, the muscle would not be suitable for use in the subsequent test. It would therefore be advisable to use another muscle such as one in the arm. To do this, place an arm straight down at the side of the body with the palm of the hands facing outwards. The partner will then use the same amount of pressure to try and move the arm outwards, again for a similar amount of time. If the person is unable to keep the arm in the same position, then it would be advisable to get in touch with a trained kinesiologist.

To undertake the allergy test, hold the left arm in the same way as for testing the muscle (*see* page 37, figure A). If, for example, the food that is suspected of causing an allergy is chocolate, a small piece of this should be put just in the mouth, there is no need for it to be eaten. This time as well as applying the pressure on the wrist as before, the partner should put his or her first two digits of the left hand below the person's right ear. Once again, the person tries to resist the downwards force and if successful, it is claimed that there is no sensitivity or allergy connected with that food. However, if this does not happen and the arm is pushed downwards or even feels slightly weak, then kinesiology would suggest that this food, if eaten at all, should never be consumed in any great amount.

It is claimed that the use of kinesiology can be of benefit to people who suffer from irrational fears or phobias. An example of this is the recommendation that the bone below the eye, just level with the pupil, is softly tapped. Neck and back pain can be treated without any manipulation of joints and some of the methods can be learnt by patients for use at home. An example of this for the alleviation of back pain is for a patient to massage the muscle situated on the inside of the thigh. This is said to be of benefit for any muscles that are weak as they are the reason for a painful back.

A number of other practitioners, such as homeopaths, herbalists and osteopaths make use of kinesiology, so if there is a problem connected with the ligaments, muscles or bones it may be advisable to contact a chiropractor or osteopath who is also qualified in kinesiology. If the problem is of a more emotional or mental nature, then it might be best to select a counsellor or psychotherapist who also practises kinesiology. It is important always to use a fully qualified practitioner and the relevant association should be contacted for information. At the first consultation, detailed questions will be asked concerning the medical history, followed by the therapist checking the muscles' ability to function effectively. For instance, a slight pressure will be exerted on a leg or arm while the patient holds it in a certain way. The patient's ability to maintain that position against the pressure is noted and if the patient is unable to do so, then the therapist will find the reason why by further examination. Once the areas in need of 'rebalancing' have been identified, he therapist will use the relevant pressure points to correct matters. It is believed that if some of the points are painful or sore to the touch, this is because there has been an accumulation of toxins in the tissues, and these toxins stop the impulses between muscles and the brain. If this is the case, the muscle is unable to relax properly and can cause problems in areas such as the neck and shoulders.

There are ways of identifying any possible problems. For example, if there is any weakness in the shoulder muscle it may be that there is some problem connected with the lungs. To test for this, the patient sits upright with one arm raised to slightly below shoulder level and the other arm lower and out to the front. The therapist grasps the patient's upper arm and presses gently downwards on the raised arm at the elbow (*see* page 37, figure B). If the mucle is functioning correctly then this downwards force should not be allowed to move the arm lower. If the patient is suffering from pain in the back, the probable cause lies with weak muscles in the stomach. To test for this, the patient sits on the floor with the knees raised, the arms crossed on the chest and then they lean backwards (*see* page 37 figure C). The therapist checks the stomach muscles' efficiency by pushing gently backwards on the patient's crossed arms. If all is well the patient should be able to maintain the position and not lean back any further.

After treatment by massage of the pressure points, there may well be some tenderness experienced for one or two days as the toxins in the tissues dissipate gradually. However, there should be an overall feeling of an improvement in health and in particular with the problem that was being treated.

Although there has been an increase in the use of kinesiology by doctors to help discover the cause of an ailment, there has been little scientific research carried out. Therefore, the majority of doctors using conventional medicine do not believe that the flow of electrical energy present in the body can be changed by the use of massage or similar methods.

Massage

Introduction
Origins

We massage ourselves nearly every day. The natural reaction to reach out and touch a painful part of the body – such as a sprain – forms the basis of massage. As long ago as 3000 BC massage was used as a therapy in the Far East, making it one of the oldest treatments used by humans. In 5 BC in ancient Greece, Hippocrates recommended that to maintain health, a massage using oils should be taken daily after a perfumed bath. Greek physicians were well used to treating people who suffered from pain and stiffness in the joints. The relaxation and healing powers of massage have been well documented over the past 5,000 years.

The therapeutic value of applying oils and rubbing parts of the body to lessen pain and prevent illness was recognized among the ancient Mediterranean civilizations. In ancient times scented oils were almost always used when giving massages, creating an early form of aromatherapy massage.

Popularity

Massage increased in popularity when, in the 19th century, Per Henrik Ling, a Swedish fencing master and academic, created the basis for what is now known as Swedish massage. Swedish massage deals with the soft tissues of the body.

Swedish massage is a combination of relaxing effects and exercises that work on the joints and muscles, but it is still based on the form that was practised in ancient times. More recently, a work was published in the 1970s called *The Massage Book,* by George Downing, and this introduced a new concept in the overall technique of massage, that the whole person's state should be assessed by the therapist and not solely the physical side. The emotional and mental states should be part of the overall picture. Also combined in his form of massage were the methods used in reflexology (*see* page 89) and shiatsu (*see* page 154), and this was known as therapeutic massage. The aim of this is to use relaxation, stimulation and invigoration to promote good health.

Uses
Massage is commonly used to induce general relaxation, so that any tension or strain experienced in the rush of daily life can be eased and eliminated. It is found to be very effective, working on the mind as well as the body. It can be used to treat people with hypertension (high blood pressure), sinusitis, headaches, insomnia and hyperactivity, including people who suffer from heart ailments or circulatory disorders. At the physical level, massage is intended to help the body make use of food and to eliminate the waste materials, as well as stimulating the nervous and muscular system and the circulation of blood. Neck and back pain are conditions from which many people suffer, particularly if they have not been sitting correctly, such as in a slightly stooped position with their shoulders rounded. People whose day-to-day work involves a great deal of physical activity, such as dancers and athletes, can also derive a great deal of benefit from the use of massage. Stiffness can be a problem that they have after training or working, and this is relieved by encouraging the toxins that gather in the muscles to disperse. Massage promotes a feeling of calmness and serenity, and this is particularly beneficial to people who frequently suffer from bouts of depression or anxiety. Once the worry and depression have been dispelled, people are able to deal with their problems much more effectively and, being able to do so, will boost their self-confidence.

Medical use
An aid to recovery
In hospitals, massage has been used to ease pain and discomfort as well as being of benefit to people who are bedridden, since the flow of blood to the muscles is stimulated. It has also been used for those who have suffered a heart attack and has helped their recovery. A more recent development has been the use of massage for cancer patients who are suffering from the after-effects of treatment, such as chemotherapy, as well as the discomfort the disease itself causes. Indeed, there are few conditions when it is not recommended. However, it should not be used when people are suffering from inflammation of the veins (phlebitis), varicose veins, thrombosis (clots in the blood) or if they have a raised temperature such as occurs during a fever. It is then advisable to contact a doctor before using massage. Doctors may be able to recommend a qualified therapist, a health centre may be able to help or contact can be made with the relevant professional body.

Psychological benefits
Along with the diagnosis element of massage there are great psychological benefits – the enjoyment of touch and of being stroked and caressed by another person. During a massage the patient is coaxed from emotional and occupational stresses and brought into the intense arena of the here and now. The importance of this kind of one-on-one nonverbal communication can never be underestimated in our increasingly impersonal and detached society.

Massage has a wide range of uses for a variety of disorders. Its strengths lie in the easing of strain and tension and inducing relaxation and serenity, plus the physical contact of the therapist. Although doctors make use of this therapy in conjunction with orthodox medicine, it is not to be regarded as a cure for diseases in itself and serious problems could occur if this were the case.

Benefits
Massage affects the whole body through rhythmically applied

pressure. Gentle pulling and stroking movements increase the circulation of the blood and cause the blood vessels to dilate. The stimulation of nerves and blood will also affect the internal organs. Lymph is a milky white liquid that carries waste substances and toxins away from the tissues via the lymphatic system. Inactivity can cause an unhealthy build-up of this substance, and as the circulation of the lymph is largely dependent on muscle contractions, so massage will help speed the lymph's progress through the system. Active people can also benefit from massage as strenuous activity burns up the muscle, producing an increase of waste products in the muscle tissue. Massage will help to balance the system in both cases and can increase oxygen capacity by 10–15 per cent.

By realigning our bodies, massage can go a long way to repairing our generally damaged postures. Inactive lifestyles and sedentary occupations have created a society of people with cramped, stooped and neglected postures. Not only does massage help to coax the spine and corresponding physiology back into position, it also makes us more aware of our bodies. Relieved of muscle tension, the body feels lighter and can therefore be borne more naturally and with more poise. Used in conjunction with postural therapies such as Pilates or the Alexander technique (*see* page 18), massage can help achieve a relaxed yet controlled posture.

Women in labour have found that the pain experienced during childbirth can be eased if massage is performed on the buttocks and back. The massage eases the build-up of tension in the muscles, encouraging relaxation and easing of labour pains. It is said to be more effective on women who had previously experienced the benefits and reassurance of massage.

Many of the benefits of massage come through the healer/patient contact. Our hands are one of the most sensitive parts of our body, and we experience much of our sense of touch through our hands. An experienced masseur is able to use his or her hands to communicate feelings of harmony and relaxation. A practised masseur will also be able to diagnose the patient through touch. He or she can 'listen' to tension and stress through the texture of the skin, knotted muscles and stiff joints. Old and current sprains, congestion and swelling should all be obvious to a good masseur. The actions of massage – the stroking, kneading and pulling – detoxify the body, improving circulation and lymphatic drainage. After tension and weaknesses in the body have been pinpointed and relieved, the patient is left feeling, relaxed and energized.

The massage session
Preparation

A session may be undertaken in the patient's home, or he or she can attend the masseur or masseuse at a clinic. At each session the client will undress, leaving only pants or briefs on, and will lie on a firm, comfortable surface, such as a table that is designed especially for massage. The massage that follows normally lasts from 20 minutes to one hour.

If performed by professionals, massage is not a technique for the unduly modest. It achieves best results if the person receiving the massage is either naked or else dressed in the scantiest of underwear. For anyone who is competent and wishes to provide some simple massage for a partner, there are some basic rules to follow. The room should be warm and peaceful. People will find it difficult to relax if they are cold, and the person performing the massage will be faced with a mass of goose pimples. The surface on which the person lies should be quite comfortable but firm. Use a mid-thigh level table or the floor. A futon (a quilted Japanese mattress) can be used, and to relieve the upper part of the body from any possible discomfort, a pillow should be placed underneath the torso. Any pressure that may be exerted on the feet can be dispelled by the use of a rolled-up towel or similar placed beneath the ankles. Both people should be relaxed, and to this end soft music can be played. All the movements of the hand should be of a continuous nature. It is suggested that the recipient always has one hand of the masseur or masseuse placed on him or her. If you wish you can buy a perfumed massage oil from a chemist or health shop, or mix your own using a blend of aromatherapy oils. Vegetable oil (about one teaspoonful) is suitable but should not be poured straight on to the person. It should be spread over the hands by rubbing, which will also warm it sufficiently for use. Should the masseur or masseuse get out of breath, he or she should stop for a rest, all the while retaining a hand on the person.

Basic techniques

Massage can be divided into four basic forms, and these are known as *percussion* (also known as drumming); *friction* (also called pressure); *effleurage* (also called stroking) and *petrissage* (also called kneading). These methods can be practised alone or in combination for maximum benefit to the patient.

Percussion (drumming or tapotement)

Percussion is also called tapotement, which is derived from tapoter, a French word that means 'to drum', as of the fingers on a surface. As would be expected from its name, percussion is generally done with the edge of the hand with a quick, chopping movement, although the strokes are not hard. This type of movement would be used on places like the buttocks, thighs, waist or shoulders where there is a wide expanse of flesh.

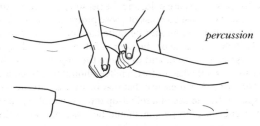

percussion

Friction (pressure)

Friction strokes are used to penetrate into deep muscle tissue. Friction is often used on dancers and athletes who experience problems with damaged ligaments or tendons. This is because the flow of blood is stimulated and the movement of joints is improved. Friction can be performed with the base of the hand, some fingers or the upper part of the thumb. It is not advisable to use this method on parts of the body that have been injured in some way, for example where there is bruising.

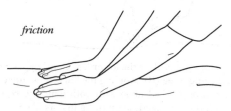

friction

Effleurage (stroking)

Effleurage is performed in a slow, rhythmical, controlled manner using both hands together with a small space between the thumbs (A). If the therapist wishes to use only light pressure he or she will use the palms of the hands or the tips of the fingers with light gliding strokes, working away from the heart. Light gliding strokes have a relaxing effect on the nervous system. For increased pressure the knuckles or thumbs will be used in an upwards stroking

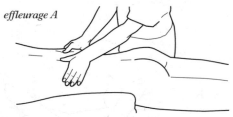

effleurage A

motion towards the heart. Stronger pressure has more of an effect on the blood circulation and the nervous system.

Effleurage can be used on the upper leg as far up as the hip on the outside of the leg. Once the person is lying face downwards (with support under the chest), continue to use effleurage

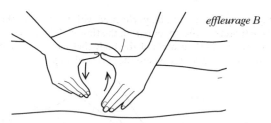

effleurage B

movements on the back of the lower leg. Continue as before but work on the upper leg (B), avoiding the knee. The muscles in the buttocks can be worked upon with both hands to squeeze but making sure that the hands are moving in opposite ways (B).

Petrissage (kneading)

Petrissage is ideal for unlocking aching or tense muscles, in particular the trapezium muscle between the neck and shoulders (A). Both hands work together in a rhythmic sequence, alternately

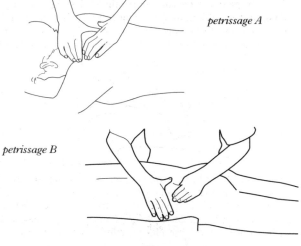

petrissage A

petrissage B

picking up and gently squeezing the tense muscle. The kneading action gets deep enough to stimulate the lymph into removing the build-up of lactic acid. As the therapist works across each section, an area of flesh is grasped and squeezed, and this action stimulates the flow of blood and enables tensed muscles to relax. People such as athletes can have an accumulation of lactic acid in certain muscles, and this is why cramp occurs. Parts of the body on which this method is practised are along the stomach and around the waist (B).

Neck and shoulder massage

What follows can be used to relieve headaches, loosen the shoulder muscles and provide a general feeling of relaxation.

Neck and shoulders – A

Stand behind your seated partner. Begin with effleurage, applying firm pressure with both hands. Start at the bottom of the shoulder blades up each side of the spine to the base of the neck. Move your hands apart across the top of the shoulders and then bring them gently down to the starting position. Repeat several times, finishing with a light return stroke.

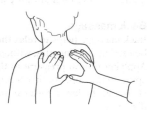

Neck and shoulders – B

Stand at right angles to the side of your partner. Locate tension spots in the shoulders using your thumbs and then work these areas with the thumbs. The pressure can approach your partner's pain threshold but not exceed it.

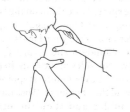

Neck and shoulders – C

Place your left hand in an 'L' shape on your partner's shoulder. Apply-ing firm pressure, move it slowly up the whole length of the shoul-der. Repeat with your other hand. Continue repeating the sequence using alternate hands. Place one hand at the base of the back of the neck and move it gently up to the hairline, gently squeezing all the time. Return with a gentle stroke. Repeat several times. Without re-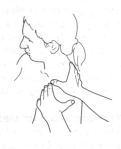
moving your hands, walk round to the other shoulder and repeat B and C. Move behind your partner and repeat A several times.

Back massage

Back massage helps to relax the whole body. The strokes should be carried out smoothly, without lifting the hands from the back. Applying thumb pressure to the channels on either side of the spine on the upper back will help respiratory problems. The same stroke on the lower back can relieve constipation and menstrual discomfort.

Back – A

Place your hands, facing each other, on either side of the base of the spine. Move them up the back, using your body weight to apply pressure. Take your hands round the shoulders and return lightly down the sides of the body. Repeat several times before stopping to knead the shoulders. Work on one shoulder and then the other. Repeat the movement.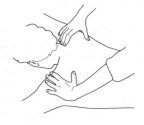

Back – B

Place your hands at waist level, with your thumbs in the hollows on either side of the spine and your fingers open and relaxed. Push your thumbs firmly up the channels for about 2 ins (6 cm), relax them, and then move them back about 1 in (2 cm). Continue in this way up to the neck. Then gently slide both hands back to the base of the spine. Repeat. Follow with the sequence in A.

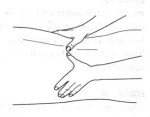

Back – C

Place your hand flat across one side of your partner's back at the base of the spine. Apply firm palm pressure and work up to the shoulders. Follow closely with your other hand. Repeat using alternate hands. Work through the same sequence on the other side of the back, then repeat on both side several times. Finish by working through A.

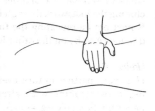

Back – D

Place your hands, facing up the back, on either side of the spine. Applying firm palm pressure, work from the base of the spine to chest level. Turn your fingers outwards and move your hands apart to the sides of the body. Repeat this stroke at waist and hip levels. Repeat the first movement in A several times.

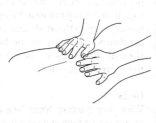

Limb massage

Limbs – A

Begin at the ankle and stroke vertically up the leg with one hand. Follow the same path with your other hand. Continue this sequence, using alternate hands.

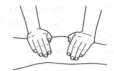

Limbs – B

Raise your partner's foot and hold it with the knee at a right angle. Using the palm of your free hand, stroke firmly down the back of the leg from ankle to knee level. Use a light stroke to return to the ankle. Repeat the whole movement several times. If including the foot, work through D and E next before repeating the full sequence (A to B) on the other leg.

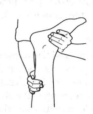

Limbs – C

Help your partner to turn over, and begin by stroking with alternate hands up the whole leg, as in A. Then put your hands on either side of the knee and, using your thumbs to apply pressure, circle around the knee cap. If including the foot, bring your hands down to the ankle and use the sandwich stroke (D) on the front of the foot. Work through the full movement on the other leg.

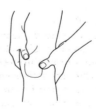

Limbs – D

With your partner lying face down, take one foot between your hands, so that the palm of your upper hand is resting in the arch. Press firmly, and slowly draw your hands down to the tip of the foot. Use plenty of pressure for this 'sandwich' stoke.

Limbs – E

Hold the foot with your thumbs lying side by side behind the toes. Pull both thumbs back to the sides of the foot, then push them forward. Repeat this zig-zag movement as you work down to the heel. Then push firmly all the way back to the toes, keeping your thumbs side by side. Repeat the whole movement several times. Work through the whole sequence (D to E) on the other foot.

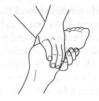

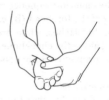

Limbs – F

Take hold of your partner's hand as in a firm handshake, and lift the arm up slightly, as far as the elbow. Gently place the palm of your fee hand across the top of the wrist and close your fingers round the raised arm. Apply firm pressure and slide your hand up to the elbow, or as far as the shoulder. Move your palm underneath the arm and use a light stroke to return to the wrist. Repeat several times.

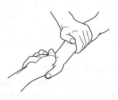

Limbs – G

Place your thumbs across the inside of your partner's wrist. Applying pressure with both your thumbs, make

wide circles around the wrist area.
Repeat F. As you finish, relax your
hold on the wrist and pull off firmly
and slowly in a sandwich stroke, as
in D. Repeat the full sequence (F
to G) on the other arm, finishing
with the hand variation of D.

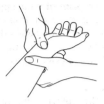

Face and head massage

The following sequence encourages deep relaxation. Gentle stroking of the forehead (B) can help to relieve stress-related tension
and headaches, while pressure applied to the sides of the nose
and along the cheekbones (C) alleviates nasal congestion and si-
nus problems. Scalp massage (D) stimulates circulation.

Face and head – A

Use alternate hands to stroke up one
side of the face, starting beneath the
chin and working up towards the forehead. Work through the same movement on the other side of the face.
Repeat several times. Finish by placing one palm across your partner's
forehead, ready for the next stroke.

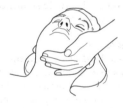

Face and head – B

Begin by stroking up the forehead
with alternate palms. Then place the
pads of the middle three fingers of
both hands in the centre of the forehead between the eyes. Draw them
gently apart across the brow and
round the outside corner of the eyes.
Lift off the middle two fingers and
use your fourth fingers only to return
under the eyes towards the nose.

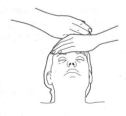

Face and head – C

Position your thumbs on your partner's forehead. Using the three middle fingers of both hands, press firmly against the sides of the nose. Continue along the top of the cheekbone, until you reach the temple. Keeping your thumbs in position, return to the nose, pressing along the middle of the cheekbone.

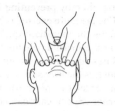

Face and head – D

Spread out the fingers and thumbs of both hands and place them on your partner's scalp. Keep them in position and begin to move the scalp muscle over the bone by applying gentle pressure and circling slowly and firmly on the spot. Stop occasionally to move to a different area, then begin again, working gradually over the whole scalp.

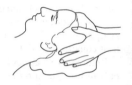

Acupressure

This is an ancient form of healing combining massage and acupuncture, practised over 3,000 years ago in Japan and China. It was developed into its current form using a system of special massage points and is today still practised widely in the Japanese home environment.

Certain 'pressure points' are located in various parts of the body and these are used by the practitioner by massaging firmly with the thumb or fingertip. These points are the same as those utilized in acupuncture. There are various ways of working and the pressure can be applied by the practitioner's fingers, thumbs, knees, palms of the hand, etc. Relief from pain can be quite rapid at times, depending upon its cause, while other more persistent problems can take longer to improve.

Acupressure is said to enhance the body's own method of healing, thereby preventing illness and improving the energy level. The pressure exerted is believed to regulate the energy that flows along the meridians,qi. As previously menntioned, the meridians are the invisible channels that run along the length of the body. These meridians are mainly named after the organs of the body such as the liver and stomach, but there are four exceptions, which are called the 'pericardium', 'triple heater', 'conception' and 'governor'. Specifically named meridian lines may also be used to treat ailments other than those relating to it.

Ailments claimed to have been treated successfully are back pain, asthma, digestive problems, insomnia, migraine and circulatory problems, amongst others. Changes in diet, regular exercise and certain self-checking methods may be recommended by your practitioner. It must be borne in mind that some painful symptoms are the onset of serious illness so you should always first consult your G.P.

Before any treatment commences, a patient will be asked details of lifestyle and diet, the pulse rate will be taken along with any relevant past history relating to the current problem. The person will be requested to lie on a mattress on the floor or on a firm table, and comfortable but loose-fitting clothing is best so that the practitioner can work most effectively on the energy channels. No oils are used on the body and there is no equipment. Each session lasts from approximately 30 minutes to 1 hour. Once the pressure is applied, and this can be done in a variety of ways particular to each practitioner, varying sensations may be felt. Some points may feel sore or tender and there may be some discomfort such as a deep pain or coolness. However, it is believed that this form of massage works quickly so that any tenderness soon passes.

The number of treatments will vary from patient to patient, according to how the person responds and what problem or ailment is being treated. Weekly visits may be needed if a specific disorder is being treated while other people may go whenever they feel in need. It is advisable for women who are pregnant to check with their practitioner first since some of the acupressure methods are not recommended during pregnancy. Acupressure can be practised safely at home although it is usually better for one person to perform the massage on another. Common problems such as headache, constipation and toothache can be treated quite simply although there is the possibility of any problem worsening first before an improvement occurs if the pressure points are over stimulated. You should, however, see your doctor if any ailment persists. To treat headache, facial soreness, toothache and menstrual pain, locate the fleshy piece of skin between the thumb and forefinger and squeeze firmly, pressing towards the forefinger. The pressure should be applied for about five minutes and either hand can be used. This point is known as 'large intestine 4'.

To aid digestive problems in both adults and babies, for example to settle infantile colic, the point known as 'stomach 36' is utilized, which is located on the outer side of the leg about 75 mm (3 ins) down from the knee. This point should be quite simple to find as it can often feel slightly tender. It should be pressed quite firmly and strongly for about five to ten minutes with the thumb.

When practising acupressure massage on someone else and before treatment begins, ensure that the person is warm, relaxed, comfortable and wearing loose-fitting clothing and that he or she is lying on a firm mattress or rug on the floor. To discover the areas that need to be worked on, press firmly over the body and see which areas are tender. These tender areas on the body correspond to an organ that is not working correctly. To commence massage using fingertips or thumbs, a pressure of about 4.5 kg (10 lbs) should be exerted. The massage movements should be performed very quickly, about 50 to 100 times every minute, and some discomfort is likely (which will soon pass) but there should be no pain. Particular care should be taken to avoid causing pain on the face, stomach or over any joints. If a baby or young child is being massaged then considerably less pressure should be used. If there is any doubt as to the correct amount, exert a downwards pressure on bathroom scales to ascertain the weight being used. There is no need to hurry from one point to another since approximately 5 to 15 minutes is needed at each point for adults, but only about 30 seconds for babies or young children.

Using the 'self-help' acupressure, massage can be repeated as often as is felt to be necessary with several sessions per hour usually being sufficient for painful conditions that have arisen suddenly. It is possible that as many as 20 sessions may be necessary for persistent conditions causing pain, with greater intervals of time between treatments as matters improve. It is not advisable to try anything that is at all complicated (or to treat an illness such as arthritis) and a trained practitioner will obviously be able to provide the best level of treatment and help. To contact a reputable practitioner who has completed the relevant training it is advisable to contact the appropriate professional body.

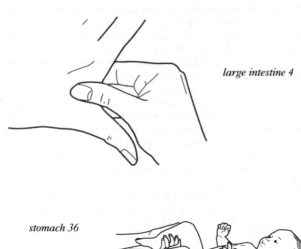

large intestine 4

stomach 36

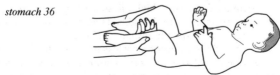

Do-in

Do-in (pronounced doe-in) is another ancient type of massage that originated in China. It is a technique of self-massage and, as in other forms of alternative therapy, it is believed that there is a flow of energy throughout the body that travels along 'meridians' and that each of these is connected to a vital organ such as the lungs, liver and heart. Do-in has a connection with shiatsu (*see* page 154), and people of any age can participate, the only stipulation being that they are active and not out of condition. Clothing should not be tight or restrictive and adequate space is needed to perform the exercises.

If do-in is to be used as an invigorating form of massage, then the best time of day is as soon as possible after rising, but not after breakfast. After meals are the only times when do-in is to be avoided. It is generally recommended that people wishing to practise do-in should first go to classes so that when the exercises are done at home they are performed correctly. It is claimed that the use of do-in is preventive in nature since the vital organs are strengthened and therefore maintained in a healthy state.

Warming up

Before starting, it is best to do some warming-up exercises so that the body is not stiff. Begin by sitting on the ground with the knees up, grasp the knees and begin a rocking motion forwards and backwards. Then sit up, again on the floor, position the legs as if to sit cross-legged but put the soles of the feet touching each other. Hold the toes for a short time. These two exercises should help to make the body more supple (A).

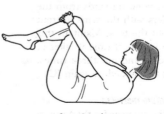

A – warming up

Spleen meridian

For the *spleen meridian* exercise, which is connected with the stomach, stand as near as possible in front of a wall. Place one hand palm-downwards high up the wall so that there is a good stretching action and with the other hand grasp the foot that is opposite to the raised arm. The neck and head should be stretched backwards, away from the wall. Maintain this stretched position, inhale and exhale deeply twice and then relax. Repeat the procedure using the other arm and leg (B).

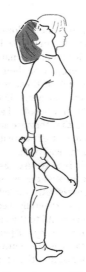

B – spleen meridien

Bladder meridian

For the *bladder meridian* exercise, and thereby the kidneys, sit on the floor with the legs straight out in front and ensure that the toes are tensed upright. The arms should then be stretched above the head and a breath taken. After breathing out, bend forwards from the shoulders with the arms in front and hold the toes. Maintain this for the length of time it takes to breathe in and out three times. Repeat the procedure again (C).

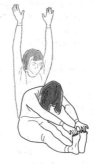

C – bladder meridien

Pericardium meridian

To do the exercise for the *pericardium meridian*, which affects the circulation, sit on the floor with feet touching, but one behind the other, ensuring that the hands are crossed and touching opposite knees. Grasp the knees and incline the body forwards with the aim of pushing the knees downwards on to the floor. Do this exercise again but with the hands on opposite knees and the other foot on the outside.

Large intestine meridian

Using the exercise that strengthens the *large intestine meridian* and in turn the lungs, stand upright with the feet apart. Link the thumbs behind the back and then inhale. Exhale and at the same time place the arms outwards and upwards behind the back. To complete the exercise, lean forwards from the hips and then stand upright (D).

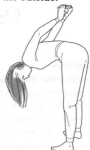

D – large intestine meridien

Gall bladder meridian

To strengthen the liver by stimulating the *gall bladder meridian*, sit upright on the floor with the legs the maximum distance apart. Then inhale, passing the arms along the length of the right leg so that the base of the foot can be held. There should be no movement of the buttocks off the floor. Maintain this stretched position while breathing deeply twice. Repeat the exercise using the other leg.

After all exercises have been accomplished, lie flat out on the floor with the legs apart and the arms stretched at the sides, palms uppermost. Then lift the head so that the feet can be seen and then put the head back on the floor again. The head and body should then be shaken so that the legs, arms and neck are loosened. To complete the relaxation, the eyes should be closed and the person should lie quietly for a few minutes.

Osteopathy

Introduction
An alternative medical treatment

Osteopathy is a technique that uses manipulation and massage to help distressed muscles and joints and make them work smoothly.

The profession began in 1892 when Dr Andrew Taylor Still (1828–1917), an American farmer, inventor and doctor, opened the USA's first school of osteopathic medicine. He sought alternatives to the medical treatments of his day which he believed were ineffective as well as often harmful.

Still's new philosophy of medicine, based upon the teachings of Hippocrates, advocated that 'Finding health should be the purpose of a doctor. Anyone can find disease.' Like Hippocrates, Still recognized that the human body is a unit in which structure, function, mind and spirit all work together. The therapy aims to pinpoint and treat any problems that are of a mechanical nature. The body's frame consists of the skeleton, muscles, joints and ligaments and all movements or activities such as running, swimming, eating, speaking and walking depend upon it.

A holistic treatment

Still came to believe that it would be safer to encourage the body to heal itself, rather than use the drugs that were then available and that were not always safe. He regarded the body from an engineer's point of view and the combination of this and his medical experience of anatomy, led him to believe that ailments and disorders could occur when the bones or joints no longer functioned in harmony. He believed that manipulation was the cure for the problem. Although his ideas provoked a great deal of opposition from the American medical profession at first, they slowly came to be accepted. The bulk of scientific research has been done in America with a number of medical schools of osteopathy being established. Dr Martin Littlejohn, who was a pupil of Dr Still, brought the practice of osteopathy to the UK around 1900, with the first school being founded in 1917 in London. He emphasized the compassionate care and treatment of the person as a whole, not as a collection of symptoms or unrelated parts. The philosophy and practices of A. T. Still, considered radical in the 1800s, are generally accepted principles of good medicine today.

Injuries and stress
Problems that prevent the body from working correctly or create pain can be due to an injury or stress. This can result in what is known as a tension headache since the stress experienced causes a contraction in muscles. These are situated at the back of the neck at the base of the skull and relief can be obtained by the use of massage. In osteopathy, it is believed that if the basic framework of the body is undamaged, then all physical activities can be accomplished efficiently and without causing any problems. The majority of an osteopath's patients suffer from disorders of the spine, which result in pain in the lower part of the back and the neck. A great deal of pressure is exerted on the spinal column, and especially on the cartilage between the individual vertebrae. This is a constant pressure due to the effects of gravity that occurs merely by standing. If a person stands incorrectly with stooped shoulders, this will exacerbate any problems or perhaps initiate one. The joints and framework of the body are manipulated and massaged where necessary so that the usual action is regained.

Athletes or dancers can receive injuries to muscles or joints such as the ankle, hip, wrist or elbow and they too can benefit from treatment by osteopathy. Pain in the lower back can be experienced by pregnant women who may stand in a different way due to their increasing weight and, if this is the case, osteopathy can often ease matters considerably. To find a fully qualified osteopath, it is advisable to contact the relevant professional body, or the G.P. may be able to help.

The treatment
The first visit

At the first visit to an osteopath, he or she will need to know the complete history of any problems experienced, how they first occurred and what eases or aggravates matters. A patient's case history and any form of therapy that is currently in use will all be of relevance to the practitioner. A thorough examination will then take place observing how the patient sits, stands or lies down and also the manner in which the body is bent to the side, back or front. As each movement takes place, the osteopath is able to take note of the extent and ability of the joint to function. The practitioner will also feel the muscles, soft tissues and ligaments to detect if there is any tension present. Whilst examining the body, the osteopath will note any problems that are present and, as an aid to diagnosis, use may also be made of checking reflexes, such as the knee-jerk reflex. If a patient has been involved in an accident, X-rays can be checked to determine the extent of any problem. It is possible that a disorder would not benefit from treatment by osteopathy and the patient would be advised accordingly. If this is not the case, treatment can commence with the chosen course of therapy.

A solution to tension

There is no set number of consultations necessary, as this will depend upon the nature of the problem and also for how long it has been apparent. It is possible that a severe disorder that has arisen suddenly can be alleviated at once. The osteopath is likely to recommend a number of things so that patients can help themselves between treatments. Techniques such as learning to relax, how to stand and sit correctly and additional exercises can be suggested by the osteopath. Patients generally find that each consultation is quite pleasant and they feel much more relaxed and calm afterwards. The length of each session can vary, but it is generally in the region of half an hour. As the osteopath gently manipulates the joint, it will lessen any tenseness present in the muscles and also improve its ability to work correctly and to its maximum extent. It is this manipulation that can cause a clicking noise to be heard. As well as manipulation, other methods such as massage can be used to good effect. Muscles can be freed from tension if the tissue is massaged and this will also stimulate the flow of blood. In some cases, the patient may experience a temporary deterioration once treatment has commenced, and this is more likely to occur if the ailment has existed for quite some time.

People who have to spend a lot of their life driving are susceptible to a number of problems related to the manner in which they are seated. If their position is incorrect they can suffer from tension headaches, pain in the back and the shoulders and neck can feel stiff. There are a number of ways in which these problems can be remedied such as holding the wheel in the approved manner (at roughly 'ten to two' on the dial of a clock). The arms should not be held out straight and stiff, but should feel relaxed and with the arms bent at the elbow. In order that the driver can maintain a position in which the back and neck feel comfortable, the seat should be moved so that it is tilting backwards a little, although it should not be so far away that the pedals are not easily reached. The legs should not be held straight out, and if the pedals are the correct distance away the knees should be bent a little and feel quite comfortable. It is also important to sit erect and not slump in the seat. The driver's rear should be positioned right at the back of the seat and this should be checked each time before using the vehicle. It is also important that there is adequate vision from the mirror so its position should be altered if necessary. If the driver already has a back problem then it is a simple matter to provide support for the lower part of the back. If this is done it should prevent strain on the shoulders and backbone. Whilst driving, the person should make a conscious effort to ensure that the shoulders are not tensed, but held in a relaxed way. Another point to remember is that the chin should not be stuck out but kept in, otherwise the neck muscles will become tensed and painful. Drivers can perform some beneficial exercises while they are waiting in a queue of traffic. To stretch the neck muscles, put the chin right down on to the chest and then relax. This stretching exercise should be done several times. The following exercise can also be done at the same time as driving and will have a positive effect on the flow of blood to the legs and also will improve how a person is seated. It is simply done by contraction and relaxation of the muscles in the stomach. Another exercise involves raising the shoulders upwards and then moving them backwards in a circular motion. The head should also be inclined forward a little. This should also be done several times to gain the maximum effect.

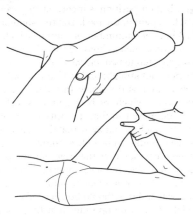

treatment of the knee by manipulation

The figure above illustrates an example of diagnosis and treatment by manipulation, in which the osteopath examines a knee that has been injured. To determine the extent of the problem, the examination will be detailed and previous accidents or any other relevant details will be requested. If the practitioner concludes that osteopathy will be of benefit to the patient, the joint will be manipulated so that it is able to function correctly and the manipulation will also have the effect of relaxing the muscles that have become tensed due to the injury.

Another form of therapy, which is known as cranial osteopathy, can be used for patients suffering from pain in the face or head. This is effected by the osteopath using slight pressure on these areas including the upper part of the neck. If there is any tautness or tenseness present, the position is maintained while the problem improves. It is now common practice for doctors to recommend some patients to use osteopathy and some general practitioners use the therapy themselves after receiving training. Although its benefits are generally accepted for problems of a mechanical nature, doctors believe it is vital that they first decide upon what is wrong before any possible use can be made of osteopathy.

Polarity Therapy

Introduction
Origins
This is a therapy devised by Dr Randolph Stone (1890–1983) that
amalgamates other healing therapies from both east and west. Dr
Stone studied many of these therapies, including yoga (*see* page
75) and acupuncture (*see* page 11), and he was also trained to
practise osteopathy (*see* page 63) and chiropractic (*see* page 26)
among others. He began to search for a cure to the problem that
he experienced with some of his patients when, although their
disorder had been cured by the use of manipulation, they subsequently became unwell. Through his studies of eastern therapies
he accepted the fundamental belief that a form of energy flows
along certain channels in the body and that to keep good health
the flow must be maintained. In India this energy is referred to as
prana and in China it was called *chi* or *qi*. The western equivalent
of this would probably be called a person's soul or spirit. It is
believed that ailments occur when this flow of energy is blocked
or is out of balance, and this could happen for different reasons
such as tension or stress, disturbances in the mind or unhealthy
eating patterns. This energy is purported to be the controlling
factor in a person's whole life and therefore affects the mind and
body at all levels. It is believed that once the flow of energy has been
restored to normal, the ailment will disappear and not recur.

The underlying belief
Dr Stone's polarity therapy states that there are three types of
relationships, known as *neutral*, *positive* and *negative*, to be

maintained between various areas in the body and five centres of energy. These centres originate from a very old belief held in India, and each centre is held to have an effect on its related part of the body.

The centres are known as *ether* (controlling the ears and throat), *earth* (controlling the rectum and bladder), *fire* (controlling the stomach and bowels), *water* (controlling the pelvis and glands), and *air* (controlling the circulation and breathing). The therapy's aim is to maintain a balance and harmony between all these various points, and Dr Stone slowly developed four procedures to do this. They are the use of *diet*, *stretching exercises*, *touch and manipulation*, and *mental attitude*, that is, contemplation allied with a positive view of life.

The treatment
Diet
To cleanse the body from a build-up of toxins caused by unhealthy eating and environmental pollution, the person will eat only fresh vegetables, fruit juices and fresh fruit. The length of time for this diet will vary according to the degree of cleansing required, but it is unlikely to be longer than a fortnight. Also available is a special drink that consists of lemon juice, olive oil, garlic and ginger. After the cleansing is complete, there is another diet to be followed that is said to promote and increase health, and finally one to ensure that the body maintains its level of good health.

Stretching exercises
Various positions may be adopted for the stretching exercises, such as on the floor with the legs crossed (A) or squatting or sitting with the hands held at the back of the head. It is believed that these exercises free the channels that carry the body's energy and strengthen the sinews, muscles, ligaments and spine. As a way of releasing any stress or tension, the person would be requested to shout out loud at the same time as exercising. For the first exercise, the person can sit on the floor cross-legged with the right hand taking hold of the left ankle and with the left hand holding

the right ankle. The eyes should then be shut and the mind relaxed and quiet.

For the squatting exercise, once in this position, clasp the hands out in front for balance and then move backwards and forwards and also in a circular motion. For people unable to balance in this position, a small book or similar item put under the heels should help (B).

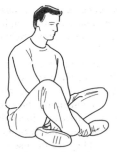

A—crosslegged

For a slight change on the basic squatting position, bend the head forward and place the hands at the back of the neck so that the head and arms are between the knees. Relax the arms a little so that they drop forward slightly and thus the backbone is stretched (C).

Another variation is to hold the hands behind the neck whilst squatting and push the elbows and shoulder blades backwards and inwards. Any tension or stress can be relieved by shouting at the same time as breathing deeply.

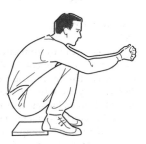

B—squatting

Another exercise in which stress can be eased by shouting is known as the *wood chopper*. This is a fairly simple one to perform, and it entails standing with the feet apart and the knees bent. The hands

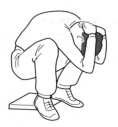

C—squatting

71

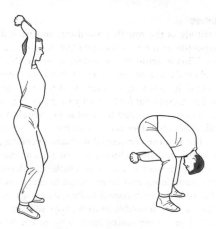

the two movements of the woodchopper

should be clasped above the head as if about to chop some wood and the arms brought down together in a swinging action ending with the arms as far between the legs as possible. As the hands are being swung downwards, the person should shout, so that any tension is relieved. This action can be repeated quite frequently as long as there is no discomfort (D).

Touch and manipulation

Touch and manipulation are used by the therapist to detect any stoppages in the flow of energy along the channels, which are believed to be the reason for disorders. It is said that by the use of pressure, of which there are three sorts, the therapist is able to restore the flow of energy. *Neutral pressure* is gentle and calming and only the tips of the fingers are used. *Positive pressure* is the use of manipulation over the whole of the body with the exception of the head. *Negative pressure* is the use of a firmer and deeper manipulation and touch.

Mental attitude

Mental attitude is the fourth procedure, and basically this encourages people to have a more positive view on all aspects of their lives. This is achieved by talking or counselling sessions, and it is believed that a negative view of things can make a person more susceptible to having an ailment. A positive attitude is regarded as being essential for harmony in the body and mind.

Polarity therapy is claimed to be of some benefit to all people who are ill, although it does not concentrate on a particular set of symptoms but is more concerned with the overall aspect of the patient's health and the achievement of internal harmony and balance. For the therapy to work successfully, each patient has to believe in it completely and be prepared to carry out the practitioner's instructions with regard to diet, exercises, and so on. It is, of course, always advisable to make sure that any therapist is fully qualified before beginning treatment. At the first consultation, the patient will be required to give a complete case history to the therapist, who will then assess the flow of energy through the body and also check on its physical make-up. Reflexes such as the knee-jerk reflex are tested, and any imbalances or blockages in the energy channels are detected by the reflex and pressure point testing. If there is a stoppage or imbalance of the flow, this will be manifested by some physical symptoms. One way in which it is believed a patient can help to speed the restoration of health is by remembering and concentrating on any thoughts, feelings or pictures in the 'mind's eye' that happen while a particular area is being treated. The patient should also have knowledge of the body's ability to heal itself. If a patient is receiving treatment on a painful knee joint, for example, he or she should focus attention on that part of the body whilst being receptive to any feelings that occur. It is believed that if the patient is aware of the overall condition, as a complete person and not just the physical aspect, this will encourage restoration of health. It is possible that a patient will need to keep details of all food consumed to enable the practitioner to detect any harmful effects, and a 'fruit and vegetable' diet may be advised (as described previously). It may be that the patient has some habit, view or manner of life that is not considered conducive to good health. If this is the case, the patient would be able to take advantage of a counselling service in order to help make a change. Other alternative therapies such as the use of herbal medicine may be used to effect a cure.

Polarity therapy has much in common with other eastern remedies that have the common themes of contemplation, exercise, touch or pressure, and diet and that can give much improvement. However, it is recommended that an accurate medical analysis of any condition is found in the first instance.

Yoga

Introduction
Origins

From its Indian origins as far back as 4000 years ago, yoga has been continually practised, but it is only in the present century that its use has become more widespread. Yoga has an effect on the whole person, combining the physical, mental and spiritual sides. The word 'yoga' is derived from a Sanskrit word that means 'yoke' or 'union', and thus reflects on the practices of yoga being total in effect. For many hundreds of years in India only a select few, such as philosophers and like-minded people with their disciples, followed the way of life that yoga dictated. The leaders were known as 'yogis' and it was they who taught their followers by passing on their accumulated knowledge. These small groups of people dwelt in caves or woods, or sometimes a yogi would live like a hermit. Yoga has had quite far-reaching effects over many hundreds of years in India.

The basics of yoga were defined by a yogi called Patanjali who lived about 300 BC. He was a very well-respected teacher and commanded great influence at that time, and his classification is one that is used now. He established the fact of yoga being separated into eight different parts. The first two concern a person's lifestyle, which should be serene with the days spent in contemplation, study, maintaining cleanliness, and living very simply and at peace with others. Anything that involves avarice or greed, etc, or is harmful to others has to be avoided. The third and fourth parts are concerned with physical matters and list a number of exercises designed to promote peace and infuse energy into both the mind and body. The remaining four sections are concerned with the advancement of a person's soul or spirit and mental faculties by being able to isolate himself or herself from outside worries and normal life, contemplation and broadening mental faculties with the ultimate knowledge known as *somadhi*. Mentally, this is a complete change that gives final realization of existence. Much more recently, yoga became available in India to everyone, in complete contrast to centuries ago. Doctors and teachers taught yoga, and it is now the rule that all schoolchildren have lessons in some of the exercises.

Modern practice

Nowadays, the practice of yoga is not restricted to India alone, with millions of people worldwide being followers. There are actually five different types of yoga: *raja*, *jnana*, *karma* and *bakti*, and *hatha*. It is this last system that is known in the west, and it involves the use of exercises and positions. The other methods concentrate on matters such as control over the mind, appreciation and intelligence or a morally correct way of life. These other methods are regarded as being of equal importance by the person completely committed to yoga as a way of life. Although people may have little or no spiritual feeling, the basic belief of yoga is the importance of mental attitudes in establishing the physical improvements from exercise. Because of media coverage of a famous violinist receiving successful treatment to a damaged shoulder by yoga, it became very popular throughout the UK. Prior to the 1960s, it was seldom practised, and only then by people who wanted to learn more of eastern therapies or who had worked and travelled in that area.

It is a belief in yoga that the body's essence of life, or *prana*, is contained in the breath. Through a change in the way of breathing there can be a beneficial effect on the general health. If a person is in a heightened emotional condition, or similar state, this will have an effect on the breathing. Therefore, if the breathing is controlled or altered this should promote joint feelings of peace and calm, both mentally and emotionally. There is a variety of exercises, and each promotes different types of breathing, such as the rib cage, shoulder and diaphragm. Some of the movements and stances in use were originally devised from the observation of animals, since they appeared to be adept at relaxation and moved with minimum effort. These stances, which are maintained for one or two minutes, aim to increase freedom of movement and make the person aware of the various parts of the body and any stress that may be present. It is not intended that they be physically tiring or that the person should 'show off' in front of others. The aim is to concentrate on self-knowledge.

The treatment
The benefits
It is recommended to follow some simple rules when practising yoga. Firstly use a fully qualified therapist, and practise daily if at all possible. It is advisable to check with a G.P. first if a person is undergoing a course of treatment or is on permanent medication, has some sort of infirmity or feels generally unwell. It is always best that yoga is undertaken before mealtimes but if this is not possible then three hours must elapse after a large meal or an hour after a light one. Comfortable clothes are essential and a folded blanket or thick rug should be placed on the ground as the base. Before commencing yoga have a bath or shower and repeat this afterwards to gain the maximum benefit. It is not advisable to do yoga if either the bowels or bladder are full. Should the person have been outside on a hot and sunny day it is not recommended that yoga is practised straight afterwards, as feelings of sickness and dizziness may occur.

Yoga is believed to be of benefit to anyone, providing that they possess determination and patience. If a person has certain physical limitations then these must be taken into account with regard to their expectation, but there is no age barrier. Teachers believe that people suffering from stress and disorder in their lives are in greater need of a time of harmony and peace. Yoga was used in the main to encourage health in the physical and mental states and thereby act as a preventive therapy. Tension or stress was one of the main disorders for which it was used, but nowadays it has been used for differing disorders such as hypertension (high blood pressure), bronchitis, back pain, headaches, asthma, heart disorders, premenstrual tension and an acid stomach. Trials have also been conducted to assess its potential in treating some illnesses such as multiple sclerosis, cerebral palsy, osteoporosis, rheumatoid arthritis and depression experienced after childbirth. Since the effects of tension are often shown by the tightening and contraction of muscles, the stretching exercises performed in yoga are able to release it. Also, being aware of each muscle as it is stretched encourages the person to mentally lose any stress or problems with which they have been beset. Suppleness is developed by the exercises through the use of the bending and twisting actions. This will help to maintain healthy joints, particularly for people who lead rather inactive lives.

There should be no strain felt and after practice some or all of them can be done in order. As mentioned previously, it is best to check with a qualified therapist if the person is an expectant mother, suffers from hypertension, is overweight or is having their monthly period.

The bow

Lie face down on the ground with the knees bent and then raised in the direction of the head. Then hold the ankles and, while inhaling,

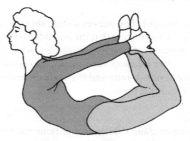

the bow

a pull should be exerted on the ankles so that the chest, head and thighs are raised up away from the floor. To start with it will not be possible to hold the legs together, but this will gradually occur with regular practice. This position should be maintained for up to ten breaths. To complete the bow, exhale and let go of the legs.

The bridge

The bridge is carried out on the floor, starting with the person lying on the back, the knees should be bent, with the legs separated a little and the arms at the side of the body. The person should then inhale and lift the torso and legs, thus forming a bridge. The fingers should then be linked under the body and

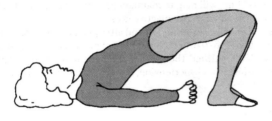

the bridge

the arms held straight. The person should then incline the body to each side in turn, ensuring that the shoulders stay underneath. To make the bridge a little bigger, pressure can be exerted by the arms and feet. After inhaling, the position should be maintained for a minimum of one minute and the body returned to a relaxed normal position on the floor.

The spinal twist

The spinal twist entails sitting on the floor with the legs outstretched. The left leg should be bent and placed over the other leg as far as possible. The person should exhale and twist the

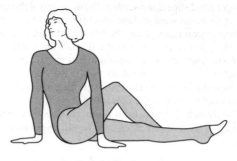

the spinal twist

body to the left. The person's right hand should be moved towards the right foot. The person should have the body supported by placing the left hand on the ground at the back but keeping the back straight. Every time the person exhales the body should be further twisted to the left. The position should be maintained for approximately one minute and then the complete action done again, but this time turning to the right. This is a gentle posture that is easy to perform.
Relax.

The spinal twist helps to strengthen the spine, improve posture and promote psychological balance.

The triangle

The triangle commences with the person standing upright with the legs apart and the arms held out at shoulder level. Extend the right foot to the side and, upon exhaling, bend over the right-hand side so that

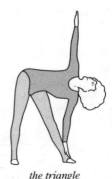

the triangle

the right hand slips downwards in the direction of the ankle. There should be no forward inclination of the body at this time. As the bending action takes place, the left arm should be lifted upright with the palm of the hand to the front. This stretched position should be kept up for the minimum of a minute, with the person trying to extend the stretch as they exhale. After inhaling, the person should then revert to the beginning of the exercise and do it again but leaning in the opposite direction.

The triangle helps to calm the nerves, acts to remove toxins from the body, and promotes good health in general.

The cat

Kneel on all fours with your hands shoulder-distance apart and your knees the same distance apart as your hands. Your elbows should remain straight throughout the entire exercise. Exhale while arching your back up high. Keep your head between your arms, looking at your abdomen. Hold this pose for a few seconds. Inhale, as you slowly hollow your back to a concave position. Raise your head and look up. Hold again. Repeat the sequence five to ten times, creating a slow flowing movement of the two postures. Relax.

The cat helps to strengthen the spine, improve posture and revitalize the whole body.

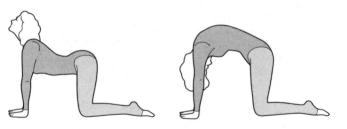

the cat

The tree

Stand with both feet together, arms loosely by your side. Focus your eyes on an imaginary spot directly ahead of you. Bring the right foot up and place the sole against the inside of the left thigh, as high as possible. When balanced, raise both arms simultaneously, placing the palms together over your head. Hold for 30 seconds. Gently lower your arms. Release your foot from your thigh. Repeat the sequence with the other foot. Relax.

The tree promotes concentration, balance and stability of body and mind.

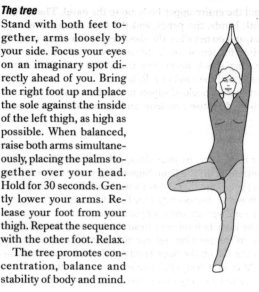

The cobra

Lie face down. Place the palms on the floor under the shoulders, fingers turned slightly inwards. Slowly lift the forehead, the nose,

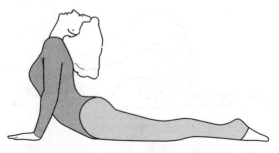

the chin, and the entire upper body, up to the navel. The weight rests on both hands, the pelvis, and the legs. Keep the elbows slightly bent, and do not allow the shoulders to hunch up towards the ears. Hold for ten seconds, focusing your attention on the lower back. Very slowly lower your trunk to the floor, then the chin, the nose, and the forehead. Relax.

The cobra increases blood supply to the abdominal organs and helps to relieve digestive problems and correct kidney malfunctions.

The plough

Lie on your back, arms by your sides, palms down. Slowly raise your legs and trunk off the floor. Supporting your hips with both hands, bring your legs slightly over your head. Keep your legs as straight as possible. Supporting your back with both hands, continue lifting your legs up and over your head until the toes come to rest on the floor behind your head. Only when you are quite comfortable in the position, release the hold on your back and place your arms flat on the floor. Hold only for ten seconds in the beginning. After your body becomes accustomed to this position, you may hold it longer. Very slowly unroll your body to the starting position. Relax.

The plough helps to reinvigorate the entire nervous system,

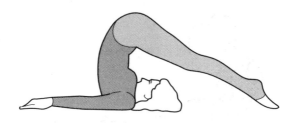

removing fatigue, listlessness and exhaustion. It is of particular benefit to the pancreas and endocrine glands.

The forward bend

Make sure you are well warmed up before attempting this posture. Sit with your legs stretched out in front of you, knees very straight. Inhale and stretch your arms above your head. Exhale and very slowly and smoothly bend forward from the hips (*not from the waist*) to grasp your toes. If at first this seems difficult, clasp instead your ankles, calves, or knees. It is important that your legs remain straight. Continue to bend forward and down, aiming to touch your knees with your head. Hold for at least ten seconds and observe your breath. Release your hold and very slowly unroll your spine, returning to a sitting position. Repeat twice.

The forward bend slows the respiratory rate to produce a calm and relaxed state of mind. It also increases the suppleness of the spine and improves blood circulation – which helps to regenerate the abdominal organs and improve digestion.

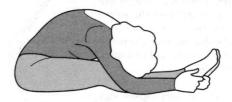

the forward bend

A salute or greeting to the sun

The following twelve stances, known as *a greeting to the sun*, have the aim of relaxing and invigorating the body and mind. This classic exercise coordinates breathing with variations of six yoga poses in a flowing rhythmic way that stretches and relaxes your body and your mind.

As suggested by its name, it was originally done when the sun rose and when it set. Although these stances are quite safe, they should not be done by pregnant women or those having a monthly period, except with expert tuition. If a person has hypertension (high blood pressure), a hernia, clots in the blood or pain in the lower back they are not recommended. Each exercise should follow on smoothly one after the other.

1 Start by facing east, standing up as straight as you can without forcing it, with your feet together. Inhale and visualize the sun just beginning to rise. Exhale and bring the palms of the hands on to your chest as if you were praying.

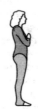

2 Then inhale and stretch the arms upright with the palms facing the ceiling and lean backwards, pushing the pelvis forward a little, and look up at your hands.

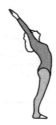

3 Exhale and, keeping the legs straight, place the fingers or palms on to the ground, ideally, your hands are touching the floor in front of or beside your feet. (Don't force this: if you can't reach the floor, let your hands hold on to the lowest part of your legs they can reach.)

4 Whilst inhaling, bend the knees and place one leg straight out backwards, with the knee touching the ground, in a long, lunging movement. Turn your toes right under and straighten your body from head to heel.

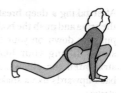

5 With both hands on the ground, raise the head slightly and push the hips to the front. At the same time as holding the breath, stretch the legs out together backwards, and raise the body off the floor supported by the arms.

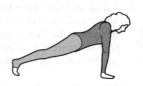

6 Exhale and fold the body over bent knees so that the head touches the ground with the arms stretched out in front, toes curled, until you are in the classic push-up position.

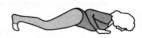

7 After inhaling and exhaling once, drop your knees to the floor, with your bottom up. Bend the elbows and bring your chest and chin to the floor. Continue breathing out and lower the whole body to the floor, straightening your legs and keeping your toes curled under with the body being supported by the hands at shoulder level and also by the toes. The stomach and hips should not be on the ground.

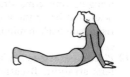

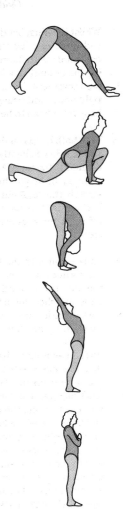

8 After taking a deep breath, stretch the arms and push the body upwards pushing down on your hands and slowly lifting your head as you straighten the elbows. Arch your back upwards like a snake before it strikes.

9 Exhale and then raise the hips upwards with the feet and hands being kept on the floor so that the body is in an inverted V-shape. The legs and back should be kept straight.

10 Breathe in and lunge forward by bending your right knee and stepping your right foot forward between your hands. When you breathe out, straighten your right leg and bring the left foot next to the right. Lift your buttocks high until you are touching your toes.

11 Inhale and slowly lift the spine, visualizing it unroll one vertebra at a time. Raise your head and look up, bringing your arms straight overhead, and bring the image of the rising sun back to mind.

12 Place the feet together keeping the legs straight. Breathe out and slowly bring your arms back to the sides, allowing the sun to glow brighter and brighter in your mind's eye.

Salute the sun six times at first, gradually increasing the number of repetitions until you are comfortably doing the routine 24 times. This whole sequence of exercises can be performed several times over if wished. If this is the case, it is suggested to alternate the legs used either forwards or backwards in two of the exercises.

As previously mentioned, yoga has recently been used to treat some illnesses such as rheumatoid arthritis, and if a person has such a severe disorder, then a highly skilled and experienced therapist is essential. Since this form of yoga, known as therapeutic yoga, is so new there is only a limited number of suitably experienced therapists available, although this situation should be remedied by the introduction of further training. For those who wish to use yoga to maintain mental and physical health, joining a class with an instructor is perhaps the best way to proceed, so that exercises are performed correctly and any lapses in concentration can be corrected. These classes last usually in the region of an hour and are separated into sessions for beginners and those who are more proficient. Proficiency and progress is achieved by frequent practice, which can be done at home between lessons. One simple exercise that helps reduce stress is quite simple to perform and does not take long. The person should lie on the floor with the arms at the side and the legs together. After inhaling, all the muscles from the toes to the thighs should be tightened in turn. As the person exhales, the muscles in the stomach up to the shoulders should then be tightened, including the hands, which should be clenched. After inhaling again, the chest, throat and face muscles should be tightened, as well as screwing up the face and this should be maintained until the next breath has to be taken. All muscles should then be relaxed, the legs parted and the arms spread out comfortably with the palms facing the ceiling. The person should then totally relax with a sensation of falling through the ground.

The majority of doctors regard yoga as a type of exercise that is beneficial, although some do recommend patients to refer to yoga practitioners. However, if a specific disorder is to be treated, it is very important that the ailment should first be seen by a doctor.

Reflexology

Introduction
Origins
Reflexology is a technique of diagnosis and treatment in which certain areas of the body, particularly the feet, are massaged to alleviate pain or other symptoms in the organs of the body. It is thought to have originated about five thousand years ago in China and was also used by the ancient Egyptians. It was introduced to Western society by Dr William Fitzgerald, who was an ear, nose and throat consultant in America. He applied ten zones (or energy channels) to the surface of the body, hence the term 'zone therapy', and these zones, or channels, were considered to be paths along which flowed a person's vital energy, or 'energy force'. The zones ended at the hands and feet. Thus, when pain was experienced in one part of the body, it could be relieved by applying pressure elsewhere in the body, within the same zone.

Subsequent practitioners of reflexology have concentrated primarily on the feet, although the working of reflexes throughout the body can be employed to beneficial effect.

Massage and energy flow
Reflexology does not use any sort of medication – merely a specific type of massage at the correct locations on the body. The body's energy flow is thought to follow certain routes, connecting every organ and gland with an ending or pressure point on the feet, hands or another part of the body. When the available routes are blocked, and a tenderness on the body points to such a closure,

then it indicates some ailment or condition in the body that may be somewhere other than the tender area. The massaging of particular reflex points enables these channels to be cleared, restoring the energy flow and at the same time healing any damage.

The uses of reflexology are numerous, and it is especially effective for the relief of pain (back pain, headaches and toothache), treatment of digestive disorders, stress and tension, colds and influenza, asthma, arthritis, and more. It is also possible to predict a potential illness and either give preventive therapy or suggest that specialist advice be sought. The massaging action of reflexology creates a soothing effect that enhances blood flow, to the overall benefit of the whole body. Reflexology, however, clearly cannot be used to treat conditions that require surgery.

Reflex massage initiates a soothing effect to bring muscular and nervous relief. The pressure of a finger applied to a particular point (or nerve ending) may create a sensation elsewhere in the body, indicating the connection or flow between the two points. This is the basis of reflexology, and although pain may not be alleviated immediately, continued massage over periods of up to one hour will usually have a beneficial effect.

There are certain conditions for which reflexology is inappropriate, including diabetes, some heart disorders, osteoporosis, disorders of the thyroid gland, and phlebitis (inflammation of the veins). It may also not be suitable for pregnant women or anyone suffering from arthritis of the feet.

The best way to undergo reflexology is in the hands of a therapist, who will usually massage all reflex areas, concentrating on any tender areas that will correspond to a part of the body that is ailing. Reflexology can, however, be undertaken at home on minor conditions such as back pain, headache, etc, but care should be taken not to over-massage any one reflex point as it may result in an unpleasant feeling. Although there have not been any clinical trials to ascertain the efficacy of reflexology, it is generally thought that it does little harm and, indeed, much benefit may result.

Some practitioners believe that stimulation of the reflex points leads to the release of endorphins (in a manner similar to acupuncture). Endorphins are compounds that occur in the brain and have pain-relieving qualities similar to those of morphine. They are derived from a substance in the pituitary gland and are involved in endocrine control (glands producing hormones, for example, the pancreas, thyroid, ovary and testis).

The reflexes
Reflexes on the hands and feet
Reflexes on the feet – the soles of the feet contain a large number of zones, or reflexes, that connect with organs, glands or nerves in the body, as shown in the figures on pages 92–93. In addition, there are a small number of reflexes on the top and insides of the feet, as shown in the figures above.

The *palms of the hands* similarly contain a large number of reflex areas, reflecting the arrangement seen on the soles of the feet, as shown in the figures on pages 94–95. The backs of the hands again mirror, to some extent, the tops of the feet, containing a smaller number of reflex areas (*see* figures above).

Use of the hands in reflexology
The hands are considered to have an electrical property, so that the right-hand palm is positive and the left-hand palm is negative. In addition, the right hand has a reinforcing, stimulating effect while the left has a calming, sedative effect. The back of each hand is opposite to the palm, thus the right is negative and the left is positive. This is important when using reflexology because if the object is to revitalize the body and restore the energy flow that has been limited by a blockage then the right hand is likely to be more effective. The left hand, with its calming effect, is best used to stop pain.

Reflexes on the body
Reflexes on the body necessarily differ from those on the feet and hands in that there is less alignment with the ten zones (the figures on pages 98–99 show some of the reflexes on the body). Also,

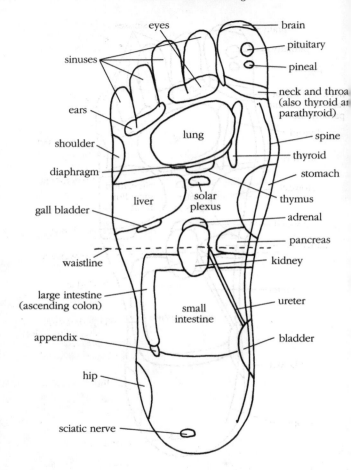

major reflex points on the sole of the right foot

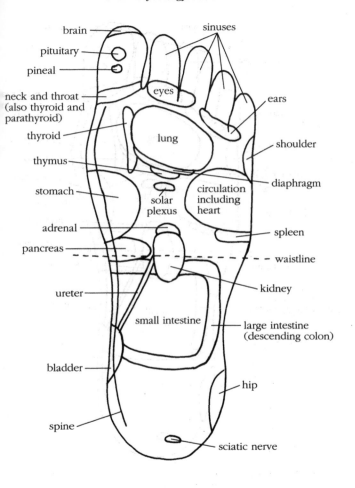

major reflex points on the sole of the left foot

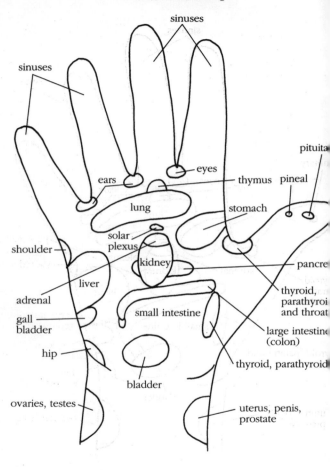

sinuses

sinuses

pituita

ears — eyes — thymus — pineal

lung — stomach

shoulder — solar plexus — kidney — pancre

liver — adrenal

gall bladder — small intestine — thyroid, parathyroi and throat

hip — large intestine (colon)

bladder — thyroid, parathyroid

ovaries, testes — uterus, penis, prostate

major reflex points on the palm of the right hand

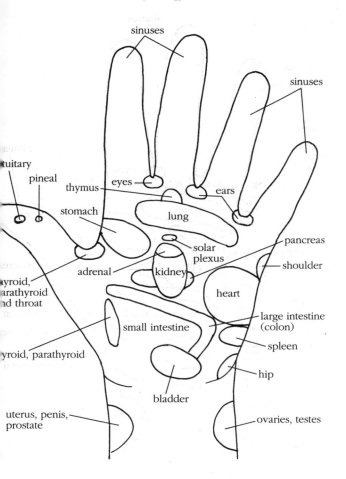

major reflex points on the palm of the left hand

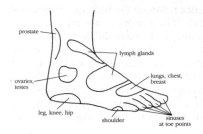

*reflex areas on the
outside of the foot*

*reflex areas on the
inside of the foot*

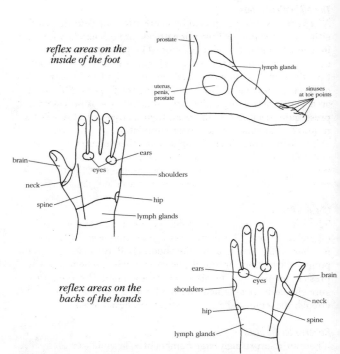

*reflex areas on the
backs of the hands*

there are a number of reflex points on the body that correspond to several organs or glands. These reflex points are sometimes harder to find accurately and may be more difficult to massage.

The middle finger is thought to have the greatest effect, so this should be used to work the reflex point. Light pressure should be applied to each point, and if pain is felt it means there is a blockage or congestion somewhere. A painful point should be pressed until the discomfort subsides or for a few seconds at a time, a shorter rest being taken in between the applications of pressure.

The abdominal reflex

A general test can be applied by gently pressing into the navel, either with the middle finger or with one or both hands, with the individual lying in a supine position. The presence of a pulse or beat is taken to mean there is a problem in this area. To combat this, the same technique is used, holding for a few seconds (six or seven), releasing slightly, and keeping the fingers in the same area, gently massaging with a circular action. If it is necessary to press quite deep to feel the beat, then heavier massage will be required to provide the necessary stimulation.

The same principle can be applied to other reflex points in the abdominal region, and the absence of a pulse or beat indicates that there is no problem. In each case, should there be a painful response, holding for a few seconds invokes the sedative action.

Chest reflexes

There are a number of reflex points on the chest relating to major organs in the body. The same massage technique can be adopted for these reflex points as for the abdomen. Because many of the points lie over bone or muscle, however, it will not be possible to press in the finger as deeply as for the abdomen. However, pressure should be maintained over tender areas, with a subsequent circular massage, and a similar effect will be achieved.

Reflexes on the head

There are a surprisingly large number of reflex points on the head,

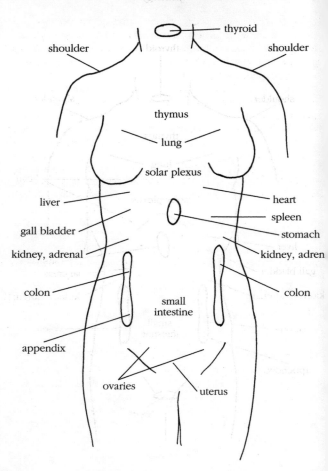

the major reflexes on the body (female)

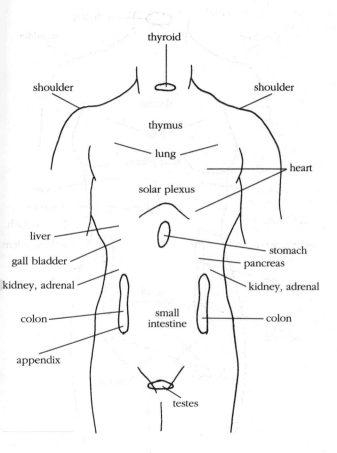

the major reflexes on the body (male)

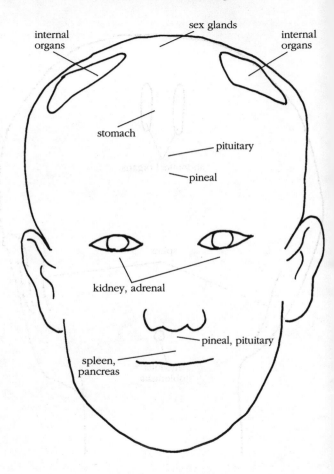

sex glands

internal organs

internal organs

stomach

pituitary

pineal

kidney, adrenal

pineal, pituitary

spleen, pancreas

some of the maor reflex points on the head

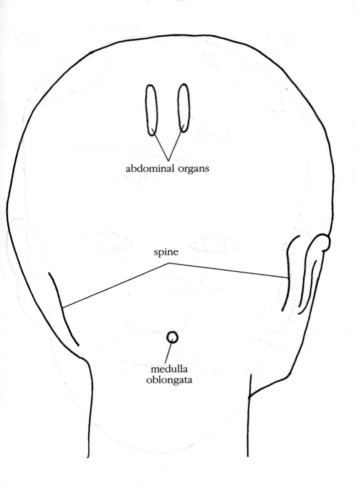

abdominal organs

spine

medulla
oblongata

the back of the head showing the medulla oblongata reflex

although all may not be apparent immediately. With time and experience, such points are often located more by touch than by sight.

There are many important reflexes on the head including the stomach, kidneys, spleen and pancreas. Again, the middle finger can be used for massage, beginning in the middle of the forehead with a gentle circular motion. The massage should go through the skin to rub the bone beneath – the skin should not be rubbed. In so doing, a sensitive point may be felt (pituitary) and another one a little lower down, which is the pineal. (The pituitary gland secretes hormones that control many body functions and the pineal body is thought to regulate the natural variations in the body's activities over a 24-hour period.) This massaging action can be continued to check other parts of the body.

The back of the head also shows a large number of reflexes. However, there are a number of ways of stimulating the body as a whole through the head. These include:

- tapping the head gently with the fists, all over and very quickly for a period of about thirty seconds
- pulling handfuls of hair
- tapping the head gently with a wire brush

Each has a specific result, for example, stimulating the hair, but also enlivening organs and glands over the whole body.

One particularly important reflex point is the medulla oblongata (*see* page 101). The medulla oblongata is the lowest part of the brain stem, which joins to the upper part of the spinal cord. It contains important centres for the control of respiration, swallowing, salivation and the circulation. This reflex point is located at the nape of the neck, towards the base of the skull. Massage of this point opens all channels within the body and generates a vitality, relieving nervous tension and producing almost instant energy. The point should be pressed and massaged to produce the desired effects.

Ear reflexes

The ear has long been used in acupuncture because, in addition to its ease of use, it contains scores of acupoints, which correspond to the reflex points in reflexology. Some of these points are shown in the figure below.

The ear is perhaps the most difficult area of the body to work with because there are so many reflexes in such a small space. It becomes essentially a question of touch, pressing and exploring, and any sore point located can be massaged and worked out. By using a gentle squeeze-and-roll method on the tops of the ears and the ear lobes a number of areas can be stimulated. It has been reported that reflexology can help ear problems such as ringing in the ears, and the condition tinnitus may be alleviated to some extent.

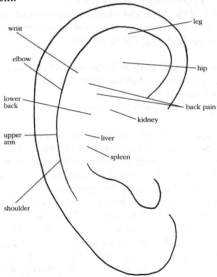

Some of the major reflex points on the ear

Techniques and practice

Some indication of the massaging, manipulative procedures of reflexology have already been mentioned, but a number of general points of guidance can also be made.

The whole process of reflexology is one of calm, gentle movements in a relaxed state. The foot is probably used most in reflexology, in which case shoes and socks and stockings, etc, should be removed. A comfortable position should be adopted on the floor or bed, in a warm, quiet room with the back supported by pillows.

To begin, the whole foot is massaged, indeed both feet should ideally be worked on. However, if working on your own feet it is thought that the right foot should be massaged first (contrary to previous practice). It is considered that the right foot is linked with the past, hence these emotions must be released before the present and future aspects are dealt with in the left foot.

Techniques of massage vary, but a simple method with which to start involves placing the thumb in the middle of the sole of the foot. The thumb then presses with a circular and rocking motion for a few seconds before moving to another reflex. Reference can be made to the diagrams to determine which reflex is being massaged. In all cases, the massage should work beneath the skin, not on the skin. Another method involves starting the massage with the big toe and then moving on to each toe in turn. In using the thumbs to effect the massage, some refinements of motion can be introduced to give slightly different movements.

1   The thumb can be rocked between the tip and the ball, moving forwards over the relevant area. This, along with the circular massage already mentioned, relieves aches and pains.
2   Both thumbs can be used alternately to stroke the skin firmly. This creates a calming effect.
3   The area can be stroked with the thumbs, one moving over the other in a rotational sense. This action is intended to soothe and allow for personal development.

In addition to the procedures already mentioned, reflexology can be used to alleviate many symptoms and help numerous conditions. The following sections provide examples of these uses. Reflexology can be approached intuitively, so that the pressure of touch and the time factor can vary depending upon response and need.

The use of reflexology
The digestive system

The *stomach* is an organ that has thick muscular walls and in which food is reduced to an acidic semi-liquid by the action of gastric juices. There are many factors that can cause an upset stomach. To assess the general condition, the stomach body reflex (above the navel) can be pressed. Around it are several related reflexes such as the liver, gall bladder, intestines and colon. The reflex should be pressed for a few seconds and then released three times to activate the reflex.

On the *hands*, the web of soft tissue between the thumb and forefinger of the left hand should be worked with the thumb of the right hand for a few minutes. The hands can be reversed but the stronger effect will be gained this way, because the stomach lies mostly on the left side.

On the *feet*, the reflexes for the stomach are found primarily on the instep of the left foot, although they are also present on the right foot. These should be massaged, but there are further factors, in addition to the use of reflexology, that will aid digestion. These include eating a sensible diet with a minimum of artificial substances, and not overeating. The use of certain essential oils (aromatherapy) can also be of benefit. In this case peppermint oil can often be particularly effective.

The *colon* is the main part of the large intestine in which water and salts are removed from the food that enters from the small intestine. After extraction of the water, the waste remains are passed on to the rectum as faeces. If this system becomes unbalanced in any way, then the water may not be absorbed or the food remains pass through the colon so quickly that water cannot be absorbed. In such cases, the result is diarrhoea, which can be painful and inconvenient.

Both body and foot reflexes should be massaged for the stomach, intestines, colon and also the liver and kidneys. The thyroid reflex should also be worked to help regulation of the body functions. A useful body reflex is to press and rotate your finger about two inches above the navel for a couple of minutes. This can be repeated numerous times, each time moving the fingers a little clockwise around the navel until a complete circuit has been made. It is important that the condition be stabilized as soon as possible as continued loss also leads to loss of vital salts and a general nutritional deficiency.

At the outset it is possible to work the colon reflexes on the hand to identify any tender areas. The right thumb should be pressed into the edge of the pad (around the base and side of the thumb) of the left palm and worked around to seek out any tender spots. Any tender reflex should be massaged and pressed for a few seconds. In each case, the tenderness should be worked out. Since there are many reflex points crowded onto the navel, it may not solely be the colon reflex that requires some attention. It is always useful to work the reflex on both sides of the body to ensure a balance is achieved.

A similar approach can be adopted for reflexes on the feet, starting at the centre, or waistline. By applying a rolling pressure, the foot is massaged along to the inner edge and then down the line of the spine and any tender points are worked through pressure and massage. It may be necessary to start with a very light pressure if the area is very tender, and then as the soreness lessens, the pressure can be increased.

Again, diet can be an important factor in maintaining the health of the body and the workings of the colon. Fibre is particularly important in ensuring a healthy digestive system and avoiding ailments such as diverticulitis.

Reflexology can be used for other conditions associated with the digestive system, notably ulcers. A peptic ulcer (in the stomach, duodenum or even the oesophagus) is caused by a break in the mucosal lining. This may be due to the action of acid, bile or enzymes because of unusually high concentrations or a deficiency in the systems that normally protect the mucosa. The result can be a burning sensation, belching and nausea.

To help alleviate the problem, which may often be stress-related, the reflexes in the feet should be massaged, as these are often the most relaxing. Obviously, the important reflexes are the stomach and duodenum, but it is also worthwhile to work on the liver and the endocrine glands (notably the pituitary). If the ulcer is a long-standing problem or if stomach complaints have been experienced for some time, then further medical help is probably needed.

The heart and circulatory system

The heart is obviously a vital organ. This muscular pump is situated between the lungs and slightly left of the midline. It projects forward and lies beneath the fifth rib. Blood returns from the body via the veins and enters the right atrium (the upper chamber), which contracts, forcing the blood into the right ventricle. From there it goes to the lungs where it gains oxygen and releases carbon dioxide before passing to the left atrium and left ventricle. Oxygenated blood then travels throughout the body via the arteries.

By using body reflexes, the heart can be maintained, and conditions can be dealt with by massaging the appropriate reflex points. A useful massage exercise is to work the muscles, rather than the reflex points, of the left arm in a side-to-side movement. This can be followed by the neck muscles and the chest muscles; in each case any tightness or tension should be massaged out. An additional preventive is a good diet, which should be low in fat and food high in cholesterol, but should contain adequate amounts of vitamins, notably the B group, C and E. Exercise is, of course, very important to maintain a good heart and circulation.

There is also a simple test that many reflexologists feel is useful in the diagnosis of possible heart problems. It may also be worth doing if strenuous activity is contemplated in the near future. Pressure is applied to the pad of the left thumb, at the top. The pressure should be quite hard. It is suggested that when this part of the pad hurts, it indicates a constriction in blood vessels, limiting supply. If the bottom of the pad hurts, this is indicative of congested arteries. If the area is too tender to touch (and there is no physical damage to the hand) then there is a possibility of a heart attack. This test thus provides advance warning and enables a medical doctor to be consulted. Should painful areas occur on both hands, this does *not* indicate a heart problem.

Many blood and circulatory disorders will benefit from the same sort of massage. In these cases the foot reflexes for the endocrine glands (hypothalamus, pituitary, pineal, thyroid and parathyroid, thymus, adrenals, pancreas, ovary or testis) should be worked well, as should those for the circulatory system and heart, lungs and lymphatic system.

Conditions that may benefit from such treatment include:

Angina

A suffocating, choking pain usually referring to angina pectoris, which is felt in the chest. It occurs when blood supply to the heart muscle is inadequate and is brought on by exercise and relieved by rest. The coronary arteries may be damaged by atheroma (scarring and buildup of fatty deposits). Of particular importance are the heart and circulatory reflexes (veins and arteries) and those of the lymphatic system.

Arteriosclerosis

A general term including atheroma and atherosclerosis (where arteries degenerate and fat deposits reduce blood flow), which results generally in high blood pressure and can lead to angina. Additional reflexes that should be worked include the liver.

Hypertension (high blood pressure)

This may be one of several types, the commonest being *essential* (due to kidney or endocrine disease or an unknown cause) and *malignant* (a serious condition that tends to occur in the younger age groups). In addition to the reflexes for the blood and circulation, those for the shoulders, neck and eyes should be worked, in combination with reflexes for the digestive system and liver.

Palpitations

An irregular heartbeat, often associated with heightened emotions. Also due to heart disease or may be felt during pregnancy. The lung and heart reflexes are particularly important, in addition to those of the circulation.

Some heart conditions are very serious and require immediate hospitalization, e.g. cardiac arrest (when the heart stops) and coronary thrombosis (a coronary artery blockage causing severe chest pain, vomiting, nausea and breathing difficulties. The affected heart muscle dies, a condition known as myocardial infarction). However, massage of appropriate reflexes may help, particularly in less serious cases. These should include the heart and circulation (veins and arteries), lungs, endocrine system and the brain. Each will have some beneficial effect in relieving stress and congestion.

Varicose veins

Veins that have become stretched, twisted and distended, and this often happens to the superficial veins in the legs. The possible causes are numerous and include pregnancy, defective valves, obesity and thrombophlebitis (the inflammation of the wall of a vein with secondary thrombosis). Phlebitis is inflammation of a vein and occurs primarily as a complication of varicose veins. Both these conditions can be treated by massaging the circulatory reflexes and also the leg and liver reflexes. In both cases, resting with the legs in an elevated position is beneficial.

The respiratory system

Asthma is one of the major problems of the respiratory system and its incidence seems to be escalating. The condition is caused by a narrowing of the airways in the lungs. It usually begins in early childhood and may be brought on by exposure to allergens (substances, usually proteins, that cause allergic reactions) exercise or stress.

There are certain body reflexes that can help in this instance. One reflex point is in the lower neck at the base of the V-shape created by the collar bones. Relief may be achieved by pressing the finger into this point with a downward motion for a few seconds. There are additional reflex points on the back, at either side of the spine in the general region of the shoulder blades. These can be worked by someone else with thumb or finger, who should press for a few seconds. Other reflexes that can be worked on the foot include the brain, endocrine glands such as the pineal, pituitary, thymus and thyroid, the lungs, and also the circulatory system. Particular attention should be paid to the lungs, which includes the bronchi and bronchioles, the branching passageways of the lungs where gaseous exchange (oxygen in, carbon dioxide out) takes place. At the point where the instep meets the hard balls of the feet, and along the base of the lung reflex area is the massage point for the diaphragm. Working the whole of this area will help alleviate symptoms of asthma. During an attack of asthma, both thumbs can be placed on the solar plexus reflexes immediately to initiate the soothing process.

The adrenal glands are found one to each kidney, situated on the upper surface of that organ. These are important endocrine glands because they produce hormones such as adrenaline and cortisone. Adrenaline is very important in controlling the rate of respiration and it is used medically in the treatment of bronchial asthma because it relaxes the airways. It is clear therefore, that the adrenal is an important reflex and it is located in the middle of each sole and palm.

Many other respiratory disorders can be helped by using massage of the same reflexes: brain, endocrine glands, lungs and diaphragm, neck and shoulders, augmented by the heart and circulatory system. Conditions responding to this regime include bronchitis, croup, lung disorders and emphysema (distension and thinning, particularly of lung tissue, leading to air-filled spaces that do not contribute to the respiratory process).

Infections of the respiratory tract leading to coughs and colds can also be helped primarily by working the reflexes mentioned above. For colds, the facial reflexes should be massaged, especially that for the nose. However, it is good practice to include the pituitary, and to work the index and middle fingers towards the tip to help alleviate the condition.

With such respiratory problems, there are complementary therapies that can help such as homeopathy , aromatherapy and Bach flower remedies. There are also many simple actions that can be taken, for example a sore throat may be helped by gargling regularly with a dessertspoon of cider apple vinegar in a glass of water, with just a little being swallowed each time. Honey is also a good substance to take, as are onion and garlic.

The endocrine glands
The major glands
Endocrine glands are glands that release hormones directly into the bloodstream, or lymphatic system. Some organs, such as the pancreas, also release secretions via ducts. The major endocrine glands are, in addition to the pancreas, the thyroid, parathyroid, pituitary, pineal, thymus, adrenal and gonads (ovaries and testes).

The endocrine glands are of vital importance in regulating body functions as summarized below:

pituitary	controls growth, gonads, kidneys; known as the master gland
pineal	controls the natural daily rhythms of the body
thyroid	regulates metabolism and growth
parathyroid	controls calcium and phosphorus metabolism
thymus	vital in the immune system, particularly pre-puberty
adrenal	control of heartbeat, respiration and metabolism
gonads	control of reproductive activity
pancreas	control of blood sugar levels

The fact that the endocrine glands are responsible for the very core of body functions means that any imbalance should be corrected immediately to restore the normality. There are some general points relating to massage of these reflex areas. It is good practice to massage the brain reflex first and then the pituitary. This is because the hypothalamus, situated in the forebrain, controls secretions from the pituitary gland. The pituitary gland then follows as this is the most important in the endocrine system. The reflexes should be gently massaged with thumb or finger for a few seconds and then gentle pressure exerted and held for a few seconds before releasing slowly.

The pituitary

An imbalance of pituitary gland secretions, often caused by a benign tumour, can lead to acromegaly (excessive growth of skeletal and soft tissue). Gigantism can result if it occurs during adolescence. There may also be consequent deficiencies in adrenal, gonad and thyroid activity. The brain and endocrine reflexes should be worked in order, supplemented by those for the circulation, liver and digestion. In addition to reflex points on the hands and feet, there is also one on the forehead. If any of these reflex areas is found to be tender, it should be massaged often to maintain the balance necessary for healthy growth.

The pineal

The pineal body, or gland, is situated on the upper part of the mid-brain, although its function is not fully understood. It would seem, however, to be involved in the daily rhythms of the body and may also play a part in controlling sexual activity. The pineal reflex points are found close to those of the pituitary on the big toes, thumbs and on the forehead and upper lip.

The thyroid

The thyroid is located at the base of the neck and it produces two important hormones, thyroxine and triiodothyronine. Under or overactivity of the thyroid leads to specific conditions.

If the thyroid is overactive and secretes too much thyroxine (hyperthyroidism), the condition called thyrotoxicosis develops. It is also known as Grave's disease and is typified by an enlarged gland, protruding eyes and symptoms of excess metabolism such as tremor, hyperactivity, rapid heart rate, breathlessness, etc. The important reflexes on which to concentrate are the brain and solar plexus, endocrine system and also the circulatory and digestive systems. The reflexes are found on the soles and palms and using the thumbs or fingers, the areas should be massaged, but in stages if the area is very tender.

Underactivity of the thyroid, or hypothyroidism, can cause myxoedema producing dry, coarse skin, mental impairment, muscle pain and other symptoms. In children a similar lack causes cretinism, resulting in dwarfism and mental retardation. The reflexes to be worked are essentially those mentioned for hyperthyroidism, and in addition (for both conditions) the liver reflexes on the right sole and palm should benefit from attention.

There are additional thyroid reflexes elsewhere on the body, notably on the neck roughly midway between jaw and collarbone and on either side. These points should be massaged gently with the thumb and fingers on opposite sides of the throat. Using a gentle gyratory motion, the massage can be taken down to the collarbone, the fingers and thumb of the other hand are then used (on opposite sides of the throat) and the procedure repeated.

Goitre is another condition associated with the thyroid and is a swelling of the neck caused by enlargement of the gland, typically due to overactivity of the gland to compensate for an iodine deficiency. The important reflexes to concentrate upon are the brain, solar plexus, endocrine system and circulatory system but working of all body reflexes will help.

The parathyroid

There are four small parathyroid glands located behind or within the thyroid. They control the use of calcium and phosphorus (as phosphate) in the body's metabolism. An imbalance of these vital elements can lead to tetany (muscular spasms), or at the other extreme, calcium may be transferred from the bones to the blood, creating a tendency to bone fractures and breaks.

The reflexes to these glands are found in the same location as those for the thyroid but it will probably be necessary to massage more strongly to achieve an effect. It is a good idea to work on these areas each time reflexology is undertaken as they are vital in maintaining the metabolic equilibrium of the body.

The thymus

The thymus is located in the neck (over the breastbone) and is a vital contributor to the immune system. It is larger in children and is important in the development of the immune response. After puberty it shrinks although seems to become more active later in life. Bone marrow cells mature within the thymus and one group, T-lymphocytes, are dependent upon the presence of the thymus. These are important cells as they produce antibodies.

The commonest disorder associated with the thymus is myasthenia gravis, which lowers the level of acetylcholine (a neurotransmitter) resulting in a weakening of skeletal muscles and those used for breathing, swallowing, etc. The thymus reflexes are found on the soles of the feet and palms of the hand, next to the lung reflexes. The thymus can also be stimulated by tapping with the finger over its position in the middle of the upper chest.

The adrenals

The two adrenals (also known as suprarenals) are situated one above each kidney and consist of an inner medulla and an outer cortex. The medulla produces adrenaline, which increases the rate and depth of respiration, raises the heartbeat and improves muscle performance, with a parallel increase in output of sugar from the liver into the blood.

The cortex of the adrenal glands releases hormones including aldosterone, which controls the balance of electrolytes in the body, and cortisone, which, among other functions, is vital in the response to stress, inflammation and fat deposition in the body.

On both the palms and soles, the adrenal reflexes are located above those for the kidneys and if this area is at all tender, it should be massaged for a few seconds. Because the kidney and adrenal reflexes are close together, the massage should be limited to avoid over-stimulation of the kidney reflexes. Disorders of the adrenal glands should be treated by working the endocrine reflexes starting with the pituitary and including the adrenal reflexes themselves, followed by the reflexes for the circulatory, liver and urinary systems.

Specific disorders include Cushing's syndrome, caused by an overproduction of cortisone, which results in obesity, reddening of the face and neck, growth of body and facial hair, high blood pressure, osteoporosis and possibly mental disturbances, and Addison's disease, which results from damage to the cortex and therefore a deficiency in hormone secretion. The latter was commonly caused by tuberculosis but is now due more to disturbances in the immune system. The symptoms are weakness, wasting, low blood pressure and dark pigmentation of the skin. Both these conditions can be treated by hormone replacement therapy but reflexology can assist, through massage of the endocrine, digestive and liver reflexes.

The gonads

The gonads, or sex glands, comprise the ovaries in women and testes in men. The ovaries produce eggs and also secrete hormones, mainly oestrogen and progesterone. Similarly, the testes produce sperm and the hormone testosterone. Oestrogen controls the female secondary sexual characteristics such as enlargement of the breasts, growth of pubic hair and deposition of body fat. Progesterone is vital in pregnancy as it prepares the uterus for implantation of the egg cell.

The reflexes for these and related organs are found near the ankles on the inside of the feet, just below the angular bone (*see* figure depicting the reflex areas on the inside and outside of the feet on page 96). The same reflex areas are also located on the arms, near the wrist. The ovaries and testes are on the outer edge, while on the opposite, inner edge, are the reflexes for the uterus, penis and prostate.

For any disorders that might involve the ovaries or testes, it is also useful to massage other systems such as the brain, other endocrine glands, the circulation and liver.

The pancreas

This is an important gland with both endocrine and exocrine functions. It is located behind the stomach, between the duodenum and spleen. The exocrine function involves secretion of pancreatic juice via ducts, into the intestine. The endocrine function is vital in balancing blood sugar levels through the secretion of two hormones, insulin and glucagon. Insulin controls the uptake of glucose by body cells and a lack of hormone results in the sugar derived from food being excreted in the urine, the condition known as diabetes mellitus. Glucagon works in the opposite sense to insulin, and increases the supply of blood sugar through the breakdown of glycogen in the liver, to produce glucose.

The primary reflexes for the pancreas are found on the soles and palms, near to the stomach. The thumb should be used, starting on the left foot, working across the reflex area and on to the right foot. If the area is tender, it should be worked until the tenderness goes. Because there are numerous reflexes in this area, there will be stimulation of other organs, to the general wellbeing of the body as a whole.

For other disorders of the pancreas, such as pancreatitis (inflammation of the pancreas) the reflexes associated with digestion should also be worked. Pancreatitis may result from gallstones or alcoholism and, if sufficiently severe, may cause diabetes.

The liver and spleen
The role of the liver

The liver is a very important organ and is critical in regulating metabolic processes. It is the largest gland in the body and is situated in the top right hand part of the abdominal cavity. Among the functions, the liver converts excess glucose to glycogen, which is stored as a food reserve; excess amounts of amino acids are converted into urea for excretion; bile is produced for storage in the gall bladder and some poisons are broken down. The liver also recycles red blood cells to remove the iron when the cells reach the end of their life; it stores vitamins and produces blood clotting substances. Due to its high chemical and biochemical activity, the liver generates a lot of heat and is the major contributor of heat to the body.

The liver reflex points

The reflex area for the liver is a large area, reflecting the size of the organ, on the right palm and right sole, on the outer edge. As a general procedure, the area should be massaged with the left thumb, searching for tender points. More massage may be required for the liver than for other reflexes.

Hepatitis is inflammation of the liver due to viral infection or the presence of toxins. Alcohol abuse commonly causes hepatitis, and it may also be due to drug overdose or drug side effects. Viral infections such as HIV and glandular fever can also cause hepatitis. There are several types of hepatitis, designated A to E, and all may persist in the blood for a long time.

To combat such disorders, after removing the source of any toxins, the reflex for the liver and digestion should be worked and the reflexes for the eyes. Dietary restraint is also important and should involve natural foods with little or no alcohol, caffeine, nicotine and a low intake of fats.

Associated with the liver, anatomically, is the gall bladder. This is a small sac-like organ that stores and concentrates bile. When fats are digested, the gall bladder contracts, sending bile into the duodenum. Sometimes stones form here, and often gallstones can cause severe pain. The gall bladder reflex is found at the foot of the liver on the right palm and foot. On the body there is another reflex just below the ribs on the right-hand side, and below the liver reflex point. A steady pressure should be held around the point, beginning near the navel and working to the right side, maintaining pressure for a few seconds on any tender point.

The role of the spleen

The spleen is situated on the left side of the body behind and below the stomach. The spleen produces leucocytes (white blood cells), lymphocytes (a white blood cell involved in the immune system), blood platelets (involved in blood coagulation) and plasma cells. It also acts as a store for red blood cells, which are made available in emergencies (when oxygen demand is greater).

The spleen reflex point

The reflex area for the spleen is found on the left palm or sole, below the reflex for the heart. If a tender point is found in this reflex, it may indicate anaemia and it would then be wise to obtain a blood test.

The kidneys and bladder
The role of the kidneys and bladder

The kidneys are important organs in the body's excretory system. They are responsible for processing the blood continuously to remove nitrogenous wastes (mainly urea) and they also adjust salt concentrations. By testing the reflexes with the thumb, tender areas can be located and worked upon. However, prolonged massage should be avoided – it is better to use shorter periods of 15-20 seconds initially as the system becomes accustomed to the treatment.

It is not surprising, considering the pivotal role of the kidneys in removing body wastes, that any interference with their normal function can lead to serious illnesses. General kidney disorders, kidney stones, nephritis and pyelitis are all best aided by massaging the kidney reflex but also the reflexes for the central nervous system, the endocrine glands (especially the pituitary and adrenal glands), liver, stomach and circulation. Kidney stones are formed by the deposition of solid substances that are naturally found in the urine but that precipitate out for one reason or another. They are commonly salts of calcium, and the alteration in pH of the urine is often a contributory factor. Nephritis is inflammation of the kidney and pyelitis is when part of the kidney, the pelvis, becomes inflamed. If the whole kidney becomes affected, it is then called pyelonephritis.

The kidney and bladder reflex points

Disorders associated with the bladder tend to be infections such as cystitis or other physical manifestation of a problem whether through stress or a medical condition. The latter category includes enuresis (bed-wetting) and incontinence. In these cases, the bladder reflex should obviously be worked upon, and the reflexes for the brain, solar plexus and endocrine system.

The reflexes for the kidneys are found just off centre on the palms of both hands and soles of both feet. They are close to the pancreas and stomach. The bladder reflex is towards the base of the palm, near the wrist and on the feet it is found on the inside edge of both soles, towards the heel. There are also body reflexes for both organs.

The body reflexes for the kidney are at the side of the body, almost at the waistline, between the hip and rib cage. They also occur on the face, just beneath the eyes.

The alleviation of back pain and other skeletal disorders
The reflex points for the spine

Within the working population of most countries, back pain accounts for millions of days in lost production. This is not unexpected as the spine is the primary part of the skeleton, hence any problem with it will inevitably upset the body and its overall well-being.

On the soles of the feet, the reflex for the spine is located along the inner edge of both feet running from the base of the big toe almost to the heel. By working this line with the fingers, any tender points can be found and worked upon. The top end of the line, near the toe, is equivalent to the spine at the level of the shoulders.

Treatment of back disorders through reflexology

With back disorders, such as lumbago, additional reflexes should be worked including the brain and endocrine system. Because the body's musculature is a complementary and antagonistic system with the skeleton, creating all the movements of which the body is capable, the muscles are also important when dealing with back pain. It will help therefore to massage muscles, rubbing quite deeply with the fingers, and moving across the muscles.

Back pain can result from a problem elsewhere in the body with posture, tight muscles or even flat feet. It is important to be aware of the possibilities and ensure that the treatment deals with the problem as a whole, and not just in part. Exercise is clearly beneficial and walking can help loosen and strengthen muscles associated with the back. A brisk walk is fine, but jogging is not necessarily the best remedy, as in some cases this can itself prove harmful.

Reflexologists often turn to the muscles in the legs to alleviate back pain, particularly in the area of the lower back. The muscles at the back of the thigh should be massaged with a pressing and pulling action, first with one hand and then the other. The whole of the thigh should be treated, from the top of the leg, to the knee. Massage of both legs in this manner, concentrating on any 'tight' areas, will help improve the overall tone and assist in eliminating causes of back pain.

Study of the diagrams for the feet and hands reveals specific reflex areas for the shoulders, hip and neck. When working on skeletal disorders in general, it is wise to undertake a thorough massage of specific reflex areas such as neck and shoulders, plus those for the brain, solar plexus, the endocrine system, remainder of the skeletal system, endocrine glands, etc. For particular conditions such as bursitis (inflammation of a joint, as in housemaid's knee), general joint pain, stiff neck and similar complaints, a common regime of reflexological massage applies. This should include working the skeletal reflexes along with those for the nervous and endocrine system, digestive and circulatory systems. It is usually the case that the specific complaint will benefit from massage of its reflex area and most of those that comprise a whole body workout. It should always be remembered that there are occasions when surgery may prove essential, e.g. in the case of a hip replacement.

The knee joint can often be the source of pain and discomfort. It may help to apply gentle pressure on either side of the knee, just where the bone ends, using the thumb and middle finger. This should be held for a few seconds, pressing as much as possible (do not press hard if it is too painful) and then the same should be done below the knee.

Relief from arthritis with reflexology

Arthritis can be a crippling disease and many people suffer from it. It is an inflammation of joints or the spine, the symptoms of which are pain and swelling, restriction of movement, redness and warmth of the skin. Two forms of the condition are osteoarthritis and rheumatoid arthritis.

Treatment of osteoarthritis through reflexology

Osteoarthritis involves the cartilage in joints, which then affects the associated bone. What often happens is that the cartilage is lost, to be replaced by osteophytes at the edges of the bones. These are bony projections that occur with the loss of cartilage or with age. The projections affect the joint function, causing pain.

Treatment of rhematoid arthritis through reflexology

Rheumatoid arthritis is the second commonest joint disease after osteoarthritis. It usually affects the feet, ankles, wrists and fingers in which there is a swelling of the joint and inflammation of the synovial membrane (the membraneous envelope around the joint). Then follows erosion and loss of cartilage and loss of bone. At its worst, the condition can be disabling.

Massage of the reflex areas for the affected areas should be worked but, as mentioned previously, it is important to massage the reflexes for the whole body to achieve a complete and balanced approach. The endocrine system is one important system in this respect.

In seeking ways to treat rheumatoid arthritis, the medical profession isolated the glucocorticosteroid hormone, cortisone, from the adrenal glands of cattle. It was found that the use of cortisone had dramatic effects on the symptoms of rheumatoid arthritis. However, the relief was only temporary, and an additional disadvantage was the occurrence of associated side effects, which could be severe, e.g. damage to muscle, bone, stomach ulcers, bleeding and imbalances in the hormonal and nervous systems. The medical use of this compound is therefore very restricted, but it is produced naturally by the adrenal cortex. Being a natural secretion, there are no detrimental side effects. There is a reflex point in the lower back, between the first and second lumbar vertebrae, which can be pressed. Finding this point will be hit and miss initially, but upon locating it (roughly 5 cm up from the coccyx or tailbone), apply gentle pressure, gradually increasing, and hold it for a few seconds. This should be repeated several times. This is helpful for other conditions, in addition to rheumatoid arthritis, such as asthma and bursitis.

As with back disorders, muscle condition is also felt to be important in the treatment of arthritis. The muscles in the area affected by arthritis should be massaged by pressing in with the fingers, either on or near to the area. The massage should be across the muscles, with a deep motion, although it may initially produce discomfort or soreness. Many practitioners regard this as an important supplementary technique in administering reflexology.

Stress and tension
The relaxing effects of reflexology

One of the additional beneficial effects of reflexology when dealing with a particular reflex area or point is that the treatment is very relaxing. If most of the body reflexes are massaged, a feeling of wellbeing is generated, and tension is released. Stress control and relief can be accomplished in a number of ways, some of which happen instinctively, such as deep breathing and, paradoxically, wringing the hands. The latter is an obvious way of working the reflex points, albeit that it is mostly done unconsciously. A related method of calming the nerves is to intertwine the fingers, as in clasping the hands, which enables all the reflexes between the fingers to be pressed. This should be done several times. Deep breathing is a common method of relaxation that ultimately can envelop the whole body, providing that the focus of attention is the attainment of the correct pattern of breathing. Mental attitude is also an important aspect of reflexology. It clearly makes sense, while undergoing massage (with or without a practitioner or partner) to imagine, or listen to, pleasing sounds, rather than worrying about the pressures of modern life. If there is no access to relaxing sounds (bird song, running water, etc) it is perfectly possible to imagine it, and thereby to augment the physical relaxation with mental calm.

Reflex points for treating stress

The *endocrine glands* are considered important in combating stress because they are responsible for the hormonal balance of the body. All reflex areas for these glands, on both soles and palms, should be massaged and special attention given to the thyroid, which controls body temperature and can help restore calm. The adrenal reflex point, almost in the centre of the hand, is also important, and, because it is so near the solar plexus, receives equal attention. (The solar plexus is a network of nerves and ganglia in the sympathetic nervous system concerned with body functions not under conscious control. It is located behind the stomach).

Quite often stress and tension can result in a sore neck or back. A number of reflex points can be worked to relieve these sorts of complaint. The medulla oblongata is important in this respect as it controls some major body functions such as the circulation. The point on the back of the head (*see* the figure on page 101) should be held with the middle finger for a few seconds and then released, and repeated several times. The reflex points of the spine should also be worked starting at the neck reflex, which is found below the base of the big toe or thumb. By moving down the side of the foot, the whole spine can be covered. To relieve a sore back completely and effectively, other reflexes to be attended to should include the shoulders, hips, and the sciatic nerve. The sciatic nerve is made up of a number of nerve roots from the lower part of the spinal cord, and pain with this origin may be felt in the back of the thigh, buttock and the foot. The reflex point may at first be painful to the touch, but through careful massage it can be worked to assist in promoting relief.

Control of the heart rate is a natural, complementary procedure in promoting stress relief. If a situation, wherever it may be, results in you feeling stressed, massaging the reflex areas for the heart will help, whether on foot or hand.

Sound, restful sleep is refreshing and also contributes to a reduction in stress. Reflexology can also help in this respect through the feeling of relaxation that it induces. The clasping of the hands, mentioned earlier, can be used to combat sleeplessness. The fingers can be clasped on the chest and then worked over each other so that the length of each finger is massaged. The fingers should remain intertwined and simply be released a little to allow each finger over the first knuckle, when the fingers are squeezed together again. This, associated with deep breathing will encourage relaxation.

Reflexology and the reproductive system
Reflex points for the reproductive system

The major reflexes of the reproductive system are those for the uterus, ovary and breast in the female, and the penis, testes and prostate in the male. The ovary reflexes are found on the outer side of the foot, just below the ankle (*see* figures on page 96). On the hand, these are found a little way beyond the wrist (*see* figures on page 96), on the outer edge. On both foot and hand, the breast reflex is found on the outer edge, a little below the base of the little toe or finger. The uterus reflex on the hand occupies a position opposite to the ovaries, i.e. just below the wrist, but on the inner edge of the arm. On the foot, this reflex mirrors that for the ovary, but it is on the inside of the foot, below the ankle.

The male reflexes

The male reflexes occupy the same positions as those of the female, thus the penis reflex is in the same position as that for the uterus and the testes is the same as the ovaries. The prostate gland reflexes are situated with the penis reflex and also at the back of the leg/foot, above the heel, (*see* the figures on page 96).

There are also reflex points on the head for the gonads (*see* sex glands on the diagram of the reflex points on the head on page 100). As well as working the various reflexes for the reproductive system, it is beneficial to pay attention to the endocrine gland reflexes as they have considerable control over the gonads (*see* endocrine glands, page 111). In particular, the pituitary, thyroid and adrenal glands and their hormonal secretions have a large influence on the reproductive system. All these points should be massaged to stimulate activity and ensure that hormone secretion is balanced and gonad activity is normal. The body reflexes can also be used to this end by pressing each point for a few seconds and repeating several times for all endocrine and sex glands.

If any of the endocrine glands are tender, it may be indicating a problem with the sex glands. By working the various reflex points, it is possible to ensure a healthy reproductive system. There are a number of reflexes to the penis and testes that can help in this respect. The sex reflex below the navel should be pressed with fingers or thumb and massaged for a few seconds. Additional reflex points on the legs, about 15 cm above the ankle on the inside of the leg, should also be massaged. Initially, massage here should be for half a minute or so, because any problems will make it tender. However, with further attention it will be possible to work out the soreness. A further point on the leg lies above the knee, in the soft area on the outer edge, above the kneecap. All these reflexes, if worked in turn, will contribute to a healthy system and lead to fewer problems, such as impotence.

Impotence itself can, however, be treated. In addition to undertaking the massage of reflex points and areas mentioned above, there are further techniques that may help. There is a particularly sensitive and stimulating area between the anus and scrotum, which should be pressed gently a number of times. It is also said that if gentle on-off pressure is applied to the scrotum, this will help.

Another problem faced by many men involves the prostate gland. This gland is situated below the bladder and opens into the urethra, which is the duct carrying urine out of the body and which also forms the ejaculatory duct. On ejaculation, the gland secretes an alkaline fluid into the sperm to help sperm motility. In older men particularly, the prostate gland may have become enlarged, causing problems with urination. Working the appropriate reflexes may help this situation as may massaging the base of the penis. However, it is advisable to check with a medical doctor to ensure that there is no other condition present.

The female reflexes

There are a number of female conditions that may be helped by reflexology. In most cases, the reflexes to be worked are very similar and the following complaints are therefore grouped in this way:

- *amenorrhoea* lack of menstruation, other than during pregnancy or pre-puberty
- *endometriosis* the occurrence of endometrial cells, normally found in the womb, elsewhere in the body, e.g. Fallopian tubes or peritoneum, causing pain and bleeding
- *fibroid* a benign tumour of the uterus that may cause pain, bleeding and urine retention
- *leucorrhoea* discharge of white/yellow mucus from the vagina, which may be normal before and after menstruation, but at other times large amounts signify an infection
- *dysmenorrhoea* painful menstruation
- *menorrhagia* excessive blood flow during menstruation

For these and related conditions, the general procedure should be to spend time on the specific female reflex, which in these cases is the uterus. In addition the endocrine gland reflexes should be massaged and to provide a balanced treatment, the reflexes for the other reproductive organs (ovary, etc) should be worked.

Further areas to concentrate upon include the urinary and circulatory systems and the central nervous system (brain) with the solar plexus.

Premenstrual tension (or syndrome) is the condition typified by headache, nervousness, irritability, depression and tiredness (in addition to physical symptoms) several days before the start of menstruation. It is advisable, before menstruation starts, to have a thorough massage of the reflexes once or twice per week. Next, the reflexes for the uterus and ovaries should be worked. The uterus reflex is on the inside of the foot in the soft area beneath the ankle. The massage should work all around the ankle, beginning with a gentle pressure, and then working back towards the heel. The other foot should then be dealt with in the same way.

To help overcome depression the endocrine glands are very important to regulate hormones, maintain body rhythms and balance the biochemical functions – all of which have some effect on emotions. Other reflexes to work, in addition to the endocrine glands, include the solar plexus, brain and liver. The liver is very important in this respect and, although the area should not be overworked, it should not be forgotten.

The *menopause* is the time when a woman's ovaries no longer release an egg cell every month, and child-bearing is no longer possible. This usually occurs between the ages of 45 and 55. It may be preceded by a gradual decline in the frequency of menstruation or there may be an abrupt cessation. There is an imbalance in the sex hormones and this can cause a number of symptoms, including hot flushes, sweats, palpitations, depression and vaginal dryness. Over a longer period there may be a gradual loss of bone (osteoporosis) leading to a greater risk of bone fractures.

In this instance, the endocrine reflexes are once again very important. In conjunction with these, the reflexes for the spine and brain should be worked, the former to promote relaxation. As a general point, the reflexes to the spine can be massaged for any length of time whereas those for organs and glands should be worked periodically and for a few seconds each time.

To help combat hot flushes, the thyroid reflex should be worked since this is the endocrine gland responsible for the control of the metabolic rate. Regulation of breathing through deep breaths will also help.

The breasts are, of course, the mammary glands that produce milk at the appropriate time, but in today's society they have also become important from a cosmetic point of view. Disorders of the breasts can include lumps or cysts, pain or tenderness. Such conditions may be due to an hormonal imbalance but in any event will benefit from a complete treatment of all the reflexes on feet, hands or head. The breast reflex is found on the top of the foot or hand, at the base of the toes or fingers, and this should be worked regularly. Since the endocrine system is of great significance in the reproductive system, all glands reflexes should receive some attention. Reflexological massage can also be used as a general technique to maintain healthy breasts. Essentially the hand should form a cup around the breast with the fingers underneath and the nipple between thumb and forefinger. Using a circular movement the breast is massaged slightly upwards. This should help retain the shape of the breast, and maintain its tone.

Diseases of the immune system
Antibodies and the lymphatic system
The human body resists infection by means of antibodies and white blood cells. Antibodies are protein substances produced by the lymphoid tissue (spleen, thymus gland and the lymph nodes) that circulate in the blood. They react with their corresponding antigens (foreign bodies that cause antibodies to be formed) and make them harmless. There are a number of immunoglobulins (large protein molecules) that act as antibodies, and each has a particular function. For example, one is responsible for allergic reactions and another is produced to fight bacteria and viruses in the body.

The lymphatic system is also important in the body's immune response. Lymph nodes are swellings that occur at various points in the system. They are found in the neck, groin and armpit, and their main function is to remove foreign particles from the lymph, and to participate in the immune response. In this latter function they become enlarged and produce lymphocytes, a type of white blood cell, which locate and neutralize antigens, or produce antibodies, depending upon their type.

The lymph itself is a colourless, watery fluid. It is derived from blood and is similar to plasma. It contains 95 per cent water, with protein, sugar, salt and lymphocytes. The lymph is circulated by muscular action, and pumped through the lymph nodes for filtering.

It is clear that the lymphatic system, and the immune system overall, are very important in maintaining good health. Any disorder or deficiency in this system will lead to illness, which in some cases may be life-threatening. Reflexology may prove useful in restoring the balance although the need for professional medical advice should always be borne in mind.

Reflex points for the immune system

A number of reflexes to the lymph glands can be worked, on the back of the hands, located over the wrists (*see* the figures on page 96) and on the top of the foot. The spleen is also an important reflex because the spleen itself produces lymphocytes (amongst other things). Associated reflexes that should be worked are those for the endocrine glands, circulation and liver.

In the case of infectious diseases, many of which occur in childhood (such as measles, mumps and chickenpox), the infection will normally run its course and as a result confer immunity to further bouts. To minimize discomfort and aid the recovery, the reflexes for the brain, solar plexus, circulation, endocrine glands and liver should be massaged.

The same applies to most infectious conditions, even autoimmune diseases where the antibodies attack their own body cells. In these cases, the lymph gland reflexes are particularly important.

Reiki

Introduction

A complementary therapy

Reiki is a complementary therapy and one of the many facets of
alternative medicine available today. It is a method of natural healing which is centred upon *universal life energy*, the meaning of
the Japanese word *Reiki*. The therapy was named after Dr Mikao
Usui, a Japanese theologist, who rediscovered the art of healing
using and by transferring this universal life energy. Following a
prolonged period of meditation, Dr Usui acquired the ability of
transferring Reiki energy. He was also able to help others to act as
channels for this energy.

To benefit fully from the technique, it is preferable to be initi-
ated into the Reiki energy. This is done by a Reiki master. A
number of Reiki grand masters brought the practice to the West
to allow many people to prepare themselves for self-discovery.
Reiki is now used to heal, either the practitioner or others, in
meditation and in conjunction with other therapies such as
aromatherapy.

In many cases traditional Reiki, as generated by Dr Usui, forms
the basis of Reiki-do, an amplification of the technique which
essentially translates into using Reiki as a way of life. This aspect
of Reiki will be discussed more fully in due course.

Reiki energy

Reiki energy is regarded as life energy at its most effective – with
the maximum vibration. It is considered to have an almost divine

130

quality and as such includes everything, in a world where problems and disorders are deemed to be due to the feeling of detachment from the world. There is no division of Reiki energy into positive and negative forms but when a person undergoes a session of therapy, they allow the energy to be taken into themselves with beneficial effects. Essentially, those receiving Reiki energy decide subconsciously just how much of the life energy is taken in.

Those who use Reiki regularly often find they are more joyful, lively and their own inbuilt energy is enhanced – almost as if their batteries had been fully charged! Existing conflicts within the person are broken down and there is a greater vitality, leading to relaxation and a stimulation of the body. As this improvement develops, the natural processes of renewal and removal of toxins are enhanced and rendered more effective, ultimately opening up more of the body to the life energy.

Body organs such as the skin, and protective systems such as the immune system are improved providing the individual is prepared regularly to undertake Reiki and in the first place to undergo an attunement or initiation into Reiki energy. The initiation is merely a means whereby the universal life energy is bestowed through the Reiki master. The master acts as a channel and a link with God to release the healing power.

An initiation is not absolutely essential but it allows the individual access to the universal life energy, which is used rather than their own life energy. Also, an initiation conveys a greater capacity for using Reiki energy, with no associated tiredness and further, it provides a protective mechanism against any negative manifestations.

The treatment
Effects and limitations

There are several inter-related effects that result from taking in Reiki energy:

- it enables the universal life energy to be received;

- it creates a feeling of deep relaxation;
- energy blockages are removed allowing a flow of life energy throughout the body;
- toxins of various sorts are removed; these and other waste products are removed from the system much more quickly.

When the toxins have been removed from the body, more energy can be received and the vital processes and functions become more highly tuned. When the body takes in more and more life energy, it is said that its frequency becomes higher, facilitating contact with the Universal Spirit and generating trust in the universal life energy.

Deep relaxation is central to Reiki therapy and this is very much dependent upon the divine quality attributed to the energy. The extent to which Reiki can work is defined by the receiver of the energy because only the necessary amount of energy is drawn in. A refusal to accept Reiki, whether or not it is made consciously, will result in no energy flowing. This is, in a way, one limitation of Reiki, albeit self-imposed. It should also be appreciated that attitude is very important and if someone attempts to use Reiki in the wrong way, it will not work. Self-discovery must go hand in hand with everyday experience of real life and it is not possible to hide from the troubles of the real world through misplaced introspection

A qualified therapist in the appropriate discipline must be sought to deal with major problems and difficulties. Of course, adopting Reiki in tandem with another therapy will be very beneficial as the Reiki will maximise the treatment being received. This applies whether the therapist is a homeopath, naturopath or medic.

The use of whole-body Reiki

Because no one part of the body exists independently, and because a disease or disorder in one area will inevitably affect the whole body, the use of Reiki is best applied in a whole-body way, to cleanse and revitalise the complete system.

Many practitioners undertake a particular routine before

commencing a regime of whole-body treatment and the main elements are briefly described below.

Preparing for whole-body Reiki

It is a good idea to prepare thoroughly for Reiki treatment to capitalise fully upon the beneficial effects. The following is a possible routine:

Remove jewellery

Most people wear jewellery of some description, whether stones of a semi-precious or precious nature, metal rings or chains, leather thongs or one of a whole variety of objects. Some metals and stones are believed to attract energies which may interfere with the life energy of Reiki. Other items such as watches create a closed circuit which reduces the flow of life energy. In a way, items of jewellery can be seen as objects which create interference in the 'signal' in much the same way that an engine or motor can generate annoying interference in the reception of a radio programme. Earrings can also be a problem because in the case of pierced ears the earrings conflict with the flow of energy – the ear is very important in other therapies such as acupuncture and must therefore be kept unencumbered.

Wash hands

The benefits of washing your hands are twofold. Firstly, there is the physical effect of cleaning which has the additional quality of making the hands pleasant to feel for the recipient of Reiki. It is essential that hot, sticky hands are not used in Reiki as this would hardly be conducive to the state of relaxation being sought.

The second benefit relates to the aura surrounding the body. This aura may be affected by contact with objects, people, etc over the course of the day and washing removes such influences which could, in sensitive people, have an adverse effect.

Say a prayer

It is helpful at this stage to recite a short prayer asking for healing and to concentrate upon and acknowledge your aims, self-perception and those of the person upon whom your hands will be placed.

Even out the aura

This is a means of gently making contact and starting the therapy, and may be carried out as follows:

- your partner/client/friend should lie down (*see* figure below)
- sitting at their side put your left hand on your sacrum
- with your right hand held about 15–25 cm (6–9 inches) above the body and palm facing down, move your hand along the length of the body from the head to the toes
- return the hand to the starting point using a circular motion along the side of the body
- repeat this three or four times

This process can be repeated after the Reiki therapy when your left hand can be placed on the sacrum of your partner/client/friend.

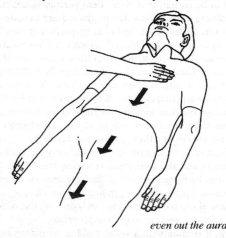

even out the aura

Energise

When each Reiki therapy session is complete the whole body may be energised via the root chakra (*see* later for chakras). The hand is held vertically above the body and then quickly moved from the pelvis to the head.

These preparatory rituals should only be performed when they are perceived to have some significance. There is little point going through the procedures if you do not see the reason why, but clearly some aspects of the procedure can be understood easily and will be accepted readily by the recipient.

The practicalities of whole-body Reiki

Before the treatment

There is great scope for variation in the number and sequence of positions used for whole-body treatment. It will depend greatly upon the practitioner and what is felt to be best for the recipient, but no one sequence can be deemed the best one for all. It is important to be certain that your client/partner is not suffering from any illness or condition that might require the attention of another health professional. Reiki has its particular uses but it is unwise to try to address problems that clearly fall beyond its scope. The client can easily ask advice from their doctor, or other professional, as to whether they should undergo Reiki therapy.

When it is clear that therapy can go ahead the next commitment to be made is that of time. It is essential that both parties agree to pledge the time to make the most of the Reiki therapy. It is likely that the practitioner will, in acting as a channel for the universal life energy, see their own status develop.

The extent of each session of Reiki will vary depending upon circumstances and the individual receiving treatment. Certain positions may be better left out of the sequence or therapy may be focussed on a particular area to help relieve blockages or deal with tension. If the recipient is currently on a regime of medication then a shorter session may be appropriate.

Similarly, if dealing with a small child or an elderly or infirm person, it is probably wise to limit the therapy to a session of 15 to

20 minutes. In all cases the Reiki practitioner should be sensitive to and aware of the condition, needs and well-being of the recipient.

Hand positions in Reiki

The hands are clearly the 'instruments' of healing in Reiki and although the position in which they are placed on the recipient is meaningful, it may not be possible, nor is it essential that the exact position is copied. Just placing the hands on the appropriate part of the body will suffice.

Reiki can be effected through clothing, as the energy will flow just as well, but many people prefer to have no material obstacles to the therapy. In this case, and particularly for partners, the Reiki can be undertaken in the nude. If there are any physical blemishes such as a burn or other wound, the hands should be held a few inches above the skin at this area, around the corresponding acupuncture point, or reflex zone.

The head

On the *head*, the basic position is shown in the figure opposite. The hands are placed either side of the nose, with the palms covering the eyes; the thumbs rest by the bridge of the nose and the fingertips cover the cheeks and reach the upper lip. This arrangement covers the sinuses, eyes, pituitary gland, teeth and is useful for dealing with colds, sinusitis, eye complaints, allergies, fatigue and general discontent.

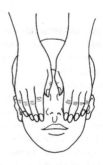

basic position for the head

In the second arrangement for the head, the hands are placed over the ears, with the fingertips extending down the jawline to the neck, encompassing the ears of course which includes the semi-circular canals, responsible for balance. The effect also extends to the pharyngeal area. Diseases and problems of these organs – colds, trouble with balance, hearing loss, etc – are dealt with in this arrangement.

If the hands are placed on the back of the head, this helps with conditions such as headaches, colds, asthma and circulatory problems. It generally promotes relaxation.

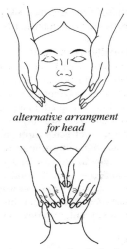

*alternative arrangment
for head*

*arrangment for the back of
the head*

The chest and abdomen

The next sequence of hand arrangements is for the chest and abdomen. Once again there are many variations, but a selection is presented here.

The arrangement for the thymus, heart and lungs is as follows: one hand is laid across the thymus and the other is at 90° starting just below and between the breasts. The thymus is a bilobed gland in the neck which is an important part of the immune system. This arrangement therefore reinforces the immune system and helps the lymphatics, the heart, lungs and counters any general debility.

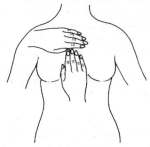

*arrangement for thymus,
heart and lungs*

The next illustration in the sequence shows the hands placed either side of the navel and slightly to one side. The stomach and digestive organs are the focus of attention here and the conditions/symptoms addressed necessarily have a link with these body systems. As such this will help digestion and the metabolism in general terms, and specifically will combat nausea, heartburn, gastro-intestinal diseases and indigestion. Because the presence of such conditions often results in tension and worry, the relief of symptoms will similarly help relieve anxiety and depression.

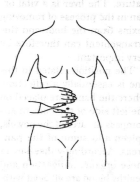

focus on the stomach and digestive organs

Next are two positions in which the hands are placed in a position similar to that shown in the arrangement used to focus on the stomach and digestive organs but further away from the body midline. One version is to approach the body from the right side of the partner/client. The left hand is placed around the base of the ribcage and in this way the gall bladder and liver are the organs to be dealt with. This position is for diseases and conditions of these important organs and associated problems of a metabolic

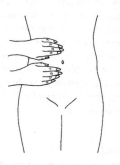

focus on the gall bladder and liver

nature. The liver is a vital organ in the process of removing toxins from the body and this arrangement can therefore be very important.

The position related to this one is essentially a reflection, where the hands are placed on the left side of the body to encompass the area of the bowels, spleen and some of the pancreas. Accordingly diseases of these organs, indigestion and healthy blood are all dealt with.

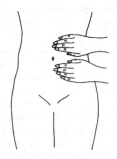

focus on the bowels, spleen, and pancreas

The position of the hands where the pelvic bones are covered and meet over the pubic area is for a number of ailments, many associated with the appendix, intestines and urinogenital organs. In addition, this arrangement is considered suitable for allergies, general debility, problems of a sexual nature and related to weight and is appropriate to reinforce the immune system.

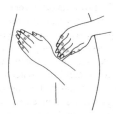

focus on the appendix, intestines and urogenital organs

The back

There are a number of arrangements which can be adopted on the back and lower back. The figure shows one such position with a number of effects but it is likely that by gently experimenting, a slightly different yet equally beneficial arrangement can be found. Here the hands are placed across the shoulder blades at mid to upper point, to influence the intestines, lung, heart and various muscles in the neck and shoulder region. This will help lung and heart diseases, muscular tension, headaches and related conditions.

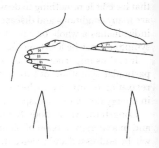

If the hands are placed lower down the back, around the midriff (on the lower ribs) this position will accommodate the kidneys and adrenal glands. (The adrenal glands are situated one each on the upper surface of each kidney and are important because they manufacture hormones that control a variety of body functions, e.g. adrenaline is one hormone produced).

focus on the back to help lungs, heart, muscular tension and headaches

In addition to these specific positions, there are many other Reiki positions to deal with a multitude of complaints and the reader is referred to a more extensive account for greater detail. It

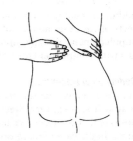

focus on lower back to help kidneys and adrenal glands

must always be remembered that serious conditions or diseases of a particular nature should be dealt with by the appropriate specialist.

The benefits of whole-body Reiki
A reinforcing effect
It is believed with Reiki, as with many similar forms of therapy, that the body cannot be treated in separate parts or as discrete organs

that have little or nothing to do with other parts of the body. There are many conditions and diseases that affect the well-being of the individual as a whole or have a knock-on effect even though the symptoms may be less tangible, such as anxiety or depression.

It is thus important that Reiki is used not just to counteract a particular symptom, but to treat the whole body to achieve the relaxation mentioned earlier and with it the removal of blockages in energy flow and the dispersal of toxins.

Long-term whole-body Reiki should be adopted in all cases, and in a therapy session of 60 to 90 minutes all parts of the body will be addressed and receive Reiki energy. Over a period of time, the general condition of the body is restored and the energy channels are opened to alow the body to deal properly and naturally with both stress and the build-up of toxins.

In cases of recovery from illness, Reiki therapy provides the additional energy to bolster recovery and will reinforce the effects of any other method of natural healing. It can be used as a supplementary therapy almost as a general, ongoing, policy as it is a truly complementary system of treatment.

Reduction of side-effects

It is well-known that the use of drugs to combat say, an infection may at first seem very effective. However, it is becoming all too obvious that the excessive use of drugs is causing its own problems. In the case of many drugs, uncomfortable, distressing and even threatening side-effects can ensue. With antibiotics, there is now the problem of drug resistance in bacteria, leading to situations where hospital patients are vulnerable to infections from so-called superbugs or killer bugs. This has resulted specifically from the overuse of antibiotics and has reached the point where hospitals now have only one or two very powerful drugs to use in these circumstances.

Reiki therapy can be a very useful adjunct for anyone taking a course of drugs. It can help reduce some side effects and generally aid the body in recovery when the course has been completed. Post-operative recovery will benefit from Reiki and it can also help after chemotherapy. In all these cases Reiki therapy supplies that extra life energy, enabling the body to bounce back more quickly from the burdens of surgery and chemicals.

In some cases, use of Reiki therapy after an operation will lessen pain and the natural healing processes will be accelerated. The key in all these examples is that the Reiki therapy must be undertaken on a regular basis. The added benefit of this is that when a person is enjoying good health, the regular therapy increases the body's inbuilt defences which manifests itself as a confidence and outward harmony in dealing with everyday events. It also bestows a greater ability to deal with stressful situations. This very positive outlook can become possible because once the blockages and toxins have been removed from the system, the scope for personal advancement and growth becomes available. In general, the better metabolic functioning afforded by Reiki therapy means that benefits and improvements may be experienced in many ways.

Reiki associations

It has already been mentioned that Reiki therapy can be undertaken in conjunction with other methods of natural healing. In addition, it can be combined with activities such as meditation and crystal therapy. The following sections consider briefly a few of these combinations which for the present purpose have been called associations.

Reiki and the use of crystals

Crystal therapy is known to many people and involves the use of precious and semi-precious stones. The stones are thought to hold positive energy and they act as a conduit for healing from the practitioner to the recipient. It is also said that the stones generate a healing vibration that acts upon the body. In some cases the stone is placed on the body where treatment is focused, in others it may be positioned on the appropriate acupuncture point. Most therapists use quartz for physical healing, amethyst for spiritual healing and rose quartz to heal emotions. Fluorite may also be used to develop awareness and knowledge of a spiritual nature.

In Reiki, three varieties of quartz are commonly used – amethyst, rose quartz and ordinary quartz (or rock crystal). The crystal structure of quartz is often taken to be related to the six chakras and the tip of the crystal to the seventh chakra. Practitioners recommend using rock crystal to avoid feeling overpowered by changes, mounting pressures and the stress of everyday life. Carrying the crystal or wearing it is meant to bring light into your workaday routines.

Rock crystal can also be used in conjunction with Reiki meditation (of which see later), being held between, or in, the hands. In this way the energy emanating from the crystal is thought to go into the palms and then the rest of the body via the reflex zones. It is recommended by some in a variety of applications such as relaxation, wound-healing with other therapy and treating particular organs.

Rose quartz, with its soft pink colouration, is used for mending emotional problems. This may be dealing with problematic emotions, such as shutting out certain desires or it may be facing trauma and stress brought about by a separation.

The use of amethyst with Reiki is varied. It can help promote the proper function of an organ that has been under treatment; placed on the Third Eye (centre of the forehead) it facilitates clearer vision in one's path through life; and it can reduce tension and fear.

Meditation with Reiki

Meditation in its own right is a useful therapy. It needs concentration and time and a will to continue with the practice. Some of the benefits may happen straight away (such as a lowering of the blood pressure) while others require some proficiency. It has been reported that it helps with insomnia, and a high blood pressure can be lowered significantly, enough to allow the dependence on drugs to be reduced. Meditation is undertaken in a quiet room and it must be at least half an hour after consuming food or drink. Sitting comfortably, the mind is then concentrated upon excluding the hustle and bustle, problems, tension and overstimulating thoughts of modern life.

Reiki assists in this concentration, with the flow of energy aiding relaxation. There are some positions that can be adopted in Reiki meditation to achieve particular goals. In the first position the legs are drawn up and the soles of the feet put together with the knees falling apart. This can be done while lying down or sitting against a wall or chair. The hands adopt a praying gesture. This is meant to complete the circuit of energy, allowing a flow around the body. The Reiki energy removes any blockages and performed regularly, this becomes a powerful meditation exercise. It can be done for short periods initially, just a couple of minutes, and then built up in small increases.

To achieve complete harmony with your partner, there is a meditation exercise which can be done together. Sitting facing each other, the legs are spread, with the knees raised slightly. Moving closer, the legs of one are put over the legs of the partner and palms are put together. This allows a joint circuit of energy which strengthens the harmonious and loving relationship between two people. Done properly, this meditation may take up to half an hour.

Group meditation is also possible with Reiki, in which the participants stand in a circle with hands joined.

Aromatherapy blended with Reiki

Aromatherapy is covered in greater detail elsewhere in this volume (*see* page 312). It is essentially a healing method that employs essential oils extracted from plants, usually in a neutral oil base (carrier oil). The oils can be used in three ways: by direct application, bathing in water to which a few drops of the appropriate oil have been added, and inhalation.

When used in conjunction with Reiki, some oils can be applied directly on particular areas of the body, or their aroma can be made to fill the room using an aroma lamp. Below a few oils are considered and their use compared to their therapeutic value in aromatherapy. It is very likely that someone with a knowledge of essential oils will be able to capitalize upon their experience and incorporate further oils in their Reiki therapy.

- *Lavender* – in aromatherapy lavender is a tonic with relaxing effects. It is also antiseptic, an antispasmodic and stimulates the appetite. It is a widely-used and versatile oil that is used for minor burns and wounds. Its soothing effects render it helpful for headaches, tension and similar conditions.

  In Reiki, lavender is associated primarily with patients/recipients who are sensitive and easily hurt, essentially introverts. It can be used in long sessions of Reiki when the lavender helps to promote the calm and confidence necessary for a period of building and strengthening of the life force energy.

- *Sandalwood* – this oil is used in aromatherapy for its relaxing and antiseptic effects. It forms a very effective oil for application to the skin (especially facial), particularly for dry or sensitive skin.

  The use of sandalwood in Reiki therapy is quite different. Its benefit seems to be in producing an ambience conducive to the Reiki therapy itself because the oil is considered to elicit trust and confidence, between practitioner and recipient.

- *Clary sage* – this is a very useful oil with a number of qualities including tonic, antispasmodic, antidepressant, anti-inflammatory, bactericidal and more. It is also used to treat colds, menstrual problems and its very low toxicity renders it suitable for general use.

  In a session of Reiki therapy, clary sage has been used to open blocked channels and to enhance sensitivity.

- *Patchouli* – apart from being accredited with some aphrodisiac qualities, patchouli is more commonly used in aromatherapy to treat skin disorders and minor burns because of its anti-inflammatory and antiseptic qualities.

  While patchouli is also used in Reiki therapy for allergies and impurities of the skin, the fundamental use and aim is to enhance the sensual qualities and aspects of life.

Other Reiki associations

Because Reiki is very much a positive therapy and benign, it can be undertaken in conjunction with other therapies with no harm. However, there are some beneficial effects of Reiki which may affect in some way the activity of other courses of treatment.

- *Prescription drugs* – many Reiki therapists believe that Reiki can readily affect the way in which such drugs work in the body. It has already been mentioned that side effects of drugs can be lessened through the use of Reiki, and in some cases it is reported that the process will be accelerated. In addition, Reiki makes the body more receptive and therefore therapy prior to a course of drugs may enhance the effect of the drug. The relaxed state engendered by Reiki may also counter, to some extent, the efficacy of an anaesthetic. However, injections such as anaesthetics can more readily and easily be released from the body with the help of Reiki.

  Although minor pains can often be remedied through the use of Reiki alone, stronger pain killers do not have their effect lessened by Reiki. The interaction between Reiki and drugs is neither well tested nor documented, but the overall positive effect of the therapy means that it is not likely to cause any problems.

- *Homeopathy* – in conjunction with this therapy, Reiki provides a reinforcing effect by rendering the treatment more effective. Reiki can help avoid strain, improve the removal of toxins and increase the body's sensitivity. After treatment, whole-body Reiki will help recovery. *See* page 485 for a full discussion of homeopathy .

- *Bach remedies* – these are named after Edward Bach, an English doctor, who in the early years of this century gave up his Harley Street practice to concentrate upon finding plants with healing qualities. He identified 38 plants, the flowers of which he floated on clear spring water. This, he believed, transferred medicinal properties to the water which could be given to patients. This practice he developed to mimic the drops of dew on the plant which in the first instance were used. Intended for home self-help, the remedies are meant for treating the whole person. Stock solutions are diluted in water and a few drops taken.

Typical examples are:

> cherry plum for fear, tension, irrationality
> holly for envy, jealousy and hatred
> pine for guilt and constantly apologizing
> sweet chestnut for despair
> wild rose for apathy

In common with many other examples, Reiki improves the effectiveness of Bach remedies.

Determining the need
Introduction

When undertaking Reiki therapy it is often necessary to determine the need for therapy in the client or partner. As therapists work with Reiki for longer, they become more sensitive and proficient and are better able to judge problem areas on what is called the subtle plane (the etheric body). Expertise comes only with experience, but it seems that there are certain reactions or feelings detected which may be indicative. Before trying to perceive a person's need, some practitioners 'sensitise' their hands. This involves holding the palms facing, about 40 to 50 cm apart and slowly bringing them together. The movement should be spread out over four or five minutes to allow an attunement and for changes to be perceived.

The following are some possible responses that may be experienced:

- *Attraction* – implies that Reiki energy is needed at that point.
- *Repulsion* – suggests a long-established blockage is present which is restricting the flow of energy. This may require a considerable period of therapy to rectify.

- *Flow* – a positive feeling representing the flow of life energy which will be enhanced by further Reiki energy, raising the entire system.
- *Heat* – if your hands feel warmer, it signifies a need for life energy. If the whole body produces such a result, Reiki energy can be applied anywhere.
- *Cold* – this is probaby due to a blockage in energy flow such that an area of the body has been deprived of energy. Such blockages may also require considerable attention and both whole-body and specific treatment will probably be required.
- *Tingling* – an inflamed area will usually produce a tingling in the hands of the therapist. The strength of the stimulus reflects the severity of the problem and additional help from a medical practitioner may be identified as being necessary.
- *Pain* – this usually represents a build-up of energy in some form. A sharp pain reflects that the energy is beginning to dissipate and in so doing is causing some conflict elsewhere in the system. In this case, whole-body therapy is beneficial before concentrating upon a particular area.

There are other methods to determine need and identify disruptions in the flow of life energy, but these are, in the main, for the more experienced practitioner. However, details can be found in a variety of publications and involve pendulum dowsing, activity of the chakras and the use of systems such as tarot or I Ching. These latter two, however, are not for novices.

When the need is answered

If Reiki is practised regularly, it can have a very positive effect and influence. One of the major problems with modern life is the very pace of life itself – every day seems to be hectic, full of demands and pressure which result in stress, discomfort and ragged emotions.

These emotional ups and downs and stressful pressures are smoothed out by Reiki. A more balanced approach to life is developed; a greater inner harmony is achieved which means that the quality of life improves and any illnesses or condition become less of a problem, responds more readily to treatment, or is cleared up seemingly of its own accord. The flow of energy from Reiki ensures that there is harmony between the Third Eye (which identifies the ideal path for the individual) and the root chakra (or energy centre). (For an explanation of the chakras *see* below).

Introduction to the significance of chakras with Reiki

Chakras are a common concept in several disciplines of alternative medicine or traditional Asian medicine. A chakra is a centre of energy, subtle energy in Reiki, which has several functions. In addition to being 'representative' of a particular organ or group of organs, a chakra also controls our being on different levels and it links these two representative states.

The chakras

In Reiki there is considered to be seven major and a number of minor chakras. The seven major chakras are shown in the figure on page 150. These are from the lowest to the highest: the root chakra, the sexual chakra, the personality chakra, the heart chakra, the expressive chakra, the knowledge chakra, the crown chakra.

The number of major chakras does vary in some instances, e.g. Hindu yoga has six centres, but the greatest variation is in the minor chakras. In some regimes of therapy ten minor chakras are identified, and these are interconnected with the major chakras. A typical system could be:

- one in the arch of each foot, connected to the first and third chakras
- one in each knee joint, connected to the fifth and sixth chakras
- one in each palm, connected to the second, third and fourth chakras
- one in each elbow, connected to the second and third chakras
- one below each shoulder, connected to the third and fifth chakras

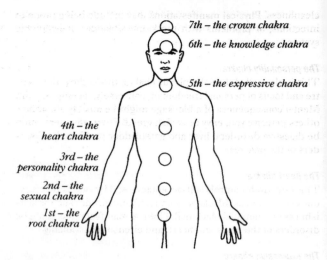

7th – the crown chakra

6th – the knowledge chakra

5th – the expressive chakra

4th – the
heart chakra

3rd – the
personality chakra

2nd – the
sexual chakra

1st – the
root chakra

Brief summaries of the major chakras are given below, followed by an indication of how the chakras interact with Reiki.

The root chakra

This is the source of strength and is essential for proper development. The other centres of energy rely upon the root chakra to perform properly. Disorders within the root chakras may result in mental problems (e.g. aggression, confusion) or physical symptoms (e.g. of the intestines, excretory systems, or bones).

The sexual chakra

This is highly influential and governs sensual and sexual factors, the means whereby experiences are felt and registered. Blockages result in a variety of phobias or conditions such as a fear of being touched, a general incomprehension or an obsessive cleanliness. Physical manifestations may include being prone to infections, or problems with the kidneys/bladder or lymphatic system.

The personality chakra

This is also called the solar plexus chakra, this is the power centre and focus of personal freedom or, conversely, feelings of guilt. Mental consequences of a blockage might be anxiety about how others perceive you, envy or selfish greed. Physically there could be digestive disorders, liver and gall bladder problems or disorders of the pancreas.

The heart chakra

This effectively controls self-acceptance and by extension everyone else around us. Blockages may result in attitudes such as selfishness or emotional blackmail. Physical manifestations could be disorders of the lungs and heart, and circulatory problems.

The expressive chakra

The expressive chakra (or throat chakra) controls overall self-expression, whether it is language or gesture. An upset in this centre could well result in an individual who becomes dictatorial while the physical signs could be growth problems, or a muscular tension leading to a lack of vocal control.

The knowledge chakra

Otherwise known as the forehead chakra or Third Eye, this is the focus of intuition, the perception of truth which enables a person to find their own course through life. Accordingly, a blockage of this chakra will culminate in a haphazard approach to life, and probably an inability to settle down to any one task for any length of time.

The crown chakra

It is generally felt that the seventh, crown, chakra is appreciated only by experience and it depends upon the other six for its development.

The practicalities of chakras with Reiki

This is quite a complicated aspect of Reiki and to develop it as an integral part of a programme of Reiki, the reader should seek a more extensive treatment of the subject. Some information is, however, presented here by way of introduction.

Some therapists use the technique of balancing chakras to completely attune the energy on the subtle plane. The chakras are paired, first with sixth, second with fifth and third with fourth by placing the hands on the relevant areas. When it feels through the hands as if the energy is balanced with the first and sixth chakras, then the second and fifth can be balanced in the same way. Other combinations may be used if it is felt that these may be beneficial.

The chakras may suffer a number of problems creating an imbalance and although considerable corrective therapy may be required, a balance can be achieved with Reiki. Many practitioners recommend sending Reiki energy through a problematic chakra. This involves placing one hand at the front of the body above the chakra, and the other hand at the back of the body. The flow of Universal Life Energy eventually corrects any defects. However, it is important to remember that due to the interconnection of the chakras, defects in one affect the whole system. Therefore the healing cannot be undertaken in isolation. It is always good practice to balance the chakras after a session of specific healing.

Higher levels of Reiki

Although it is possible to progress beyond the level of proficiency implied so far, second and third degree Reiki are really for the experts. This is particularly so with third degree Reiki, the details of which are not written down.

Available power is increased with second degree Reiki but should only be accessed by someone working with a Reiki master. The greater flow of energy means that the effect of Reiki therapy is greater and also its effect on a mental and emotional level is enhanced. Further, it is said that Reiki at this level can be transmitted over distances, to one or a number of people. This is, of course, highly specialized and advice should be sought from a Reiki master by anyone wishing to pursue this goal.

Reiki-do

In Japanese, *do* means path, hence Reiki-do is concerned with a way of life in which Reiki figures very prominently. Reiki-do is, of course, founded on the Reiki therapy described in the preceding pages and it consists of three aspects which enable personal growth. The three categories of Reiki-do are:

- *Inner* – based upon meditation as described earlier, and can be augmented by one of the methods outlined, such as the scents of aromatherapy. It adopts a whole-body system of treatment leading to a greater awareness and vitality.
- *Outer* – the application of Reiki energy forms the basis of this part of Reiki-do, with the chakras, crystals and other subsidiary therapies.
- *Synergistic* – as the word implies, this is the combination of parts which have, when used together, a greater effect than their combined individual effects; that is a merger of inner and outer Reiki-do which exceeds the anticipated combined effect. It is particularly appropriate for anyone who has reasonable experience in this therapy and can appreciate the non-exclusive nature of pleasure and success.

Conclusions

Reiki is a technique of healing available to anyone. It can lead to a more relaxed approach to life and greater harmony with the total environment. It can also be applied to plants and animals, for example your household pets, and for this and further information about the therapy, the reader is advised to seek more detailed treatments.

Shiatsu

Introduction

Origins

Shiatsu originated in China at least 2000 years ago, when the earliest accounts gave the causes of ailments and the remedies that could be effected through a change of diet and way of life. The use of massage and acupuncture was also recommended. The Japanese also practised this massage, after it had been introduced into their country, and it was known as *anma*. The therapy that is known today as *shiatsu* has gradually evolved with time from anma under influences from both East and West. It is only very recently that it has gained recognition and popularity, with people becoming aware of its existence and benefits.

Although East and West have different viewpoints on health and life, these can complement one another. The Eastern belief is of a primary flow of energy throughout the body, which runs along certain channels known as meridians. It is also believed that this energy exists throughout the universe and that all living creatures are dependent upon it as much as on physical nourishment. The energy is known by three similar names, *ki, chi* and *prana* in Japan, China and India respectively. (It should be noted that the term 'energy' in this context is not the same as the physical quantity that is measured in joules or calories.) As in acupuncture, there are certain pressure points on the meridians that relate to certain organs, and these points are known as *tsubos*.

The applications of shiatsu

Shiatsu can be used to treat a variety of minor problems such as insomnia, headaches, anxiety, back pain, etc. Western medicine may be unable to find a physical cause for a problem, and although some pain relief may be provided, the underlying cause of the problem may not be cured. It is possible that one session of shiatsu will be sufficient to remedy the problem by stimulating the flow of energy along the channels. A regime of exercise (possibly a specific routine) with a change in diet and/or lifestyle may also be recommended. Shiatsu can encourage a general feeling of good health in the whole person, not just in the physical sense. After some study or practice, shiatsu can be performed on friends and relatives. There are many benefits for both the giver and the receiver of shiatsu, both on a physical and spiritual level.

Energy or ki
Auras

There are believed to be a number of *auras*, or energy layers, that surround the physical body and can be detected or appreciated (*see* the figure on page 156). The first layer, the *etheric body*, is the most dense and is connected with the body and the way it works. An exercise is described later that enables this layer to be detected. The *astral body* is much wider, is affected by people's feelings and, if viewed by a clairvoyant, is said to change in colour and shape depending on the feelings being experienced. The next aura is the *mental body*, which is involved with the thought processes and intelligence of a person. Similarly, this can be viewed by a clairvoyant and is said to contain 'pictures' of ideas emanating from the person. These first three auras comprise the personality of a person. The last aura is known as the *causal body*, *soul* or *higher self*. This is concerned more with perceptive feelings and comprehension. It is believed in reincarnation that the first three auras die with the body, but the causal body carries on in its process of development by adopting another personality. As a person grows in maturity and awareness, these different auras are used, and energy is passed from

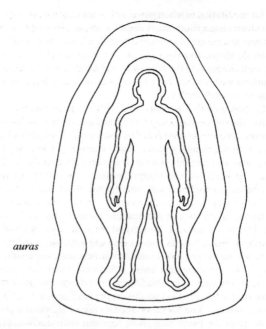

auras

one layer to another. It therefore follows that any alteration in the physical state will, in turn, affect the other layers, and vice versa. (*See also* Aura therapy, page 211.)

Seven centres of energy, or chakras

It is believed that there are seven main *chakras* (a chakra being a centre of energy) found in a midline down the body, from the top of the head to the bottom of the torso (*see* figure on page 150 of Reiki) . They are situated along the *sushumna*, or spiritual channel, which runs from the crown of the head to the base of the trunk. Energy enters the channel from both ends. Since the flow is most efficient when the back is straight, this is the ideal posture for meditation or when powers of concentration are required. Each chakra has a component of each aura, and it comprises what is known as a centre of consciousness. Each aura is activated as a person develops, and the same occurs with the chakras, beginning with the lowest (the *base* or *root chakra*) and progressing to the others with time. There is also a change of energy between the *auras* of each chakra.

The *crown chakra* is concerned with the pineal gland, which controls the right eye and upper brain and affects spiritual matters. The *ajna* , *brow or forehead chakra* also known as *the Third Eye*, is linked with the pituitary gland, which controls the left eye, lower brain, nose and nervous system. It has an effect on the intellect, perception, intuition and comprehension. The *throat* or *expressive chakra* is concerned with the thyroid gland and governs the lymphatic system, hands, arms, shoulders, mouth, vocal cords, lungs and throat. It affects communication, creativity and self-expression. The *heart chakra* is concerned with the thymus gland and controls the heart, breasts, vagus nerve and circulatory system, and affects self-awareness, love, humanitarian acts and compassion. The *solar plexus* or *personality chakra* is concerned with the pancreas. It controls the spleen, gall bladder, liver and digestive system and stomach, and has an effect on desire, personal power and the origin of emotions. The *sacral* or *sexual chakra* affects the gonads and controls the lower back, feet, legs and reproductive system. This affects physical, sexual and mental energy, relationships and self-worth. The *base* or *root chakra* is concerned with the adrenal glands. It controls the skeleton, parasympathetic and sympathetic nervous systems, bladder and kidneys, and affects reproduction and the physical will. As an example of this, if a person is suffering from an ailment of the throat, it is possible that he or she may also be unable to voice private thoughts and feelings.

Zang and fu organs
Energy storage and production

According to traditional Eastern therapies, organs have a dual function – their physical one and another that is concerned with the use of energy and might be termed an 'energetic function'. The twelve organs mentioned in the traditional therapies are split into two groups known as *zang* and *fu*, and each is described below.

Zang organs are for energy storage, and the fu organs produce energy from sustenance and drink and also control excretion. The organs can be listed in pairs, each zang matched by a fu with a similar function.

Although the pancreas is not specifically mentioned, it is usually included with the spleen. The same applies to the 'triple heater' or 'triple burner', which is connected with the solar plexus, lower abdomen and the thorax.

The lungs are a zang organ and are concerned with assimilation of energy, or ki, from the air, which with energy from food ensures the complete body is fed and that mental alertness and a positive attitude are maintained. This is paired with the fu organ of the large intestine, which takes sustenance from the small intestine, absorbs necessary liquids and excretes waste material via the faeces. It is also concerned with self-confidence.

The spleen is a zang organ and changes energy or ki from food into energy that is needed by the body. It is concerned with the mental functions of concentration, thinking and analysing. This is paired with the fu organ of the stomach, which prepares food so that nutrients can be extracted and also any energy, or ki, can be taken. It also provides 'food for thought'.

The zang organ of the heart assists blood formation from ki and controls the flow of blood and the blood vessels. It is where the mind is housed and therefore affects awareness, belief, long-term memory and feelings. This is paired with the fu organ of the small intestine, which divides food into necessary and unnecessary parts, the latter passing to the large intestine. It is also concerned with the making of decisions.

The kidneys are a zang organ and they produce basic energy, or ki, for the other five paired organs and also for reproduction, birth, development and maturity. They also sustain the skeleton and brain and provide willpower and 'get up and go'. They are paired with the fu organ of the bladder, which stores waste fluids until they are passed as urine and also gives strength or courage.

The zang organ of the 'heart governor' is concerned with the flow of blood throughout the body. It is a protector and help for the heart and has a bearing on relationships with other people (although there is no organ known as the 'heart governor' it is connected with the heart and its functions). This is paired with the 'triple heater' or 'burner', which passes ki around the body and allows an emotional exchange with others.

The liver is the sixth zang organ, and it assists with a regular flow of ki to achieve the most favourable physiological effects and emotional calmness. Positive feelings, humour, planning and creativity are also connected with it. The gall bladder is the sixth fu organ, with which the liver is paired, and this keeps bile from the liver and passes it to the intestines. It concerns decision-making and forward thinking.

The meridian system

The meridians, as previously mentioned, are a system of invisible channels on the back and front of the body along which energy, or ki, flows. There are twelve principal meridians plus two additional ones, which are called *the governing vessel* and the *conception* or *directing vessel*. Each meridian passes partly through the body and partly along the skin, joining various chakras and organs (the organs as recognized in traditional Eastern medicine). One end of every meridian is beneath the skin while the other is on the surface of the skin on the feet or hands. Along each meridian are acupressure or acupuncture points, which in shiatsu are called *tsubos*. These points allow the flow of energy along the meridian to be altered if necessary (*see* the figures on page 160). The meridians receive energy from the chakras and organs (as described previously), from the meridians with ends located on the feet and hands and also via the pressure points, or tsubos. Energy, or ki, can pass from one meridian into another as there is a 'pathway' linking each meridian to two others. The energy passes in a continuous cycle or flow and in a set order from one meridian to another. By working on the meridians, and particularly the pressure points, a number of beneficial effects can be achieved with

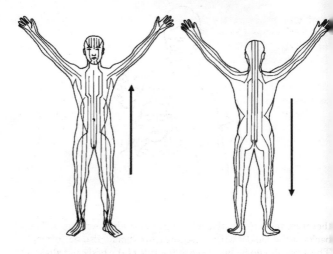

the flow of energy along the meridiens

problems such as muscle tension, backache and headache. Since the flow of energy is stimulated by working on the meridians this will in turn affect the joints, muscles and skin and thereby ease these complaints. Since a person's mental state, feelings and moods are also altered by the flow of energy, this can induce a more positive frame of mind.

A person in good health should have a constant flow of ki, with no concentrations or imbalances in any part of the body. It is believed that the greater the amount of ki there is within a person's body, the greater the vitality, mental alertness and overall awareness that person will possess.

Feeling ki

It is possible for a person to 'feel' ki, and the following exercise helps demonstrate what it is like. Stand upright with the feet apart and the arms stretched upwards. Rub the hands together as if

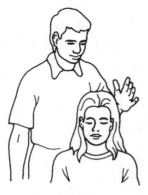

feeling ki

they were very cold, so that a feeling of warmth is generated. The backs of the hands, wrists and forearms should also be rubbed. The arms should be put down at the side of the body and shaken vigorously. This should then be repeated from the beginning, with the arms above the head and concluding with the shaking. Then hold the hands out to the front – they should have a pleasant feeling of warmth and vitality, which is due to the circulation of blood and energy that has been generated. The hands should be placed to the sides, then after inhaling deeply concentrate on relaxing as you exhale. This procedure should be done several times, and then it should be possible to feel the ki. The hands should be placed about 1 m (3 feet) apart, with the palms of the hands facing inwards. After relaxation, concentrate your thoughts on the gap between your hands and then gradually reduce the space between them – but they must not touch. It is likely that when the hands come quite close, about 15-30 cm (6-12 inches), a feeling of tingling or warmth may be felt, or the sensation that there is something between the hands. This will be when the auras that surround the hands touch. To reinforce the sensation, the hands should be taken apart again and then closed together so that the feeling is experienced again and becomes more familiar.

The following exercise also enables ki to be felt, but this time it is the etheric aura around another person's head and shoulders. The previous procedure to generate ki should be repeated, but this time the hand should be placed near to another person's head, within 60 centimetres-1 metre (2-3 feet). This person should be sitting upright on the floor or on a chair. The hand should be moved gradually nearer to the seated person's head, concentrating attention on the gap between your hand and his or her head. If no sensation is felt, the hand should be moved back to its original position and the process should be repeated. Again, a feeling of tingling or warmth will probably be experienced as the person's aura is felt. When this has been achieved, the hand can progress round the head and down to the shoulders, noting the edge of the aura at the same time. If the person has no success in experiencing the aura, it is likely that the mind is not clear of other thoughts, so relaxation is suggested prior to any further attempt.

It is also possible for a person, by concentrating his or her thoughts and by a slight change of position, to alter the flow of ki in the body. This will have the effect of either making him or her feel a lot heavier or lighter, depending on which is desired. Taken to extremes, someone who is skilled at the control of ki will prove too heavy to be lifted by four people.

Basic rules

There are some basic rules that should be followed before the practice of shiatsu. Clothing should be comfortable, loose-fitting and made of natural fibres since this will help with the flow of energy or ki. The room should be warm, quiet, have adequate space and be neat and clean. If not, this can have an adverse effect on the flow of ki. The person receiving the therapy should ideally lie on a futon (a quilted Japanese mattress) or similar mat on the floor. If necessary, pillows or cushions should be ready to hand if the person does not feel comfortable. Shiatsu should not be given or received by someone who has just eaten a large meal – it is advisable to delay for several hours. No pressure should be exerted on varicose veins or injuries such as cuts or breaks in bones. Although shiatsu can be of benefit to women while pregnant, there are four areas that should be avoided and these are the stomach, any part of the legs from the knees downwards, the fleshy web of skin between the forefinger and thumb, and an area on the shoulders at each side of the neck. Ensure that the person is calm and relaxed. It is generally not advisable to practise shiatsu on people who have serious illnesses such as heart disorders, multiple sclerosis or cancer. An experienced practitioner may be able to help, but a detailed and accurate diagnosis and course of treatment is essential. A verbal check on the person's overall health is important and also to ascertain if a woman is pregnant. If there is any worry or doubt about proceeding, then the safest option is not to go ahead.

Although the general feeling after receiving shiatsu is one of wellbeing and relaxation, there are occasionally unpleasant results, such as coughing, generation of mucus or symptoms of a cold; a feeling of tiredness; a headache or other pains and aches; or feeling emotional. The coughing and production of mucus is due to the body being encouraged to rid itself of its surplus foods (such as sugars and fats) in this form. A cold can sometimes develop when the mucus is produced, usually when the cells of the body are not healthy. Tiredness can occur, frequently with a person who suffers from nervous tension. After therapy has removed this stress or tension, then the body's need for sleep and rest becomes apparent. A short-lived headache or other pain may also develop, for which there are two main reasons. Since shiatsu redresses the balance of ki in the body, this means that blockages in the flow of energy are released and the ki can rush around the body, causing a temporary imbalance in one part and resulting in an ache or pain. It is also possible that too much time or pressure may have been applied to a particular area. The amount needed varies considerably from one person to another. If a pain or headache is still present after a few days, however, it is sensible to obtain qualified medical help. Emotional feelings can occur while the energy is being stimulated to flow and balance is regained. The feeling may be connected with something from the past that has been suppressed and so, when these emotions resurface, it is best for them to be expressed in a way that is beneficial, such as crying. There may, of course, be no reaction at all. Some people are completely 'out of touch' with their bodies and are aware only that all is not well when pain is felt. If this is so, then any beneficial effects from shiatsu may not register. Because of a modern diet that contains an abundance of animal fats, people become overweight through the deposition of fat below the skin and around the internal organs. The body is unable to 'burn off' this fat, and this layer forms a barrier to ki. The flow is stopped, and overweight people do not tend to benefit as much because of the difficulty in stimulating the flow of ki in the body.

Exercises and the three main centres

The body is divided into three main centres – the *head*, the *heart* and the *abdominal* centres. The head centre is concerned with activities of a mental nature, such as imaginative and intellectual thought processes, and is concerned with the brow chakra. The heart centre is concerned with interactions among people and to the world in general, including the natural world. It is related to the chakra of the throat and heart. The abdominal centre is related to the base, sacral and solar plexus chakras and is concerned with the practical aspects of life and physical activity. Ideally, energy should be divided equally among the three but because of a number of factors, such as activity, education, diet, culture, etc, this is frequently not so. In shiatsu, more importance is attached to the abdominal centre, known as the *hara*. The following exercise uses abdominal breathing and, by so doing, not only is oxygen inhaled but also ki is taken into the hara where it increases a person's vitality. Once the technique is mastered, it can be practised virtually anywhere and will restore composure and calmness.

Sit on the floor with the back straight and, if possible, in the position known in Japan as *seiza* (*see* figure opposite). The hands

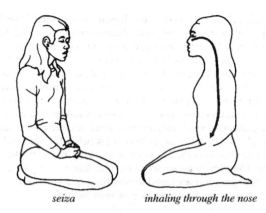

seiza   *inhaling through the nose*

should be placed loosely together in the lap and the mind and
body should become relaxed after some deep breathing. One hand
should be put on the stomach, below the navel, and the other on
the chest. When inhaling, this should not be done with the chest
but with the abdomen, which should increase in size. As the person exhales the abdomen should contract, and this procedure
should be practised for a few minutes. After a rest it should be
repeated, inhaling quite deeply but still the chest should not be
allowed to rise. Some people may not find this exercise at all difficult while others may need more practice. It may be that there is
stress or tension in the diaphragm. Once the technique has been
mastered and the hands do not need to be placed on the chest
and abdomen, imagine that ki is being inhaled down into the hara.
Sit in the same position and inhale slowly via the nose and imagine the ki descending (*see* figure above). (It may aid concentration if the eyes are closed.) The breath should be held for about
four seconds and concentration should be centred on the ki. Then
exhale gradually through the mouth and repeat the process for a
few minutes.

The next exercise is known as a centred movement, which practises movement of the ki, since it is one person's ki that should

have an effect on another. After practising shiatsu on a partner, you should not feel tired but refreshed and exhilarated. This is a benefit of the extra ki in the body. The exercise should be begun on hands and knees (a body width apart), and it is most important that you are relaxed and comfortable with no tension. This position is the basis for other movements that are practised on others. While the position is maintained, begin to move the body backwards and forwards so that you are conscious of the transfer of weight, either on to the hands or knees. The body should then be moved slowly in a circular way, again being aware of the shift of weight from the hands, to hands and knees, to knees, etc, returning to the original position. You should also realize that as the whole body is moved, the abdomen is its 'centre of gravity'. Practise maintaining a position for about five seconds, registering the increase in weight on the hands when you move forwards and the reduction when you rock backwards. Then return to the original position. It is important that the body weight is always used at right angles to the receiver as this will have the maximum effect on the flow of ki. The reason for holding a particular position is that this has the effect of making the person's ki move.

The centred movement previously described can be practised

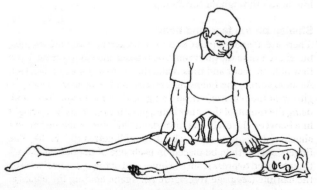

a centred movement

on a partner in exactly the same way, following the same rules. The right hand should be placed on the sacrum, which is between the hips, and the left hand midway between the shoulder blades. As before, you should rock forwards and hold the position for about five seconds and then repeat after rocking backwards on to the knees (*see* figure on page 166). This basic procedure can be repeated about twelve times, and if you are not sure whether too much or too little pressure is being used, check with your partner. You will eventually acquire the skill of knowing what amount is right for a particular person.

To summarize, there are some basic rules to be followed when practising shiatsu. A person should make use of body weight and not muscular strength, and there should be no effort involved. At all times a calm and relaxed state should be maintained, and the weight of the body should be at right angles in relation to the receiver's body. The person's whole body should be moved when altering weight on to the receiver, maintaining the hara as the centre. Any weight or pressure held should be for a short time only and both hands should be used equally. It is best to maintain a regular pattern of movement while giving shiatsu, and always keep in physical contact with the receiver by keeping a hand on him or her throughout the therapy.

Shiatsu on the face and head

There are a large number of different exercises and techniques, but at each time the giver must be relaxed and calm to enable the flow of ki to occur and thus make the shiatsu work to full effect. As an example, the following exercise on the face and head begins with the receiver's head being held firmly in one hand and, using the thumb of the other hand, pressing upwards in a straight line between the eyebrows towards the hairline. Each movement should only be quite small, about 12 millimetres (0.5 inch). The fingers should then be placed on each side of the head and both thumbs used to press from the inner end of the eyebrows towards the hairline (*see* page 168, figure A). Again, holding the hands at each side of the head, the thumbs should then be used to press

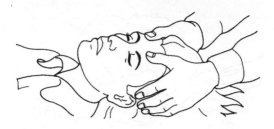

A – press from between the eyebrows towards the hairline

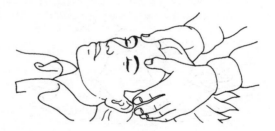

B – press from the eyebrows across the brow

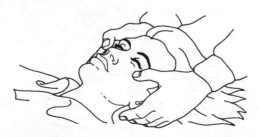

C – work the thumbs across the bones below the eyes

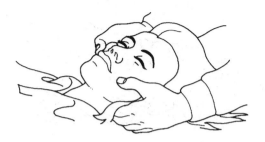

D – press across the face below the cheekbones

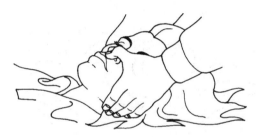

E – press the area between the bose and upper lip

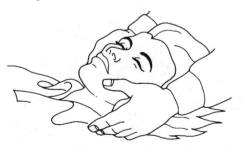

F – press the thumbs outwards over the upper jaw

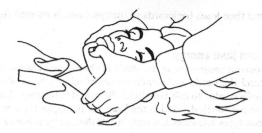

G – press outwards on the lower part of the jaw

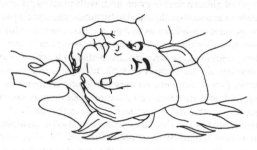

H – place fingers beneath the jaw and lean back

from the start of the eyebrows across the brow to the outside (figure B). With the fingers in place at each side of the face, work the thumbs across the bone below the eyes, moving approximately 6 millimetres (0.25 inch) at a time (figure C). Commencing with the thumbs a little to one side of each nostril, press across the face below the cheekbones (figure D). Press one thumb in the area between the top lip and nose (figure E) and then press with both the thumbs outwards over the upper jaw (figure F). Next, press one thumb in the hollow below the lower lip and then press outwards with both thumbs over the lower part of the jaw (figure G). The giver then puts all fingers of the hands beneath the lower jaw and then leans backwards so that pressure is exerted (figure H).

Kyo and jitsu energy

As a person progresses in the study of shiatsu and comes to understand the needs and requirements of others, he or she will gradually be able to give beneficial therapy. It is believed that energy, as previously defined, is the basis for all life, and it is divided into two types known as *kyo* and *jitsu*. If the energy is low or deficient, it is known as kyo, and if there is an excess or the energy is high, it is known as jitsu. These two factors will therefore affect the type of shiatsu that is given and, with practice, it should be possible to assess visually and also by touch what type a person is. A few general guidelines as to how a person can vary his or her shiatsu to suit either kyo or jitsu types are given below. As the person progresses, however, it is likely that an intuitive awareness will develop of what is most suitable for a particular person. For kyo types (low or deficient in energy), a gentle and sensitive touch is required, and any stretched positions can be maintained for a longer time as this will bring more energy to that part of the body. Pressure, held by the thumb or palm, can also be maintained for an increased length of time, approximately 10-15 seconds. For jitsu types (high or excess energy), the stretches can be done quite quickly so that the energy is dispersed, and also shaking or rocking areas of the body can have the same effect. The pressure that is exerted by the thumbs or palms should also be held for a shorter length of time, so that excess energy is dispelled.

Yin and yang

As previously mentioned, a change in diet may also be recommended by a shiatsu practitioner. From the viewpoint of traditional Oriental medicine, food can be defined in an 'energetic' way. This differs from the Western definition of foods consisting of protein, minerals, fats, carbohydrates, fibre and vitamins. It is believed that, according to its 'energetic' definition, food will have differing physical, mental, spiritual and emotional effects. This energy is split into two parts known as *yin* and *yang*. Yin is where energy is expanding and yang where it is contracting. They are thus opposites and, from traditional beliefs, it was thought that interactions between them formed all manner of occurrences in nature and the whole of the world and beyond. All definitions of yin and yang are based on macrobiotic food (a diet intended to prolong life, comprised of pure vegetable foods such as brown rice), this being the most usual reference. Food can be divided into three main types – those that are 'balanced', and some that are yin and some that are yang. Foods that are defined as being yin are milk, alcohol, honey, sugar, oil, fruit juices, spices, stimulants, most drugs (such as aspirin, etc), tropical vegetables and fruits, refined foods, and most food additives of a chemical nature. Yang foods are poultry, seafood, eggs, meat, salt, fish, miso and cheese. Balanced foods are seeds, nuts, vegetables, cereal grains, beans, sea vegetables and temperate fruits (such as apples and pears).

The balance between yin and yang is very important to the body, for example, in the production of hormones such as oestrogen and progesterone, and glycogen and insulin and the expansion and contraction of the lungs, etc. A 'balanced' way of eating, mainly from the grains, beans, seeds, nuts and vegetables, etc, is important as this will help to achieve the energy balance in the meridians, organs and chakras, as defined previously. When these two opposing forces of yin and yang are in harmony and balanced, physical and mental health will result.

Body reading

It is possible for practitioners of shiatsu, as they become increasingly experienced, to assess a person's physical and mental state of health by observing the body and forming accurate observations. If the traditional ways of Eastern diagnosis are studied, this can assist greatly. The Eastern methods were based on the senses of hearing, seeing, smelling and touching and also by questioning people to obtain information leading to an overall diagnosis. This is known as body reading.

Makko-ho exercises

Makko-ho exercises are six stretching exercises, each of which affects one pair of the meridians by stimulating its flow of energy. If the complete set of exercises is performed, all the body's meridians will have been stimulated in turn, which should result in increased vigour and an absence of tiredness. Before beginning the exercises, you should feel calm and relaxed. It may prove beneficial to perform some abdominal breathing first (as previously described). One example is the triple heater and heart governor meridian stretch. Sit on the ground with either the feet together or crossed. The right hand should grasp the left knee and the left hand the right knee, both quite firmly (*see* figure A below). Then inhale and, as you exhale, lean forwards and downwards with the top half of the body so that the knees are pushed apart (*see* figure B below). Hold this position for approximately 30 seconds while breathing normally, and then, after inhaling, return to the upright position. After completion of all exercises, lie flat on the ground for several minutes and relax.

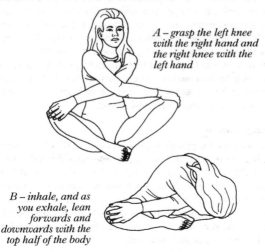

A – grasp the left knee with the right hand and the right knee with the left hand

B – inhale, and as you exhale, lean forwards and downwards with the top half of the body

Explore Your Inner Self

A state of confusion

The second part of the 20th century has seen a great many radical changes, changes that have had a dramatic effect on our way of life. Many of the changeswere for the better in that towards the end of the century more people had a comfortable lifestyle than they ever did at the beginning of the century. Some of the effects, however, were not so good. People began to feel stressed and confused, to the extent that they began to question their whole way of life and even their own identity.

'Who exactly am I and why on earth am I doing this?' became a common *cri de coeur*, if not actually spoken then at least thought. Some who felt a desire to know more about themselves toyed with the idea for a bit, but set it aside and got on with their rat-race lives to the best of their ability. Others again felt that 'Know thyself' was a good maxim for the remainder of their lives and set about putting the knowing of themselves into action.

Exploring one's inner self is obviously no mean task. Even thinking of a way to approach the task is daunting. Different people find different courses of action helpful, and differences in situation can affect the nature of the approach. This section describes some of the ways that people explore in order to get a clearer picture of themselves.

In the 20th century stress and speed are key words, and many feel that they are on a kind of relentless treadmill from which it is impossible to escape. Everything is in a state of hurry and hassle, and there is no time to stand and stare – let alone to think.

It is understandable that this sort of pressure causes some

people to have what are known to the lay person as nervous breakdowns. In the case of others, it is their physical health that breaks down. In yet other cases, it proves to be marriages and relationships that cannot stand the strain. In less dramatic cases, some people simply opt out of what they have previously been doing.

People speak of experiencing a personal crisis – a moment of truth when some kind of decision about their lives has to be made. Others speak of requiring space. Many simply want to get off the roundabout of life, which they feel is somehow hurtling round almost out of control, and to stand still for a while.

Certainly the closing years of the 20th century have found many people feeling lost, as though they have completely strayed from the way on which they had intended to set out. It is a set of circumstances very likely to induce people to try to seek inner strength and inner knowledge in an attempt to improve their lot in some way, and many are doing just that.

It is often something specific that triggers off such a response, some circumstance or life event that makes someone stop in his or her tracks and think. What exactly the crisis point is does, of course, differs from person to person and from circumstance to circumstance.

People who have suffered from mental breakdowns, or who have suffered from severe reactive clinical depression in response to some form of life crisis, often begin to explore their inner selves as they begin to recover. Having been seriously ill, they often take a new look at life and at themselves, and sometimes alter their entire lifestyles. Those who have been seriously physically ill, such as those who have had a near-death experience during a heart attack, often have a similar response.

It is not always something obviously tragic or unfortunate that leads people to embark on a journey of self-discovery. Sometimes it is a particular age, often the age of forty in men, that triggers it. Sometimes it seems to be nothing in particular that acts as a trigger, just a sudden realization that life is going nowhere and some reappraisal is necessary.

Even a happy event can lead people to try to explore their inner selves. The birth of a baby to a high-powered woman executive might find her suddenly wondering what she really wants out of life and who she really is. Likewise, the marriage of a daughter might find a mother wondering about her role in the family and looking within herself to find out to what extent she has done what she really wanted to do.

The reasons why people embark on a journey of self-discovery are many and varied. The ways in which they set out to explore their inner selves are also many and varied. The following sections deal with these various ways.

A helping hand
Help yourself by seeking help
It may seem something of a contradiction in terms to speak of seeking another's help when one sets out to discover one's inner self. Surely only the person involved can bring about such a personal revelation?

To some extent this is true, but some people need a little help, at least to get started on their journey of discovery. Whether or not they do need some assistance will depend partly on the personality of the individual concerned and perhaps partly on the set of the circumstances that led him or her to look at the inner self.

Dealing with depression
Some life changes are too difficult to make without the help of others, although the wish to change must come from within the person his or herself. Clinical depression, or what is popularly known as a nervous breakdown, is too serious a condition to be treated without some form of medical treatment .

The nature of the medical treatment will vary according to the severity of the illness. If, for example, clinical depression is diagnosed early on it can be treated by the patient's general practitioner, but it is the nature of the disorder that, even today, when a great deal more is known about the condition, it is frequently not identified until it has become quite severe, when psychiatric treatment and sometimes hospitalization become necessary.

Drug treatment is often extremely effective in the treatment of clinical depression, and there is a variety of drugs available today. It is recognized, however, that depression is a condition where the person suffering from it needs to talk to someone, to discuss the life event, such as bereavement or divorce, that led to the onset of the condition or the set of circumstances that led the person to be a depressive personality. Psychiatrists are skilled in the art of drawing people out to talk about themselves and by so doing can obtain some idea of what has led to their mental health problems.

In the course of their talks with their psychiatrists, often when they are in a stage of recovery and so more appreciative of what is going on, patients frequently feel that they have learned much more about themselves. While trying to explain their concerns and reactions to their doctors, and to set these in the context of the background to their illness, they have given themselves an insight into their true selves.

Some people continue with their self-exploration as a do-it-yourself exercise after having been discharged by their psychiatrists. After they have been shown the way, they feel confident about continuing on their journey of self-discovery on their own. Frequently, self-knowledge acquired in this way leads people to change their lives, or at least to appreciate certain aspects of life more. Some realize, for example, that it was their high-pressure, low-satisfaction jobs that were at the heart of their breakdowns, and they look for a career more in line with what they now see as their true personalities, or indeed decide to opt out of the career structure altogether. Perhaps they are country people at heart, who have been forced to live in a hectic urban environment, and they now revert to type.

It is an unfortunate feature of very severe clinical depression that it can lead to patients suffering from suicidal tendencies. When they have been cured of the feelings of black despair that induces such tendencies, they begin to feel that life is worth living again, and their newly discovered selves begin to think about what is best for them. Nothing much has changed about the world, or about their place in it, but their illness has been a learning experience that has made them see both themselves and the world in a different light.

Psychotherapy

Therapy involving discussion between therapist and client need not be organized by a doctor specializing in mental illness, and the client undergoing the therapy need not be mentally ill. He or she may just feel that there is something wrong with life and be seeking help, or someone who knows the person well may have recommended such a course of action. The person in charge of the therapy programme will not be a psychiatrist but a psychoanalyst or psychotherapist.

Many people find psychotherapy a very useful and rewarding step on their way to self-discovery. At the very least they have talked about things that they would never have dreamt of speaking about before and have learned to face up to them. They have been helped to come to terms with the past and have been able to achieve some understanding of how the past, with its suppressed fears and emotions, had affected the present and prevented them living life to the full. In a very real sense, many people discover who they really are through psychotherapy. Now they are ready to build a future.

There are some who see drawbacks in psychotherapy. The process of psychotherapy, as we have seen, aims to release blocked and negative emotions by getting clients to talk about things that had happened in their lives but had been subconsciously blocked out by them. Some sceptics are afraid that some of the psychotherapists' clients are talking not only about terrible things that had happened in their lives but about terrible things that had not happened at all but are the products of the clients' imagination.

This phenomenon, the existence of which is denied by many, is known as 'false memory'. Cited examples of it include people who suddenly claim that they were abused in some way, often sexually abused, when this seems highly unlikely in the light of evidence put forward by parents, other family members, neighbours, and so on. There are stories of parents being completely rejected by their grown-up children after therapy, when previously they had seemed to enjoy a very happy relationship – although it has to be borne in mind that only two people need to know the truth about abuse, onlookers being often ignorant of the truth.

Not enough is yet known about 'false memory', although the argument about it rages on. What is the case is that more and more people are turning to psychotherapy. People nowadays are considerably better informed, and they have a much better idea of when to seek help and where to find it. Many know the importance of being put in touch with themselves and with their own feelings, and many choose to do so by means of psychotherapy.

Counselling

If people have a particular problem that is having a harmful effect on their lives, they may care to seek help not from a psychiatrist or a psychotherapist but from a counsellor. Counselling has become a very important part of our lives in the late 20th century, although it is quite a recent phenomenon.

Counselling tends to seek to help someone deal with a particular experience rather than delve into the subconscious, as psychotherapy does, but the simple fact of talking to someone about a specific problem can have a wider therapeutic effect. We have become increasingly aware of the trauma, both long-term and short-term, that can be caused by some life events, and counselling is very often recommended to someone who has just experienced such an event.

Talking about a problem to someone and working our way through it can make us start thinking more closely about our emotions and thoughts generally. The net result is often that we find we have gone through a learning experience that has left us wanting to know more about ourselves.

Counselling is appropriate in a wide range of life events such as bereavement and post-traumatic stress. For example, someone who has been involved in a car accident in which others have been killed may be advised to seek counselling. Couples who have suffered a miscarriage and are having difficulty in coming to terms with the situation may be advised to seek counselling to try to deal with the potential long-term effects of such bereavement.

Public bodies are also becoming aware of the need for counselling for people who have potentially traumatising jobs, such as the police, paramedics and those in the fire service. Before, it was assumed that coping with traumas was part of the job. Now, for example, police officers who have watched a colleague being shot to death, or a firefighter who has failed to rescue a child from a blazing building, may well be offered counselling, and it has been suggested that this also be offered to soldiers who have experienced trauma in battle. People who undergo trauma and who do not receive counselling are thought to be in danger of what is known as post-traumatic stress syndrome or disorder.

Schools often offer counselling to schoolchildren if one of their number is suddenly killed. It is recognized now that the other children in the school need to be able to grieve and so are offered counselling to try to obviate any ill effects in a later life.

When someone seeks counselling about a problem, he or she will be put in touch with a professional who will discuss the situation from a sympathetic point of view and often offer practical advice. Frequently the object of counselling is to talk through the problem in such a way that the discussion will enable the person seeking counselling to discover for himself or herself the solution to the problem. It is often this working-through process that puts the person concerned in control of his or her own life again.

There are some extremely effective counsellors around, some of them attached to a particular body or organization. As is the case with psychotherapists, however, there are some counsellors practising who have minimal skills and minimum training, partly because it very rapidly became rather a trendy profession with no very obvious basic qualifications. Again it is wise to seek guidance from your general practitioner or hospital, or from a friend with some experience of the field of counselling.

Hypnotherapy

Some people, in an effort to help them sort out their problems, turn to a hypnotherapist. These problems range from trying to break an addiction, such as smoking, to trying to slim by receiving help in controlling the appetite, from trying to increase one's level of confidence, to trying not to be so self-conscious, or to trying to help solve some emotional problems.

We will see later in this section how hypnotherapy can be used in several ways, such as helping people to stop smoking. Hypnosis can, however, be used specifically to get us to be more in touch with ourselves. Sometimes called hypnoanalysis in this context, it was used by Freud before he went on to practise psychoanalysis. By means of hypnotic suggestion, the person seeking help through hypnosis can move backwards in time, in a kind of regression, and relive memories that would not be recoverable by ordinary memory or an act of will. This can add to our self-knowledge in a similar way to psychoanalysis. However, many people prefer psychoanalysis or psychotherapy to hypnoanalysis since they feel that they are more in control, although this might not be the case. There is sometimes a vague feeling among people in general that to undergo hypnosis is to put oneself entirely in someone else's power, although this is not in fact true.

There is another way that hypnosis can help us on our journey of self-discovery. If cure by hypnosis is effective in cases of addiction, it helps to put the addict back in charge of his or her life instead of being under the control of the addictive substance. Addiction often results in alienation from one's self. By the same token, breaking free from addiction frees the self and is instrumental in allowing former addicts to get to know their real selves.

Self-help groups for addicts

This section is dealing with people who can help others on a journey of self-discovery, usually by helping them cope with some problem or disorder that is having an effect on their lives. It may seem like a contradiction in terms, therefore, to mention self-help groups, such groups being a set of people who have the same kind of problem and who meet together to work through this, and to offer advice and support to each other. These groups are included in this section, simply because, as is the case with counselling, someone has to point the person seeking help in the right direction, and the other members of the group have to give any new member a great deal of support. Only then can he or she learn to begin to cope with the problem involved and begin to contribute effectively within the group.

The first self-help groups began in the United States in the 1930s to help people suffering from alcoholism to cure themselves. Alcoholics Anonymous was the first well-known self-help group, and it is probably still the best known. They hold regular meetings to help members face up to their drink problem, to help them break the habit, and to help them fight the temptation to start again. The meetings provide a forum where you can share your problem with others, knowing that they too have first-hand experience of the problem. People who are trying to break free of their addiction know that they are in no danger of being patronized by do-gooders or of being in receipt of contempt or condemnation. They are among their own.

A similar group is Gamblers Anonymous, which provides the help for those addicted to gambling that Alcoholics Anonymous does for those addicted to alcohol. The extent of gambling addiction in this country has increased greatly in recent years, partly because the potential for gambling has increased so much. Formerly it was only betting on horses that was the problem, but there is concern, particularly with reference to the young, about addiction to fruit machines, and now there are worries that the National Lottery, particularly in its scratch-card versions, will add to gambling tendencies, especially in people who are too poor to indulge such tendencies with equanimity. Those of us who buy the occasional lottery ticket have no idea of the forces that are at work in someone spending the week's housekeeping on scratch-cards. It is all too easy to condemn without appreciating the problem. At Gamblers Anonymous this ready condemnation is unheard of.

Self-help groups for those with some form of addiction are extremely important because they not only help addicts to keep away from their particular form of addiction but they also help them to rebuild their lives and give them back their self-esteem and self-control. Addicts are never in control of their own lives until they can relinquish their addiction, because to be addicted to something is to be controlled by it. Thus it is that alcohol, gambling, or whatever form the addiction takes, rules the addicts, and they themselves are virtually powerless.

The source of the addiction alienates addicts from their true selves. While they are in its grip they cannot really know themselves, as their true selves have become submerged and subjugated. Coming to terms with addiction and ceasing to be the slave of the addictive substance means that the former addicts can come terms with themselves and embark on what is a very important journey of self-discovery, to find the lost self.

The self-help groups for addicts that have so far been mentioned have been large groups designed either for people suffering from alcohol abuse or from gambling addiction. There are, of course, other addictions – one very obvious and very serious one being that of drug abuse – and there are self-help groups for some of these, some local groups and some branches of larger groups.

Addicts need all the help they can get, although of course they first have to want to break free from the addiction. It is frequently maintained that addicts are never really cured, that the most that they can hope for is that they will stay away from the addictive substance or habit, although that is in fact a major achievement. Being able not actually to involve themselves with the addiction to a large extent puts them in charge of themselves again, although many of them need the support of the self-help group for life.

Self-help groups for non-addicts

Self-help groups do not exist simply for addicts. They have proved of enormous help to many others and deal with a wide range of problems or experiences. For example, parents whose children have been the victims of cot death often find great comfort from being with people who have been in the same terrible situation. They realize that they are not alone and that they are in no way to blame for the tragedy, although some of them will have been torturing themselves with this thought.

Another well-known self-help group is Al-Anon, which provides help and understanding for the members of the family of someone who is suffering from alcohol abuse. This is a particularly useful group since alcohol destroys not only individuals but whole families, coming, as it often does, accompanied by violence, poverty and loss of self-esteem. Often family members feel, usually quite wrongly, a sense of blame and a sense of failure if they have been unable to get the alcoholic to stop drinking.

Other self-help groups include those formed by people who have been raped, suffered sexual abuse, people who are suffering from Aids or who are HIV-positive, people who are part of the adoption triangle and people who suffer from depression. Obviously, the nature of the groups will vary, but they have in common the fact that the members all know what other members are going through, and they know exactly what to do to help. Being part of a group takes away the terrible sense of isolation that is often felt by people who are suffering in some way. 'Why me?' they often ask, and it is something of a comfort that God or fate has not selected them alone to undergo tragedy or disorder.

We have seen how self-help groups for people fighting an addiction can help the members lose their sense of alienation and discover more about themselves while helping them to fight the addiction. Whatever traumatic experience members of other groups are recovering from, it will have left its mark. The help and support that they receive from fellow group members will enable them to recover enough from the trauma to be able to stop and think, and to use the learning experience in a positive way so that it may well in some way enrich their lives. The whole experience will certainly tell them a good deal about themselves, their strengths and weaknesses, and will be a major stage in any journey of self-discovery.

Women's self-help groups

There are some organizations that aim to encourage self-help among women with particular needs. Such organizations, of which Women's Aid is a well-known example, provide refuges for battered wives and encourage the women to take charge of their lives. The location of the refuges is kept strictly secret so that husbands who have acted violently towards their wives will not be able to track them down and attempt to take them back.

As has been indicated, the aim of these women's organizations is to get women who have suffered at the hands of violent partners to take charge of their own lives and to try to make new and independent lives for themselves away from the tyranny of violence. To some extent, however, the self-help is the second part of this aim. First the women have to feel assured that there is somewhere safe to go before they take the huge step of leaving their home and partner. Organizations like Women's Aid provide such assurance, with their refuges and staff providing backup support and advice on benefits, childcare, job opportunities and many other areas of concern.

Women, particularly women with children, never leave violent partners lightly. Most of them keep hoping for some form of miraculous change in the man concerned, who may ordinarily be very charming. When they eventually face the fact that this is not going to happen, when they start to become terrified for their children as well as for themselves, indeed when they begin to fear for their very lives, they often still hesitate before leaving, even if they know about the work of the women's organizations and the refuges.

The recurrent violence, which will often have been accompanied by verbal abuse, will very likely have left the women with very low self-esteem. They have probably been told repeatedly that they are useless, and they have begun to believe what has been said. Worse, they frequently feel that they are responsible for what is happening to them. A woman may feel that if her partner is so charming to everyone else then it must be something in her that is inviting the blows.

A woman who leaves her partner and then returns to him feels even less self-esteem, since she has tried and failed. The failure may well have been no fault of her own, but she will not see it that way. Many battered women go to their parents or other family members and return because the partner turned up at their house, made a scene and offered violence to her family. They sometimes return because their families do not have the space to accommodate her and the children, or the money to support them, or sometimes are not willing to offer them either financial or emotional support. Sadly, they frequently return when their violent partners tell them that they will take the children from them if they do not return.

The woman who has heard about one of the agencies that help battered wives – such agencies, fortunately, are now much better known than they were formerly – and decides that there is no hope other than to leave and seek their help, has already embarked on a journey of self-discovery as well as one of self-help. When she leaves she realizes that she has more strength than she thought she had – the sheer act of leaving is testament to this. After she has received help and advice she will realize that she has far greater potential than she felt she ever had before, and this will in turn lead to greater self-confidence. When she has been out on her own for a bit, and coping with children and home on her own, she may well begin to take stock and really begin to discover even greater depths in herself.

For some women their new-found liberation from violence and their new independence will have been part of a journey of self-discovery, but for others they may be a part of a journey of rediscovery. They may have been quite different people, when they married, from the frightened, shivering, worthless-feeling wrecks that they became. The incidence of domestic violence is not related to class, education or money, and some women might have had quite good jobs before marrying jealous men and giving up their jobs. As she re-establishes her life independently of her violent husband she will probably also end up on a journey of discovery as she reflects on how far she can come and on how far she can go.

Thus we have seen how some people who have been rendered vulnerable in some way, or who have suffered some form of trauma, can achieve some degree of self-discovery in the course of seeking help with their problems.

There can be benefits from the experience of trauma, and these benefits are enhanced by the help given in the various ways described above. Thus psychiatry, psychotherapy, counselling and self-help groups can not only help people towards a greater sense of wellbeing and a greater sense of being at peace with themselves, but they can also help them to have a greater understanding of their inner selves.

Religious support

In a way, the professionals involved in the processes described in this chapter so far are the priests of the modern world. In earlier centuries, or even in the earlier decades of the 20th century, people with some of the problems described above would seek the help of a priest or minister of the church. Particularly in the second part of the 20th century, however, the number of people taking part in organized traditional religions diminished considerably, and so this was no longer an option for them.

Of course the priest or minister would not have the range of professional expertise of some of today's advisers. In earlier times, the kind of trauma and emotional problems that are now generally acknowledged as affecting the lives of people were simply not known or not recognized as such. Problems were seen in more simplistic terms, and members of the clergy were expected to be able to deal with these.

Things were often seen in moral or ethical terms, and clergymen were judged to be eminently qualified to deal with such issues. Spiritual issues, such as crises of faith, were obviously also adjudged to be part of their remit, and many more issues than were strictly relevant to the spiritual topic were included under its umbrella. There may well have been objections to this kind of blanket coverage of problems by the clergy, but there was little alternative.

At least in the case of families whose members had tended to stay much in the same place for some time, the relevant clergymen had a background to go on when offering advice. He probably had a very real idea of the weaknesses and strengths of the various family members, and this might well have proved useful when trying to show someone the way forward to a greater contact with his or her inner self. No one exists in a vacuum, and the past often has a very powerful influence on the present and even on the future.

So much for the influence of the clergy on the family, which in time waned dramatically as it became no longer the norm in Britain for people to attend church regularly, whether or not they were members of the Church of England, the Roman Catholic Church, the Church of Scotland, the Methodist Church, the Baptist Church or any of the others. There are still some people who do not attend church regularly but who still opt to get married, to be buried and to have their children baptised under the auspices of the church – some may even feel a nostalgic desire to attend church at Christmas and Easter.

On the other hand, secular arrangements for the major events in life are becoming more and more common in Britain all the time. More and more people are choosing to be married in registry offices, and efforts are being made to make civil wedding ceremonies more civilized, welcoming and considerably less bleak. In any case, more and more couples are opting to live together instead of getting married, some for part of the time that they are together, some for all of the time that they are together, even after they have children. The net result is that many couples are relinquishing even the tenuous connection that they had with the church. Even so there are still brides who think that a church is a better backdrop for their wedding photographs than a registry office.

Even people who declared themselves to be agnostics or even atheists in life used to be buried under the auspices of the church. In recent years, it has become common for the burial service to be a cremation service, churchyards and cemeteries being no longer able to cope with the sheer volume of corpses and cremation becoming a more compact acceptable alternative. For a long time the cremation ceremony was still very much a 'service'. Although the ceremony would take place in a crematorium rather than a church, the person who usually officiated at such a ceremony was a minister or priest of the church.

Gradually the secular impression created by the often rather bleak crematorium got people used to dissociating the idea of interment and the church. Frequently the relatives of the person being cremated had to make a lot of enquiries in order to find a minister or priest to officiate, and even then the cleric had a great deal of difficulty finding something complimentary and truthful to say about someone whom he or she had hardly known – if at all. Many people began to feel that the whole thing was becoming a bit hypocritical and sought to make the whole cremation ceremony more secular. This has become particularly easy to organize if the person who has died was a member of the Humanist Society, as they will provide for someone to officiate at a secular ceremony.

For many, the church baptismal service has long been something that does not reflect the beliefs of those participating. Either godparents or parents, or both, are required to promise to bring the child up according to the dictates of the church and to be responsible for his or her spiritual and moral welfare. This many of them have done – and never been near a church after the baptismal service or seen to it that the child has. Gradually the secularization of marriage and burial ceremonies has spilled over into baptismal ceremonies. Formerly, there was a general feeling that children were not quite legally registered if they were not baptised in church, there being some confusion between civil registration of the birth, compulsory by law, at the local registry office, and baptism in church. In time more people became aware that the civil registration was enough.

Certainly, by the very late decades of the 20th century, the church had ceased to play a major part in many people's lives. If births, marriages and deaths could be officially recognized without benefit of clergy then many people had little use for the church. Of course this is by way of being a generalization. Many people, particularly those of an older generation, have gone on attending church regularly, and some others have gone on paying lip-service to the church by using it for family marriages, births and deaths, and perhaps have graced it occasionally at Christmas and Easter. Another point worth making is that many of the churches have tried valiantly to modernize themselves, indeed have even made themselves trendy, in an effort to attract more people, particularly younger people, back to the church. Alas, in many cases the effort has not been totally successful. Perhaps one could say in all charity that the efforts were a classic case of too little, too late.

What has been missing for some considerable time is the emphasis placed on pastoral care by the clergy in the average community. Many families would feel extremely embarrassed, and even encroached upon, if a member of the clergy called, even if the family was going through a bereavement or other family crisis, and even if its members were still technically members of the church. On the other side of the clerical fence, so to speak, the clergy, although coping with fewer church members, are probably also trying to cope with larger workloads, fewer clerical colleagues and an ageing church membership, which makes more demands on their time, not least in terms of bereavement. They may have very little time to experience the embarrassment they might encounter if they enter a house of church membership, but not of churchgoers, or even a house of agnostics or atheists that happens to be situated in their parish.

This represents a complete turnaround. There was a time in the relatively recent past when pastoral care was of major importance in the community. If something major went wrong in the life of a member of the family, the local minister or priest was likely to be among the first to be consulted. Thus, if a husband died, or a child was stillborn, or a daughter became pregnant while unmarried, or a son ran away from home, then both spiritual comfort and practical help would be sought from the relevant local cleric. Before the advent of a higher general standard of education and while literacy levels were quite low, the local clergyman was also the person to whom people turned if some kind of official letter had to be written or even read.

The standing of the clergy in the average community has fallen drastically, although the extent of this falling-off has obviously differed from church to church, area to area, and even person to person. With this reduction of importance of church and clergy in the average family's life has come an inevitable decrease in pastoral care. When the family members could no longer turn to the parish minister or priest for help or comfort, then they had to look elsewhere – to psychotherapists, counsellors and self-help groups in fact.

The fact that a great many people have abandoned the church as a source of solace, and even of self-discovery, does not mean that this is true for everyone. There is still a significant number of people in Britain who are staunch members of the church and who regard religion as a spiritual quest and thus a journey of self-discovery.

Furthermore, there are many people who were not brought up in the ways of organized religion but who seek membership of a church to help them find a faith, often in an attempt to help them find themselves, or at least to help them come to terms with themselves. Some of these speak of suddenly seeing the light, as though their lives up to the point of their conversion to religion had been deep in darkness. Such people may be seen as being against the trend, but there are others who, to some extent, might be seen in the same context.

These include people who, in their early years, were brought up to be regular churchgoers and believers in religion but who somehow let such habits and such beliefs lapse, only to find that at the point of some crisis in their lives they felt a need to revert to these and began to attend church regularly, and to consult priests and ministers of religion. They frequently feel that they have somehow lost themselves along life's way and have a deep conviction that the only way to get back in touch with themselves is through the church. Some of these turn to a church other than the one in which they were brought up. For example, a member of the Church of England might feel that he or she wishes to join the Roman Catholic Church.

Often people who either join the church or revert to regular churchgoing are seeking help, sometimes consciously, sometimes unconsciously, with a problem, whether this be an emotional, mental or spiritual one. Whatever the problem, they are probably also seeking to find spiritual enlightenment or fulfilment, and by so doing to extend their knowledge of themselves.

They see their parish minister or priest as a source of help, support and enlightenment, someone to whom they can entrust their deepest thoughts and feelings without fear of these being passed on without consultation. Often by talking these through with the cleric, the problem-ridden people can find their own answers to what is bothering them, while at the same time adding a spiritual dimension to their lives that enriches and extends them.

This is all very well for people who have a religious faith or for people who are working their way towards a religious faith. They have someone trustworthy on hand to whom they can confide their innermost secrets and thoughts, and by so doing they can explore their inner selves. People without religious faith and without a church connection do not have such an outlet. That is why they seek help from other sources, which take on the mantle of a religious confessor and confidant and which can help them on their path to greater self-knowledge. Thus the need for psychotherapists, counsellors and self-help groups.

In our multicultural society it is not uncommon for people to seek solace in one of the eastern religions, although they were not born into one of these. At school many people learn something about other religions as well as Christianity, and some feel drawn to these. The eastern influence on some people's religious feelings was very prominent in the 1960s, when a good many people, particularly young people, went off to India in search of spiritual fulfilment and often in search of a guru, a spiritual teacher, who would bring them such fulfilment. The guru took the place that a clergyman would once have held in their lives but had the advantage of being considerably more exotic in their eyes. This trend towards eastern religions was increased by the interest of the Beatles, the British pop group that leapt to extraordinary fame in the 1960s. John Lennon in particular was drawn towards the East and influenced other young people.

For many young people, looking towards the East for spiritual satisfaction was an attempt to get in touch with their inner selves, the guru being a guide to show the way. It was also an attempt to give expression to their dissatisfaction with the materialistic way of life of the West, often the way of life of their middle-class or upper-class relatives. This dissatisfaction was also displayed by people who embraced the Hippie culture in the 1960s and later by people who embraced the New Age philosophy in the late 1980s and 1990s. These movements are treated in greater detail in the next section.

Of course not everyone who felt drawn towards the religions and philosophies of the East went to India in search of a guru – neither did they all seek out one of the gurus who came to the West. Indeed, many more people than embraced the whole panoply of a religion such as Hinduism or Buddhism simply adopted parts of these. Thus they came to be drawn towards meditation and yoga, and these activities often took the place that Christian prayer would once have done in their lives.

As has been mentioned, many people in the 1960s felt drawn to gurus in the hope that they would give them spiritual leadership and help them to a greater realization of their inner selves. Later in the 20th century there was an increased tendency for people to join religious cults and to look towards the cult leader for the same kind of guidance that some had looked for in gurus in the 1960s, and countless others had looked for in clergymen throughout the centuries. Cult members were often looking for some kind of inner fulfilment or realization and looked to the cult leader to help them in their journey towards this. Religious cults were more common in the United States than in Britain, but in both countries fears were expressed that members of the cults were being brainwashed, although there is often a danger that someone vulnerable, seeking emotional or spiritual help, will form too great an attachment to the person seeking to provide such help.

There is a very real need in many of us to find spiritual fulfilment, whether or not we would categorize the need as such, and in order to do this we often feel that we have to find ourselves or to reach a clearer understanding of ourselves. This often involves seeking help from someone professionally concerned in some way with this kind of work, and such a person is personally central to the success of the other person's search for self. Such help has been described in this section, but there is also help to be provided in a less central, more peripheral way, by other people. This kind of help, together with the kind of help that people embarking on a journey of self-discovery might provide for themselves, is described in the next section.

Self-help

The previous section dealt with situations in which other people, at least at first, play a major part in our attempts to seek out our inner selves. This section explores the attempts made by people themselves to undertake a journey of self-discovery. Although again they may receive help and encouragement from other people, the other people do not play such a major role as, for example, a psychotherapist.

There are many different ways in which people seek to become more in touch with themselves and to find out more about themselves. Some people find a method that suits them right away, although the actual self-exploration might take a considerable time. Others try various methods before hitting on the one that contributes to their self-discovery.

Solitary self-exploration

Some seek solitude in which to create the right kind of atmosphere for communing with themselves. This can be quite informal and might take the form of a quiet holiday in which the person on a journey of self-exploration goes off alone, often somewhere solitary, such as a remote cottage, to find time and space to think and reflect, and to provide an opportunity for self-analysis. People who opt out of their usual worlds in this way, whether for a short or long time, often do so to give themselves the opportunity to look at their lives and to consider the past, present and what seems to be the likely future. Some go back refreshed by such self-analysis others, on the basis of it, decide to change their whole lifestyles.

They may, for example, have been pressurized by their parents to follow some formally-structured career while they themselves would rather have done something quite different, such as write poetry or paint pictures. At this point in their lives, having taken time to find out more about themselves, and their thoughts and feelings, they may decide to be true to themselves and their personal aspirations and turn their backs on their careers to do something that will bring them more fulfilment.

Some decide not only to leave the work they have been doing but the whole environment in which they have been living. Reflection on their lives has brought them a realization of the futility of their existence and a dislike of the materialism that has brought so much stress into their lives. They feel a need not only to get back to themselves but to get back to nature and a simpler way of life.

It is in such circumstances that, for example, a London stockbroker, used to a highly paid job and an affluent city lifestyle, might abandon his way of life and buy a croft in some remote part of Scotland with a view to living off the land and leading a virtually self-sufficient life. Of course, such dramatic changes do not always work out, and it is likely that he would discover that the whole thing was a wild romantic dream, hastily selling up the croft to return to the affluence of Surrey. Still, at least he would have learnt something about his true self, even although it might have proved an expensive venture.

New Age travelling

The desire to lead a simple, non-materialistic life does not necessarily involve a solitary life. The later decades of the 20th century have seen the evolvement of the New Age travellers. These are people who seek a less materialistic, simpler, more golden age, but they wish to do so in the company of others who share their philosophy. There are often various other aspects to their philosophy, such as a concern for the environment and animal rights, a preference for natural remedies rather than formal medicine, and a leaning towards more ancient religions. New Age travellers are also intent on finding themselves, but they choose to do so in a communal, peripatetic way, moving on in vans and caravans from place to place and in so doing frequently falling foul of landowners or the police. Their desire to shake off the shackles of materialism and to lead a freer, less restricted life has something in common with the Hippies of the 1960s.

Retreats

Of course, not everyone who feels the need to take time out changes an entire lifestyle, whether to go off alone or as part of a group. As we have seen, many people simply want to be alone for a while to sort themselves out. This can be done in quite a structured, formal way as well as in the informal way described above. One example of this more formal way of taking time for reflection and self-exploration is the retreat; a place, as the name suggests, where one can get away from it all.

Retreats vary quite a bit. Some are extremely Spartan, encouraging one to concentrate on the mind, soul and spirit, rather than on the needs and delights of the body. Others are less basic, providing at least a minimum standard of comfort, although one should obviously not expect pampered luxury from a retreat. Some retreats are more organized and structured than others and provide lectures, discussions and workshops on various subjects for those who wish to attend. Others leave people more to their own devices, leaving them to meditate or pray and reflect as they wish.

Many retreats are religious in nature. Some of these relate to one of the Christian denominations, and people attend them to spend time in prayer and Bible study as well as to spend time in reflection. Other retreats of a religious nature relate to one of the eastern religious movements rather than to Christianity. In such retreats people tend to spend a good deal of time in meditation.

Yet other retreats of a religious nature may be based on the teachings on one of the sects that have become popular in the later decades of the 20th century. Retreats may differ widely in their nature, but they have one important thing in common – they provide the opportunity for people to get out of the world for a while, to have time for self-exploration and perhaps to achieve a degree of spiritual and mental refreshment.

For some people a short time spent at a retreat proves not to be enough. They feel the need to get out of the world for a longer time in order to spend time communing with themselves, and often with God. Such people sometimes choose to join religious communities for a time in order to find themselves and come to terms with themselves.

Personal growth and women's groups

Some people feel that they might be more inclined to initiate an exploration of their inner self, and to persist with it, if they had some support from a group. In particular the later years of the 20th century has seen the rise of a number of what are known as personal growth societies, which are in many ways a later form of the consciousness-raising groups popular in the 1970s.

Such societies often attract people who feel that they have not achieved what they should have achieved in life. They feel stunted in some way or feel that they have taken a wrong direction somewhere along the path of their lives. The members of such societies, in their efforts to achieve their aims, often begin with an attempt to get to know their true selves and to find out how they have become what they are. Until they do so they feel that they cannot come to terms with themselves or maximize their potential by finding out their true capabilities.

There are groups, other than personal growth societies, that people join in order to find out more about themselves. We have seen in the previous section that many people join self-help groups, but these tend to be people who have a particular problem for which they seek the help of group-members. Other people, for example, might join a women's group.

Such groups became very popular in the later decades of the 20th century with the rise of feminism and the interest in the Women's Movement. The initial aim of a women's group is not specifically to enable the members to explore their inner selves. Many are formed with the aim of discussing issues that are important to women which are many and varied. They include such issues as equal opportunities in the workplace, equal pay, health issues, such as screening for breast cancer, childcare, domestic violence. Several such groups were formed initially simply to discuss women's literature.

Although women's groups were not necessarily started with the intention of leading their members to explore their inner consciousness, they often have this effect. When women begin to discuss the role of women in society and how it has changed in recent years, it often leads them to begin to think about their own individual roles in society and within the family, and to reassess themselves, their achievements and aspirations. They have, in fact, begun a journey to find their inner selves, although the original journey was designed to explore the standing and potential of women in the world.

For hundreds of years women were totally underestimated, and the struggle to assert themselves and to establish even a relatively fair position for themselves in society has been an extremely hard one. The fact that they had to put up a joint fight in order to achieve this, however, brought them together in a spirit of sisterhood and raised their consciousness of what it means to be a woman and the problems that this can bring. This encouraged the habit of joint discussion over women's issues.

In the closing years of the 20th century things are beginning to change with respect to men's group. More men are beginning to feel the need to meet to discuss joint issues with other men and to receive support. These issues are often very specific ones. For example, men who are single parents sometimes form groups, or men who are separated or divorced and feel the need to fight for their rights as fathers sometimes do likewise. In addition, men are beginning to become aware of health problems that are specific to the male sex, and it is extremely feasible that this concern may give rise to the formation of more specifically male groups.

Another reason why men are beginning to group together in a

way that has been common in women for some time relates to their concern for their rights and for their standing in society, the very issues that first drew women together. Because of women's success in the workplace, and because of the lack of employment opportunities generally, men have begun to feel threatened and to think that the assertion of women's rights has gone too far at the expense of their own.

Men's groups
More men are beginning to feel the need to discuss joint issues with other men and receive support. These issues are often very specific ones, divorce, being a single parent, the rights of fathers and men's health problems. If the formation of purely male groups continues to increase, it will certainly encourage individual men to explore their inner selves simply because such groups will set them thinking about their individual lives and roles in the same way that they set women thinking about theirs.

Thus, some people find the way to self-exploration through membership of some kind of discussion group, whether or not they had that specific intention when they became members. Others feel that self-exploration is a more solitary pursuit.

Relaxation and healing-related therapies
There are many ways in which we can develop and expand the five senses to which we are limited in order to become sensitive to the energy vibrations that surround us somewhere where physics and mysticism meet. By tuning in to the rhythms of the universe we can learn to co-operate with nature's innate healing capacity

Here are several therapies, all of which respond to the vibrations of the life-energy around us.

Relaxation
An increasingly common method of getting in touch with one's inner self using one's own resources is through meditation. Mention has been made in the preceding section of how an interest in

eastern religions and spiritual movements arose in the West in the 1960s. This in turn inspired an interest in meditation, which is often an essential part of such religions, even among people who do not embrace the whole religion.

An essential part of meditation is relaxation. Some people begin with relaxation and move on to meditation. Others find that relaxation alone fulfils their needs. They find that through relaxation they can unwind totally and free themselves from a buildup of stress. By devoting time and space to completely relaxing themselves and to making their minds completely free of the accumulation of thoughts and worries that usually occupy our 20th-century minds, they feel that through relaxation alone they can commune with themselves and so explore their inner selves. In screening out the world, they give themselves the chance of looking into their subconscious, in the way that other people achieve through meditation.

Of course, there are degrees of relaxation, and some people use relaxation techniques simply to de-stress themselves. It represents a therapeutic pause in an overcrowded life. Others, again, see it as an opportunity to make time for themselves, to clear the mind of all the impediments that have built up there, and to unleash emotions and memories. For this second group, relaxation is a stage on a journey of exploration, even a final stage.

Relaxation techniques vary with the preference of the individual, and it is important for everyone who is interested in relaxation to find the method that is right for him or her. Some people, even if they lead highly stressed lives, find it easy to relax. Others find it extremely difficult, often thinking that they have no time for such a pursuit and often imagining that they will find it boring since they assume, quite wrongly, that deep relaxation is essentially a zombie-like state in which your level of consciousness is markedly dimmed.

It is usually the case that to relax, people like to find a comfortable position, although not a position that induces sleep. This applies especially to those who are just begining to learn relaxation techniques. Such a position varies from person to person.

For example, some like to lie on the floor and others prefer to lean back in a comfortable chair. As long as you are comfortable, but not too comfortable, it really does not matter. People who have mastered the art of relaxation after much practice can go into their relaxation routine anywhere, but there is no point in putting obstacles in your way to begin with.

Comfort should also be considered when choosing clothes for relaxation sessions. Loose and comfortable clothing is considerably more conducive to relaxation than the rather tight suit that you may have worn to the office. If you are trying to slough off the worries of the day, you are less likely to achieve your aim if you are constantly aware of the tightness of your waistband.

It is important deliberately to set aside some time each day for your relaxation session. We all know how easy it is to have good intentions but somehow never find the time to carry these out. A little self-discipline is necessary to make some time for oneself, and it is easier to do this on a regular basis, rather than simply snatch a few minutes at a different time each day, at least until your relaxation session becomes a central part of your life. Again, people who are experienced in relaxation techniques can snatch a few minutes anywhere to go into their routine and relieve their stress, but it takes some considerable time to achieve such expertise.

If you are just embarking on a relaxation programme, it is also important to provide yourself with somewhere quiet and private to set about the process. Until you have learnt something about the art of switching off, it is not fair to yourself to try out your relaxation technique in busy or noisy surroundings. It is all too easy to become distracted and then to assume that you are not a suitable candidate for relaxation. In time you may become one of those lucky people who can go into a relaxation programme anywhere, no matter how noisy or stressful your surroundings are, but it is rather foolish to assume that you will be able to do this right away.

Physical considerations must be thought of if you are contemplating a relaxation programme. Not only do clothing, place and time have to be considered but also the state of one's stomach. If you have just eaten a very heavy meal and go into your relaxation technique, you are very likely to fall asleep. On the other hand, if you have not eaten all day and are absolutely ravenous, you will very likely find it difficult to take your mind off your hunger long enough to concentrate on your relaxation technique.

Time, space, clothing and the state of the stomach are important to the person embarking on a relaxation programme, but there are other things that will help would-be relaxers to achieve their aim. One of these is a concentration on breathing techniques. Most of us, although we are probably unaware of the fact, have a shallow, erratic breathing pattern, in keeping with our busy, erratic lives. Controlled, regular breathing, however, is important both in relaxation and meditation. Apart from anything else, it induces a sense of calm that is central to both of these.

In order to master the breathing techniques used in relaxation and meditation programmes, it is worth becoming aware of the timing of the four-second breath, which is the basis of many breathing techniques. You breathe in to a count of four and breathe out to a count of four, often holding the breath at the top of the lungs to a count of two in between breathing in and breathing out, and holding the lungs empty to the count of two in between breathing out and breathing in again. If you practise this a few times by the clock, you will learn to judge the timing without recourse to a clock or watch and will be able to perform automatically the breathing techniques based on the four-second sequence.

Concentration on breathing directs one's thoughts away from the day's concerns and problems and enables one to concentrate purely on oneself. Perhaps the best-known example of using breathing techniques to induce relaxation and to divert concentration from problems, or in this particular case pain, is its use in natural childbirth. Expectant mothers are taught a series of regular breathing techniques at antenatal classes so that they might put these into practice during labour and so decrease their pain levels and the levels of drugs that are otherwise necessary.

Breathing techniques are thus an important part of thought-control or concentration-direction. Another effective way to accomplish this is by muscular relaxation techniques. This involves concentration on parts of the body in turn, for example, on the legs, and on how to recognize tension and relaxation in the muscles related to these. Total relaxation occurs when you are able to concentrate on the whole body part by part, getting each part to relax. More information on relaxation of body parts is given further on in the chapter in the discussion on meditation. As with concentration on breathing, concentration on relaxed muscles or parts of the body helps to direct one's concentration away from the problems and pressures of one's life.

Obviously, there is more to advanced relaxation and meditation techniques than are described here. For anyone interested in the subject, however, there is a great deal of help available. There are various books on the subject obtainable either from your public libraries – although these are so popular now that you may have to reserve them – or from bookshops. Also there are various classes and courses run throughout the country so that people can acquire the essential techniques of relaxation that they can then practise by themselves.

Whether or not you join a class is a matter of personal preference. Some people find that it helps them to get started on something if they make the commitment to join a class. Others find it more difficult to follow written instructions given in a book than spoken instructions given by a teacher or class leader. Both such groups will obviously opt for a class, but many others are quite happy to follow written instructions at home at their own pace, perhaps seeking the advice of a friend with some knowledge of the subject.

Some people who opt for the home-based situation find that relaxation tapes are extremely helpful. These are readily available, and many of them talk would-be relaxers through relaxation techniques or a whole relaxation programme. A degree of self-discipline and concentration is required to get started on such a tape scheme As with most things in life, the tapes tend to vary in quality.

Ordinary music tapes are often just as helpfl in a relaxation programme. Such tapes should not be too stimulating, or they will defeat the purpose, or too soporific, or they will send the would-be relaxer to sleep. Something reasonably quiet and re-petitive is usually wha is required, but choice of music is very much a matter of personal taste and preference.

Massage

Other people associate relaxation with massage. Although to some extent this can be self-administered, in that one can massage those areas of the body that one can reach with ease, such as the legs, arms and feet, it is one area in this section where a little outside help should be used to augment the self-help. Massage by a friend or family member, or by a professional, is more common and prob-ably more relaxing.

See also Massage page 42.

Aromatherapy

Some people performing – or receiving – massage prefer to use some form of lubricant, although this is not an essential part of massage. In the later years of the 20th century massage with aromatherapy oils became extremely popular, and aromatherapy generally became associated with relaxation and the removal of the effects of stress as well as with natural healing and alternative medicine. Aromatherapy is a kind of holistic therapy that uses essential oils. It aims not only to achieve relaxation and healing but also to achieve and maintain physical and mental equilibrium. The use of aromatic oils in healing is an ancient one. They were used in ancient Egypt almost 3000 years before Christ for me-dicinal as well as cosmetic purposes and for embalming their dead. The Greeks also made use of plants and herbs in medicine, as did the Arab physicians later. Knights who had taken part in the Crusades brought back from the East to Europe perfumes and the knowledge of how to distil them. The Europeans did not have many of the aromatic, gum-yielding trees that were common in the East, but they used the aromatic shrubs that were native to the Mediterranean, such as lavender, rosemary and thyme, together with other herbs and plants.

Many forms of plant medicine were used in Europe throughout the Middle Ages and during the Tudor era. By the 17th century, however, chemical compounds were beginning to replace the use of plants in medicine, although many of the active ingredients of medicinal plants, such as quinine, morphine and atropine, found a place in the new medicine. The plant-based substances, especially in the 20th century, began to be replaced by synthetic drugs.

Then, in the later decades of the 20th century, there came a movement towards natural things generally and a movement towards natural things in medicine in particular. There was a reaction against formal medicine, and various forms of alternative medicine began to be popular. These included acupuncture, homeopathy , herbal medicine, hypnosis, and so on, and particular attention was placed on holistic medicine, to treating the body and the mind as a whole.

As part of the movement towards natural, non-drug-based forms of medicine, aromatherapy has become very popular, and the essential oils have become generally available, although these tend to vary in quality.

Not everyone uses aromatherapy to cure or relieve medical disorders. Others use it because it gives them a sense of wellbeing, and many use it for purposes of relaxation. It is now common for people to combine massage and aromatherapy to help them relax by having a massage with essential oils either from a friend or family member or from a professional masseur or masseuse. When combined with base oils to dilute them, the essential oils are very readily absorbed through the skin, and so they make the ideal massage oil. The person applying the massage will choose a blend of oils to suit the particular client, and a great deal of skill is required to get this right. Essential oils should not be used neat.

People who regularly have massage sessions with a blend of oils especially designed to relax them often indicate that they are left after the massage sessions with a great sense of calm and peace, which is an excellent frame of mind for exploring one's deeper self. The essential oils, however, need not be used just as a massage lubricant to achieve relaxation. Many people use a few drops of essential oils in a bath to rid themselves of stress and become more relaxed. Others prefer to use them as an inhalation. In both these cases, as with massage, it is important to find out about the properties and uses of the various essential oils because by no means all of them make you feel relaxed, some having the effect of stimulating you.

As has been indicated above, the extent to which relaxation helps people to explore their inner selves depends to a great extent on the degree of relaxation achieved. The deeper degree of relaxation the more likely it is that you will be able to get more in touch with yourself.

See also Aromatherapy, page 312.

Yoga

Many people either add a yoga component to their relaxation programme or take up yoga as a regular pursuit to increase the degree of their relaxation. There are several forms of yoga, the word being a general term for various spiritual disciplines followed by devotees of Hinduism to attain a higher consciousness, and also the name of one of the six orthodox systems of Indian philosophy. It is an integral part of Hinduism, and its name derives from the 'yoke' that binds the individual self and universal self together. A common form practised in the West is Hatha yoga, which emphasizes physical control and postures.

Yoga is now very popular in this country. It is based on a system of physical exercises and postures and of controlled breathing. You will find many classes on yoga throughout the country, but many of them do not concentrate on the spiritual aspect of yoga. Of course, this is by no means always the case, and you may well be fortunate enough to find a teacher who will bring this extra dimension to the class.

Whether or not you are looking for a teacher who will be able to impart the Hindu principles of yoga, or whether you are simply

ooking to it as a potential aid to relaxation or to reduce your stress
evels, you should spend some time taking advice so that you may
ind someone competent. As with other areas of alternative therapy
.nd medicine, where there are few hard and fast qualifications
equired, not everyone who has set up as a yoga teacher is truly
ompetent. It is important to be taught by someone with training
.nd experience, if only so that you may adopt the relevant pos-
ures without in any way injuring yourself. Yoga is certainly one
method of relaxation that needs to be taught, although after you
ave mastered the basic techniques you can practise them alone
t home.

Even if the spiritual content is either missing or not very strongly
emphasized, yoga is for many people an excellent way of achiev-
ng relaxation and a sense of wellbeing and peace. Partly because
f the degree of concentration involved, many people also find
yoga a good way of blocking out the world, bringing them calm
nd inner peace and giving them the opportunity and means of
exploring their inner selves.

See also Yoga, page 75.

Meditation

Meditation is yet another way in which people set out to rid themselves of stress and perhaps embark on a journey of self-discovery. As we have seen above, relaxation is one of the components of
his, and many people who successfully establish a relaxation programme for themselves go no further, seeing relaxation as an end
n itself. Others, however, go on to master, or to try to master, the
rt of meditation. Although meditation is the cornerstone of many
religions and cults, and in many cases corresponds to prayer, peo-
ole who decide to practise meditation do not necessarily adopt
the other aspects of the religion or cult.

The verb 'to meditate' can mean simply to think deeply about
something, but meditation in its true meaning is more than just
deep thought. Like thought, meditation is a mental discipline,
but it requires even more concentration than our usual thought
processes. It is a state of mind in which all thoughts are

concentrated on a single point or subject. Such concentration is very difficult to achieve and takes time, patience and persistence. Our minds have a tendency to wander from subject to subject, and concentration on one point has to be worked at.

Many people give up on meditation at an early stage since they lack the patience and commitment to come anywhere near achieving the degree of concentration that is necessary to reap its benefits. People who do persist with the practice of meditation, however, often say that the benefits that meditation has brought to them have been very great indeed, one of the most important being that it has brought them inner peace and inner knowledge, which has in turn brought self-realization, central to any journey of self-discovery.

Some people say that they meditate to bring the mind into a state of calmness and concentration so that it can explore its consciousness. Others view it as a way of achieving a greater clarity of perception, or of finding a new way of perceiving the world and of relating to it. Others again feel that through it they can come into contact with their very soul or even with God. This sounds extremely interesting, but how do you set about meditating? As has already been pointed out, the physical conditions that are conducive to deep relaxation tend also to be conducive to meditation.

One of the purposes of meditation is to make space in our minds, leaving room for higher thoughts and for communication with one's inner or higher self. If the desire to know yourself has been one of the reasons why you have taken up meditation, then you can use this as the focus of your meditation, starting with a phrase such as 'Know yourself' and the meaning and implications of that. You can then move on to focus on different aspects of your being, using your memories of the different stages of your life, the different emotional states you have known, and so on. You might even consider using the phrase 'Who am I?' as a starting point for one of your meditation sessions, hoping that in the course of the meditation you will find your true self.

This kind of meditation, performed in a structured way, has been called 'self-inquiry' by Ramana Maharishi. If this form of meditation is carried out on a strictly structured question-and-answer basis it is said to be very difficult to achieve and to require several months of practise in other structured forms of meditation.

There are people who are cynical about meditation, and most of us are very ill-informed about it. It is quite common, for example, to think of people who are meditating as rather weird people who go into self-imposed hypnotic trances. People who have been successfully meditating for some time, however, often speak of the inner knowledge that meditation has brought to them, and so, clearly, someone interested in exploring the inner self should try to master the techniques of it.

What must be remembered is that meditation is a rigorous discipline of the mind, which requires practice, time and steady, regular hard work. Anyone seriously thinking of taking up meditation should be prepared for this and should be prepared for setbacks. It is not an easy path to sudden enlightenment.

Dance movement therapy

Dance movement therapy is aimed at helping people to resolve deep-seated problems by communicating with, and relating to others through the medium of physical movements and dance. The ability to express deep inner feelings in 'body language' and physical movements is innate in human beings. Young children express themselves freely in this way and without inhibition, and dancing would appear to be common to all past and present races and tribes. However, in modern industrial societies, many people find themselves unable to communicate their problems and fears either verbally or physically and may repress them to such an extent that they become ill. Dance movement therapy aims to help people to explore, recognize and come to terms with feelings and problems that they usually repress, and to communicate them to others. This therapy can help emotional, psychological and stress-related disorders, anxiety and depression, addiction, problems related to physical or sexual abuse, and learning disabilities. Children with behavioural or intellectual problems, autism or other mental and physical disabilities are often very responsive to this therapy.

People of any age can take part in dance movement therapy as the aim is to explore gently physical movements that are within each person's capabilities. The therapist may suggest movements, but hopes to encourage patients to learn to take the initiative. Eventually some groups learn to talk over feelings and problems that have emerged through taking part and are better able to resolve them.

Dance therapy sessions are organized in some hospitals and 'drop-in' and day-care centres.

Music therapy

Making music has always been important in all cultures and societies, as a means of self-expression and communication. Many people have experienced the powerful effects of music, which may stimulate feelings of excitement, tranquillity, sadness or joy. Music therapy consists of creating music, using a range of different instruments and the human voice, as a means of helping people to communicate their innermost thoughts, fears and feelings.

Music therapy can help people with a variety of different disorders. It is especially valuable in helping people with intellectual impairment or learning difficulties. However, those who are physically disabled in some way may also benefit, especially people who need to improve their breathing or extend their range of movements. The sessions are conducted by a trained therapist who has a qualification in music, and the treatment may be available at some hospitals. Many therapists work in residential homes and schools and the demand for the service greatly exceeds the number of people working in this field. The approach taken depends upon the nature of the patient's problems. If the person is a child who is intellectually impaired and who perhaps cannot talk, the therapist builds up a relationship using instruments, vocal sounds and the shared experience of music-making. With a patient who is physically disabled or who has psychological or emotional problems, a different approach with more discussion is likely to be adopted.

Since most people react in some way to music and enjoy the experience of music-making, this form of therapy is usually highly beneficial and successful. Anyone can benefit and the person need not have any previous musical ability, knowledge or experience. Music therapy is especially helpful for children with intellectual and/or physical disabilities.

Aura therapy

Many healers believe that as well as a physical body, we all possess a psychic 'body' that extends beyond our corporal form. This is believed to be a force field of spiritual energy that surrounds all living things and connects individuals through a universal source.

The aura, as this force field is called, is thought to comprise all the radiations from the actions and interactions of cells and chemicals in the body, and therefore reflects the state of health of the individual. If the body is suffering from illness, the radiations from the affected organ will be weak, and subsequently dull patches in the aura are perceived.

The aura can stretch up to several metres from the body, or merely several centimetres, and consists of bands of different coloured light, all the colours of the spectrum as well as black, white and grey. Each person's aura is different in shape, colour and definition, and those who can perceive auras say that they can tell a lot about an individual's character and mood as well as the state of his or her physical, emotional and spiritual health.

Practitioners of aura healing are so sensitive to tuning into auras that the colours and shapes of a patient's aura are actually visible to them, not just sensed. Then they can interpret the order and the intensity of these colours, as each colour signifies different emotions, characteristics and disposition to illness. In a proper interpretation of someone's aura, the positioning of the colours in relation to each other is very important, but here is a basic outline of what each colour may signify:

- *Red* – red is the colour of vitality, passion and energy, and someone with a lot of red in his or her aura will be outgoing, physically vigorous and generous of spirit, although an excess indicates selfishness and materialism. Dark red in the aura may be indicative of anger or malice, whereas light red shows anxiety and tension.

- *Orange* – bright orange denotes a strong, ambitious personality and is also associated with good health and energy. A slightly lighter shade of orange signifies a compassionate, considerate and well-adjusted nature, but too much orange in the aura indicates overambitiousness to the detriment of others

- *Yellow* – yellow in the aura shows mental agility and is apparent when someone is concentrating. As well as intellect, yellow also highlights optimism, and gold-yellow shows spirituality and perception. A murky yellow in the aura may indicate weakness, indecisiveness, frustration or suspicion.

- *Green* – gr een is a healing colour as it is the colour of nature and rebirth. In the aura it shows a vibrant sociable personality and may mean that the individual has the healing gift. A preponderance of green, on the other hand, signifies a lack of empathy with others.

- *Blue* – blue is a very positive colour, associated with idealism, inspiration and integrity. Dark blue indicates specifically religious inspiration and a deeply spiritual nature while pale blue shows a predisposition to scholarship. A dingy blue, however, means negativity.

- *Indigo* – indigo is also a spiritual colour, denoting strong moral values and the search for a higher truth. A lot of indigo in an aura signifies inner calm, serenity and good-naturedness. If it shows up blotchy or weak, this could indicate moodiness and irritability.

- *Violet* – violet is a devotional colour signifying love and spiritual enlightenment. Not everyone possesses a noticeable amount of violet in his or her aura, but those who do have profound insight and spiritual awareness.

- *White* – white represents perfection, the attainment of the highest possible spiritual enlightenment. It signifies truth and purity.

- *Black* – black in the aura shows an emotionally damaged individual. Black represents negative thoughts, destruction and despair.
- *Grey* – grey in the aura usually signifies illness or depression. In rare cases it can denote an individual devoid of personality.

As stated previously, these colours are present in different combinations in every individual and can appear mixed, layered or patchy, depending upon the ailment. Aura healing is not only a diagnostic but a curative therapy. Once the therapist has defined and interpreted the state of a patient's aura, and feels that he or she fully understands the problem, there are a number of ways in which the patient can be treated.

As with other forms of spiritual healing, the therapist acts as a channel through which universal spiritual energy can flow. Rather than use energy from their own auras, practitioners harness this greater energy and 'feed' it into the patient's aura. This could involve increasing the amount of colour that has become depleted in a particular area of the aura, or introducing a complementary colour that will even out any imbalances in the intensity of another colour.

The role of the patient in his or her own healing is heavily emphasized in this form of therapy. Patients are encouraged to take an active part in the healing process through self-awareness and positive thinking. Meditation and visualization exercises can be used to tune into and strengthen the aura.

Some auric practitioners believe that everyone has the ability to sense auras, if not actually see them. We subconsciously pick up the vibrations that another person's aura sends out, and this is the basis on which we place our impressions of him or her and gauge his or her personality and mood. If an individual makes you feel uneasy it could be because the aura is vibrating in conflict with your own, creating disharmony.

There are ways in which you can develop your ability to sense, or even see, auras. This means adopting a completely open mind and attitude, and setting aside any scepticism about the existence of auras. Watch people closely and listen very carefully to what they say, with as much empathy as possible. Notice their movements and mannerisms, and observe how they relate to their environment. It is a question of learning to notice and understand the subliminal messages that people continually send out about themselves and their situation.

Of course, there is no scientific evidence to support the existence of auras, although Kirlian photography shows that the body does emit some kind of electromagnetic energy. It could be said that the way in which auric therapists sense moods, emotions and disorders is through a form of observant intuition, itself as intangible as the idea of the aura.

Colour therapy

Colour therapy is closely linked to aura healing, and the two are often practised in conjunction. The idea of colour therapy goes back to ancient civilizations, as the Greeks and Egyptians are believed to have chosen the colours of their temple adornments for their beneficial effects on the mind, body and spirit. Colour therapy is also still practised in Tibet and India, where Buddhist monks wear orange robes because of the colour's spiritual properties. It has been proven that people are affected both psychologically and physically by different coloured light. What colour healers do is work with the various principles of certain colours to bring about effective healing.

Recent investigation has shown that there is a close correlation between certan colours and states of mind. Colour can affect people's mood, perception of time and temperature, and their ability to concentrate and function effectively. Some colours can induce anxiety and unease while others create a tranquil, restful state of mind. For example, greens and blues are commonly used in the decoration of hospitals and prisons because they have been found to have a relaxing effect, counteracting aggression and anxiety. Even fast-food restaurants know the significance of colour psychology and use the colour red to encourage people to eat quickly and move on. The strength of the colour induces a feeling of urgency and discourages the desire to linger.

Colour therapists go beyond psychology and believe that specific maladies can be treated and cured by adjusting the colour input to the body. As with aura therapy, it is believed that the body absorbs the electromagnetic energy of light and gives out its own aura of energy, which vibrates in a specific pattern. An unhealthy body creates an imbalance in this pattern, and the colour therapist strives to restore the balance through the stimulation of bodily reactions by colour. Colour healing is said to be based on the principle of attraction„the vibrations of the colour attract similar vibrations in the human body and extract the vibrations that are causing imbalance and illness.

The main colours used in colour therapy are red, orange, yellow, green, turquoise, blue, violet and magenta. Each colour is considered to be effective in the treatment of specific ailments.

- *Red* – red can be helpful in the treatment of circulatory problems, low blood pressure and anaemia.
- *Orange* – orange is effective on complaints involving the chest and the digestive system.
- *Yellow* – yellow can be used to help sufferers of skin complaints and nervous conditions.
- *Green* – green can treat stress, headaches and emotional disturbances.
- *Blue* – blue also calms the mind and can be used to help ease fevers and complaints of the nervous system.
- *Violet* – violet is helpful in the treatment of rheumatism, epilepsy and nervous disorders.

When making a diagnosis, a colour therapist will ask about your colour preferences as well as for details of your medical history and lifestyle. Most therapists will also employ an element of intuition or extrasensory perception to assess any imbalances in your aura.

Then the therapist will concentrate on your spine, stroking the length of it while focusing on your condition. Each vertebra relates to a part of the body as well as to one of the main eight colours listed earlier, which are repeated in sequence down the twenty-four vertebrae of the spinal column. In this way, any vibrations from an individual vertebra are picked up and interpreted to reveal where the colour balance is upset.

Once the balance or imbalance has been established, the practitioner will know which colours are required for effective treatment. Treatment involves the beaming of different coloured lights onto the patient by a special colour therapy instrument. Sometimes the whole body is bathed in the healing light, and at other times the colour will be focused only on a specific part of the body, depending on the patient's condition. The main colour used in the healing will usually be interspersed with a complementary colour, apparently increasing the efficacy of the former.

A session of this treatment will usually last around twenty minutes, and the patient should undergo at least seven or eight sessions over several weeks in order to receive the full beneficial effects. In addition to this formulaic treatment, the practitioner will advise the patient on what colours to wear and use around the home in the form of furnishings or lighting. Self-help techniques will also be taught and encouraged, to reinforce psychologically the benefits of the colour treatment. The therapist will guide the patient by visualization exercises, which he or she may then practise at home. These exercises may include visualizing a particular colour penetrating the body and suffusing it with coloured light, or the visualization could be based on a narrative and involve the patient imagining himself or herself enacting a journey through fields of specifically coloured flowers.

There is no doubt that colour can indeed affect mood and perhaps alter behaviour patterns, but the curative powers of colour therapy are yet to be scientifically proven. Even colour therapists recognize that this form of treatment should not replace orthodox medical diagnosis and treatment, but should be complementary.

Healing with crystals
Crystals and gemstones can be used to aid healing when used in

conjunction with other alternative therapies, particularly colour therapy because of the obvious links of colour and refracted light. Some people believe that crystals are actually the tools of healing and can be used in isolation, although practices of meditation and visualization are usually also employed. As with the previous two therapies, crystals act on energy vibrations and are believed to emit their own vibrations, which amplify and focus the natural energies of the recipient's mind and body.

Crystals are believed to alleviate blockages in the flow of energy around the body, which may be causing physical or spiritual distress. It achieves this by working on the chakra points.

The chakra is a concept of Indian origin, literally meaning wheel, and its system is used in many different types of healing. The chakras are subtle points of focused energy in the human being and are believed to be the source of physical, mental, emotional and spiritual energy. They are sometimes described in physical terms as whirling vortices that can easily become blocked, but, of course, this is merely a symbolic representation of an abstract concept.

There are seven major chakras, each relating to different functions of the mind and body. Each chakra also relates to specific colours and different gemstones. Here are the seven chakras, beginning at the bottom of the body and working up:

Root or base chakra
This chakra is located at the base of the spine, near the reproductive organs. It relates to sexual activity and feelings, and links us to our basic instincts. The root chakra is associated with the elimination of waste from the system and the regeneration of cells and tissues in the body. Its colour is red, and its stones are rubies, garnets and bloodstones.

Abdominal or sacral chakra
This chakra relates to the digestive system and the reproductive system, as well as controllig the body's production of adrenaline. This chakra also signifies happiness and openness towards others.

Its colour is orange, and its gemstones are coral, carnelian and amber.

Solar plexus chakra

Situated at the level of the naval, this chakra relates to the internal organs, such as the liver, spleen, pancreas and intestines. It is also to do with the intellect and communication. Its colour is yellow, and its stones include citron, topaz and yellow amber.

Heart chakra

This chakra is connected to the heart, circulation and immune system. It is also the centre of love and emotions. The colour of the heart chakra is green, and its corresponding stones are emeralds, jade and green tourmaline.

Throat chakra

Located just below the vocal chords, this chakra is connected to sound and the larynx. It is also associated with the thyroid gland and the lymphatic system. The throat chakra's colour is blue, and its stones include turquoise, sapphires and aquamarine.

Brow chakra

Situated between the eyebrows, this chakra relates to psychic or spiritual matters, and governs the perpetuity gland and certain parts of the brain. The brow chakra coordinates all the other chakras, and its colour is indigo, its stones being amethyst, dark sapphires and lapis lazuli.

Crown chakra

This last chakra is located at the top of the head and is associated with the functions of the brain and spiritual aspirations. Its colours are violet and white-gold, and its stones include amethyst, rose quartz, clear crystal quartz and diamonds.

In order to unblock a chakra, a charged crystal is held above or placed directly on the area where the affected chakra is located. (*See also* Reiki, page 130, and Shiatsu, page 154.)

There are different ways in which a crystal can be charged with energy. One method is to sit quietly holding it in your palm, concentrating on positive thoughts and visualizing spiritual energy entering into it. Some people like to sleep with a crystal under their pillow, so that they can absorb their own special psychic power during dream sleep.

Another popular method of charging is to leave the crystal in direct sunlight (or moonlight) for at least six hours, or, even better, leave it outside during an electric thunderstorm.

Once a crystal has been used for healing it will have absorbed a lot of negative energy and must be cleansed before being recharged. An easy way of cleansing a crystal is to leave it to soak overnight in a bowl of spring water and sea salt, or, if there is a handy stream nearby, just give it a good dip.

When it comes to choosing a crystal, as well as bearing in mind what function you wish the stone to fulfil, you must use your intuition to guide you to what you are looking for. If you feel towards a particular stone, pick it up and handle it to see if you can sense its energy. Always inspect every crystal carefully for chips or cracks, as any imperfection may result in a dramatic loss of energy and healing sensitivity.

Here is a small selection of some of the most widely available stones and their uses:

Quartz crystal

Quartz crystal is the most easily recognizable type of healing crystal. It is the rough-cut clear stone that you will find in most New Age boutiques. Quartz is highly suitable for healing as it is believed to unblock the energy centres, allowing the body to respond and heal itself. It is a good all-round crystal to use for meditative and healing purposes as it promotes mental and spiritual wellbeing.

Rose quartz

Rose quartz is a beautifully coloured version of clear quartz, with its soft pink glow. This is another very important stone of healing as it deals with love and emotions. It is also a comforting stone and can ease distress in someone who has suffered trauma, as well as relieving everyday stresses and tensions.

Amethyst

Amethyst is thought to be a highly spiritual stone, associated with heightened perception and psychic insight. It is believed to have protective properties and is therefore a good stone to carry about with you. Amethyst is also said to relieve insomnia and provoke inspired dreams if placed under the pillow.

Carnelian

Of a warm red colour, this stone is believed to help with circulatory problems. Carnelian can also help to ease feelings of anger and frustration, and induce contentment and fulfilment.

Sodalite

Sodalite is a blue stone often speckled with white. It is believed to help those suffering from neuroses and irrational thoughts by balancing the mind and lowering the blood pressure.

Tiger's-eye

This also belongs to the quartz family and is golden brown in colour. Tiger's-eye is thought to increase confidence and reduce nervousness. On a physical level it can aid the digestive system.

There is no harm in experimenting with crystal in order to find out what feels right for you. Meditation with crystals is a good way to introduce yourself to the types of energy emitted, before trying to achieve healing effects. It must also be stressed that using crystals can neither diagnose illness nor provide miracle cures. If in doubt, see a doctor.

These then are some of the ways by which people might help themselves towards a greater understanding of themselves. Some of these ways may depend, at least initially, on the help and guidance of others, but the onus is on the person seeking this understanding to make the time and effort – often considerable – to enable this to come about. Many have found that the effort and time involved were a small price to pay for the self-knowledge that they were able to uncover.

The Natural Way to Combat Stress

The body's internal reaction to external pressure

Stress is the 'wear and tear' our minds and bodies experience as we attempt to cope with our continually changing environment. People often think of stress as pressure at work, a sick child or rush-hour traffic. These events may be triggers, but stress is actually the body's internal reaction to such factors. Stress is the automatic 'fight-or-flight' response in the body, activated by adrenaline and other stress hormones, which stimulate a variety of physiological changes, such as increased heart rate and blood pressure, faster breathing, muscle tension, dilated pupils, dry mouth and increased blood sugar. In simple biological terms, stress is the state of increased arousal necessary for an organism to defend itself when faced with danger.

Whenever we feel anxious, tense, tired, frightened, elated or depressed, we are undergoing stress. Few aspects of life are free from the events and pressures that generate such feelings, and stress has become an acceptable and unavoidable part of normal everyday existence. In fact, contrary to popular assumptions, stressed lifestyles are not an exclusively modern phenomenon – stress has *always* been intrinsic to human existence, and life without stress would be unbearable. For example, certain types of stress, such as physical and mental exercise, sex, and intense creativity, are actually very desirable. It is only when real or perceived change overwhelms the body's ability to cope, that stress becomes harmful (distress), leaving us prone to unwanted physical, mental or emotional reactions and illnesses.

Types of stress

The causes of stress ('stressors') are multiple and varied, but they can be divided into two general categories – external and internal:

External stressors

- *physical environment* – noise, bright lights, heat, confined spaces
- *social interaction* – rudeness, bossiness or aggressiveness by others
- *organizational* – rules, regulations, 'red tape', deadlines
- *major life events* – death of a relative, lost job, promotion, new baby
- *daily hassles* – commuting, misplacing keys, mechanical breakdowns

Internal stressors

- *lifestyle choices* – caffeine, not enough sleep, overloaded schedule
- *negative self-talk* – pessimistic thinking, self-criticism, over-analysing
- *mind traps* – unrealistic expectations, taking things personally, all-or-nothing thinking, exaggerating, rigid thinking
- *stressful personality traits* – type A, perfectionist, workaholic

These factors generate various symptoms of emotional and mental stress, the most common including: anger, anxiety, worry, fear, and depression.

Negative stress

Excessive, prolonged and unrelieved stress can have a harmful effect on mental, physical and spiritual health. If left unresolved, the feelings of anger, frustration, fear and depression generated by stress can trigger a variety of illnesses. It is estimated that stress is the most common cause of ill health in modern society, probably underlying as many as 80 per cent of all visits to family doctors. Stress is a contributory factor in relatively minor conditions such as headaches, digestive problems, skin complaints, insomnia and ulcers, but also plays an important role in the leading causes of death in the western world – cancer, cardiovascular disease, respiratory disorders, accidental injuries, cirrhosis of the liver and suicide.

Positive stress

Stress can also have a positive effect. It is essential in spurring motivation and awareness, providing the stimulation needed to cope with challenging situations. Tension and arousal are necessary for the enjoyment of many aspects of life, and without them existence would be pretty dull. Stress also provides the sense of urgency and alertness needed for survival when confronting threatening situations, such as crossing a busy road or driving in poor weather conditions. An overly relaxed approach in such situations could be fatal.

Stress and the individual

There is no single level of stress that is optimal for all people. Everyone is different, with unique perceptions of, and reactions to, events: what is distressing to one person may be a joy to another. A person who loves to work alone would be stressed in a job that involved high levels of social interaction, whereas the person who thrives as part of a team would very likely be stressed in a job that involved working from home.

Even when we agree that a particular event is distressing, we are likely to differ in our physiological and psychological responses to it. Some individuals are more sensitive to stress than others, owing to experiences in childhood and the influence of teachers, parents, religion, etc. It is also important to note that most of the stress that we experience is actually *self-generated*. How we perceive life – whether an event makes us feel threatened or stimulated, encouraged or discouraged, happy or sad – depends to a large extent on how we perceive ourselves.

Self-generated stress is something of a paradox, because so many people think of external causes when they are upset. Recognizing that we create most of our own upsets is an important first step towards coping with them.

The stress response

It is tempting to think that mental and physical stress is an ailment only of modern civilization; that our fast-paced urban lifestyles, straining under the relentless pressure of greater competitiveness and automation, has created a culture that lives on its nerves and feeds off crisis. This is a misconception; stress has been part of the human condition since the beginning of time. Like the air we breath, stress is an integral factor in human survival. Think about any challenge or stimuli, and stress has been a factor in our response. It is an active force that helps us rise to meet whatever everyday life throws at us and we thrive on taking up challenges, meeting that deadline and adapting to difficult situations.

How our bodies respond to stress was first described in the 1930s by two American doctors, Walter B. Cannon and Hans Selye. They found that the first reaction to severe stress is what is known as the 'fight-or-flight' response, which activates the body's protective mechanism either to fight (confront the stressor) or flee (act to avoid the stressor or threat of it). Initially, the fight-or-flight response alerts us to danger and is, in fact, beneficial – providing the strength, speed and stamina necessary for survival.

The stress response is controlled by the endocrine system, which regulates various bodily functions, including the reproductive system, the immune system, growth, metabolism, allergic response and stress tolerance. Any unusual demand on the body's physical and mental resources stimulates the endocrine glands – mainly the adrenal, pituitary and hypothalamus – to secrete chemical messengers, called hormones, into the blood stream. These stress hormones include powerful stimulants, such as adrenaline,

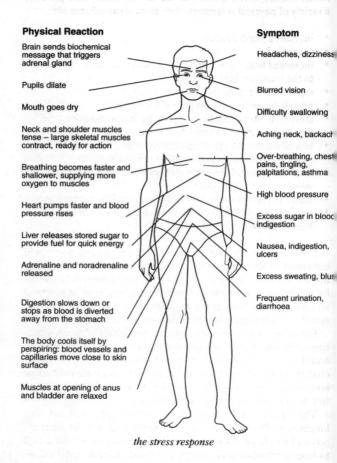

Physical Reaction

Brain sends biochemical message that triggers adrenal gland

Pupils dilate

Mouth goes dry

Neck and shoulder muscles tense – large skeletal muscles contract, ready for action

Breathing becomes faster and shallower, supplying more oxygen to muscles

Heart pumps faster and blood pressure rises

Liver releases stored sugar to provide fuel for quick energy

Adrenaline and noradrenaline released

Digestion slows down or stops as blood is diverted away from the stomach

The body cools itself by perspiring: blood vessels and capillaries move close to skin surface

Muscles at opening of anus and bladder are relaxed

Symptom

Headaches, dizziness

Blurred vision

Difficulty swallowing

Aching neck, backach

Over-breathing, ches pains, tingling, palpitations, asthma

High blood pressure

Excess sugar in bloo indigestion

Nausea, indigestion, ulcers

Excess sweating, blus

Frequent urination, diarrhoea

the stress response

noradrenaline, cortisol, testosterone and thyroxin, which produce a variety of physical responses. The most common include:

- increased pupil dilation
- perspiration
- increased heart rate and blood pressure (to get more blood to the muscles, brain and heart)
- rapid breathing (to take in more oxygen)
- muscle tenseness (in preparation for action)
- increased blood flow to the brain, heart and muscles (the organs that are most important in dealing with danger)
- less blood flow to the skin, digestive tract, kidneys and liver (where it is least needed in times of crisis)
- increased mental alertness and sensitivity (to assess the situation and act quickly)
- increased blood sugar, fats and cholesterol (for extra energy)
- a rise in platelets and blood-clotting factors (to prevent haemorrhage in case of injury)

Unfortunately, although this natural physical response would have been invaluable at an earlier stage in human evolution, fighting and running away are rarely appropriate responses to stressful situations in the modern world. Under long term, unrelieved stress our bodies remain in a constant state of arousal, which can result in the gradual onset of various health problems.

Primitive human beings frequently faced life and death situations, when alertness, strength, speed and performance were vital and the primary, instinctive response was to survive. The type of challenges we all meet with today, however, are rather different and, as they rarely require a physical response, the body's reaction to the situation is often inappropriate.

The stresses of modern life are more complex and last over longer periods of time. In the past, challenges were instantaneous and had to be resolved instinctively; today, we are subjected to long-term emotional, occupational and environmental anxieties, which demand that we maintain a certain level of mental and physical health. We also have to prepare ourselves for times of crisis and events that test us to our fullest, such as divorce, redundancy, bereavement or illness. This means that we have to be poised to 'fight or flight' at another level and in a completely different way from our forebears.

The rapid way in which our society now changes and constantly throws up fresh challenges places an unhealthy strain on a system that may be struggling to keep up. The extra mental exertion we all expend just to keep 'on top of things' can create a bottleneck of energy as pressure builds up with nowhere to go. If nothing is done to relieve the situation the mechanisms we have for dealing with stress will eventually fail us, causing illness and exhaustion. It is vital, therefore, that we make a priority of finding ways of easing our bodies and minds out of 'fight or flight' mode and put ourselves on a better footing to be able to deal with the ever-changing pressures of the modern world.

In order to do this we need a greater understanding and awareness of how our bodies work. Our automatic physical response to danger or stress involves an intricate chain reaction of bodily and biochemical effects, involving the brain, the nervous system and hormones. As soon as we perceive a threat, our body explodes with energy and strength, and thousands of messenger hormones flood into the bloodstream to call the alarm. Our minds and bodies instantly become clear, alert and poised – ready for action. In this alarm reaction the main players are the lungs, brain, nervous system, muscle systems and hormones. Arousal is initially registered by the hypothalamus – a tiny crowd of cells at the base of the brain – which controls all automatic bodily functions and reactions. It releases chemicals called endorphins, which act as natural painkillers. They dull the perception of pain and mental turmoil and help us to deal with the situation by blocking out factors that may otherwise prevent us from giving less than our peak performance.

Adrenaline, also helps us rise to the situation. It causes a quickening of the heart rate, a raising of blood pressure and a release of vital nutrients. It also creates muscle tension and affects breathing patterns, making them faster and shallower. But it is only one of the arousal hormones released by the adrenal gland near the kidneys. Noradrenaline, associated with positive ecstatic arousal, is also released into the bloodstream. The hormone cortisol is the agent involved in converting glycogen, stored in the liver, into blood sugar, creating instant energy and alerting the brain. The required surge of strength and effort comes from the male hormone testosterone. The thyroid gland also plays a part in our body's arousal response. It releases thyroxin, a hormone that stimulates the metabolic system, increasing its work rate and regulating oxygen consumption. This is vital, as the body anticipates that it will need increased resources of energy. Our digestive system also slows down during this process, as blood is diverted from the skin and stomach. We instinctively shut down the unnecessary systems in order to concentrate on mobilizing those vital for survival. As the digestive system is not deemed essential in a life or death situation it slows down and is effectively put on hold.

The body has undoubtedly evolved an efficient and prompt survival response but, as already mentioned, the goalposts have moved slightly. The things that cause stress today are more complex and require more sophisticated solutions over a longer period of time. Our hormonal system suffers if it stays in 'fight' mode, as lengthy periods with our bodies on red-alert are not healthy for our mental or physical wellbeing. What begins as a positive range of responses, therefore, can eventually have a negative effect on our health.

Research shows that we put our bodies on challenge alert without realizing it. Emotions such as anger, anxiety and impatience produce the same chemical reactions in the body as standing in front of a speeding car – our nervous systems and hormones will still be poised for 'fight-or-flight'. But the same physiology that leaves us feeling poised and alert can create havoc over a long period of time. A build-up of energy can lead us to become stress addicts, who become hooked on the adrenaline rush that stressful situations create. Or we can become so used to living on such a psychological and physical 'tilt' that we don't realize the harm it is causing.

Overdoses of adrenaline can cause irritability and agitation, while too much noradrenaline can leave us feeling disconnected and high. If arousal continues, the adrenal glands create anti-flammatory chemicals to speed tissue repair, but cortisol will also suppress the immune system, leaving it vulnerable to illness and disease. Extra sodium is retained, endangering the performance of the cardiovascular system by causing fluid retention, raising the heart rate, increasing blood pressure and possibly inducing blood clots. Stomach ulcers are a classic symptom of stress, as the stomach cannot deal with the extra secretion of acid that occurs during times of turbulence. Acute and cumulative stress over a period of time can even cause death.

General Adaptation Syndrome

How the body adapts to prolonged stress is described by Dr Hans Selye in terms of the General Adaptation Syndrome. Selye divides the stress response into three phases: the Alarm Response, Adaptation, and Exhaustion. The Alarm Response is the fight-or-flight response that prepares the body for immediate action. If the source of stress persists, then the body prepares for long-term protection through the secretion of further hormones that increase blood sugar levels to sustain energy and raise blood pressure. This Adaptation phase, resulting from exposure to prolonged periods of stress, is common, and not necessarily harmful, but without periods of relaxation and rest to counterbalance the stress response, sufferers become prone to fatigue, concentration lapses, irritability and lethargy as the effort to sustain arousal slides into negative stress. Under persistent chronic stress, sufferers enter the Exhaustion phase: mental, physical and emotional resources suffer heavily, and the body experiences 'adrenal exhaustion', where blood sugar levels decrease as the adrenals become depleted, leading to decreased stress tolerance, progressive mental and physical exhaustion, illness and collapse.

Symptoms of stress

Exposure to excessive stress results in hormonal imbalances, which can produce a variety of symptoms:

Physical symptoms
- changes in sleep patterns
- fatigue
- changes in digestion – nausea, vomiting, diarrhoea
- loss of sexual drive
- headaches
- aches and pains in different areas of the body
- infections
- indigestion
- dizziness, faintness, sweating and trembling
- tingling of hands and feet
- breathlessness
- palpitations
- missed heartbeats

Emotional symptoms
- deterioration in personal hygiene and appearance
- bouts of depression
- impatience and irritability
- fits of rage
- tearfulness

Mental symptoms
- lack of concentration
- memory lapses
- difficulty in making decisions
- confusion
- disorientation
- panic attacks

Behavioural symptoms
- appetite changes – eating too much or too little
- eating disorders – anorexia, bulimia
- increased intake of alcohol and other drugs
- increased smoking
- hypochondria
- restlessness
- fidgeting
- nail-biting

Stress-related illness
Cardiovascular disease

The term 'cardiovascular' refers to the heart and to the body's system of blood vessels. Cardiovascular disease is probably the most serious health problem that can be linked to stress – it is the most common cause of death in Britain and the USA. The primary causes of heart disease include smoking and high-fat diets, but stress is a significant contributory factor.

Adrenal hormones act to increase blood pressure; temporary rises in blood pressure present no threat to health, but a frequent or perpetual state of high blood pressure can have a serious effect on health in the long term. High blood pressure is linked with the development of arteriosclerosis, or hardening of the arteries. Arteriosclerosis is the result of the development of blood plaque in the arteries, which progressively narrows the pathway through which the blood flows. Eventually an artery can become blocked, leading to angina, stroke and heart failure.

The immune system

The immune system protects the body from infection. It fights foreign invaders (such as viruses and harmful bacteria) and cancer. Excessive stress can damage the immune system by affecting the thymus gland. This manufactures white blood cells, called T-cells, for regulating immunity and also produces various immune-related hormones. The stress reaction diverts resources to the main parts of the body that need to deal with stress, mainly the brain, heart and muscles. Other systems are deprived of resources, including the immune system. Hormones produced by the adrenal glands can cause the thymus gland to shrink and also degrade the activity of white blood cells, causing damage to the body's ability to fight infection. As a result high stress can result in reduced resistance to common infections, such as colds, influenza and herpes (cold sores). Because certain types of white blood cells produced by the thymus are active in preventing the development of cancer cells in the body, any damage to the thymus may effect the body's ability to resist cancer.

Asthma

Asthma is a respiratory disorder marked by the temporary constriction of the bronchi, the airways branching from the trachea to the lungs. Attacks usually are brought on by allergic reaction to antigens, such as grass and tree pollens, mould spores, fungi, animal dander, and certain foods, but may also be caused by chemical irritants in the atmosphere or by infections of the respiratory tract. Susceptibility to an asthma attack is based on hyperactivity of the bronchial muscles, which constrict on exposure to one or other of these agents. Chronic stress reduces the efficiency of the adrenal glands, reducing the output of anti-inflammatory and anti-allergic adrenal hormones, which may make an asthma attack more likely.

Diabetes

Diabetes is caused by the inability of the body to metabolize sugar correctly, leading to excessively high levels of sugar in the blood. Sugar metabolism is the responsibility of the hormone insulin, which is secreted by the pancreas. Most diabetics can produce insulin, but various factors limit the hormone's efficiency, known as 'insulin sensitivity'.

As we know from the physiology of the stress response, the release of adrenal hormones under stress can have significant impact on blood-sugar levels. Adrenaline causes sugar in the liver to be dumped into the blood stream, and cortisol acts to reduce metabolism of glucose by cells. Large amounts of cortisol act to decrease insulin sensitivity. High blood-sugar levels are not dangerous in normally healthy individuals, but chronic stress, combined with other factors such as obesity, act to increase the likelihood of developing diabetes.

Ulcers

Ulcers are frequently associated with stress, although no conclusive link has yet been demonstrated. Normally the lining of the stomach is covered with a layer of mucus to protect it from the digestive acids and enzymes used in the breaking down of food. Over time, chronic stress can stimulate the overproduction of gastric juices, which break down the protective mucus and act upon the walls of the digestive tract, resulting in ulceration. Ulcers usually occur singly as round or oval lesions; the erosions are usually shallow but can penetrate the entire wall, leading to haemorrhage and possibly death.

Digestive disorders

Many problems with the digestive tract, such as constipation, diarrhoea and irritable bowel syndrome, are linked to stress. The nerves in the digestive tract receive messages from the brain in the form of hormones, which tell the intestinal muscles to expand or contract. Hormonal imbalances can cause alterations in intestinal function, such as spasms, constipation and diarrhoea. Chronic stress tends to shut down the digestive system altogether, exacerbating intestinal problems.

Skin complaints

Stress increases levels of toxicity in the body and contributes to hormonal imbalances, both of which have an effect on the skin. The visible effects of stress on the skin include:

- acne
- spots
- eczema
- psoriasis
- excessive pallor
- skin diseases

Headaches and migraines

Headaches are one of our most common afflictions. Millions of people seek medical help for this problem every year, and millions of pounds are spent on headache remedies annually.

Most headaches are caused not by disease but by fatigue, emotional disorders, or allergies. Intermittent tension headaches are caused by worry, anxiety, overwork, or inadequate ventilation. The most common type – a chronic tension headache – is often caused by depression. Brain tissue itself is insensitive to pain, as is the bony covering of the brain (the cranium). Headache pain results from the stimulation of such pain-sensitive structures as the membranous linings of the brain (the meninges) and the nerves of the cranium and upper neck. This stimulation can be produced by inflammation, by the dilation of blood vessels of the head, or by muscle spasms in the neck and head. Headaches brought on by muscle spasms are classified as tension headaches; those caused by the dilation of blood vessels are called vascular headaches.

Almost 90 per cent of all persons seeking medical help for headaches suffer from tension headaches. These are characterized by a diffuse ache that either spreads over the entire head or feels like a tight headband. Tension headaches are often usually associated with poor sleep and persistent tension in the muscles of the neck, shoulders and forehead. These muscles must relax before the pain eases.

Migraine is the most common from of vascular headache. About 60 per cent of all migraine sufferers are women, and most sufferers first develop symptoms between the ages of 10 and 30. In approximately 30 per cent of all cases, migraine attacks are preceded by warning signs such as blind spots, zigzag flashing lights, numbness in parts of the body, and distorted visual images. Migraine pain almost always occurs on only one side and is usually accompanied by nausea. Many things seem capable of triggering migraine attacks, including stress, fatigue, changes in the weather, fasting, menstruation, drugs, such as birth control pills, that contain oestrogen, and foods, such as cheese, alcohol, and chocolate, that contain substances that affect the blood vessels. Many migraine patients have family histories of the problem.

Many of the relaxation techniques and alternative therapies outlined later in this book will help to alleviate headaches. However, chronic headaches may be physical symptoms of depression or other kinds of severe emotional problems. If you suffer from persistent headaches, then be sure to consult your doctor for professional treatment.

Premenstrual Syndrome (PMS)

Stress has a debilitating effect on the nerves in general, and certain premenstrual symptoms may be aggravated by stress. Many sufferers of PMS have abnormal levels of the adrenal hormone aldosterone, which may account for some of the problems of excessive fluid retention and weight gain, breast tenderness and abdominal bloating. Further release of aldosterone caused by stress will exacerbate these problems.

Depression

Chronic stress can produce severe depression, because of its debilitating psychological effects. The physiological changes produced by stress can also contribute to depression. Adrenaline and noradrenaline are not only adrenal hormones but also chemical messengers in the brain. Deficiencies of noradrenaline have been linked to depression in certain individuals, and so adrenal exhaustion through chronic long-term stress may be a contributory factor in depressive illness.

The causes of stress
Environmental stress

Urban decay and deprivation are a major source of distress for large sections of the population. Inadequate housing, noise, pollution, crowding, violence and poverty create some of the most cumulative and pervasive forms of stress. These factors affect how we live, work and play. Their impact depends on the infrastructure of the location, transport requirements, and availability of opportunities to spend time away from the environment.

We all have different reactions to stress, and experience helps us to develop our own methods of dealing with it. While some of us may lead *less* stressful lives, it is impossible to lead a completely stress-free life, as things happen to all of us unexpectedly and 'out of the blue'. The trick comes in weeding out as much of the trivial stress as possible and learning how to control our response to unavoidable, accumulative stress. If we can do this then we can be better prepared for the surprises life springs on us and learn to enjoy rising to the challenges they present.

All of us will have times in our lives that cause us great distress and leave us feeling unable to go on. Bereavement, family break-up and redundancy are devastating events, but even moving house or changing jobs, usually seen as happy occasions, can produce high levels of stress. This is because stress doesn't just occur when we feel angry or are in grief. Welcomed events can be just as stressful if they create self-doubt or anxiety. Any sort of change, with relationships, homes or occupations, can induce stress, as human beings are essentially creatures of habit. The fight for homeostasis – internal and physiological equilibrium – is a relentless process and is made more difficult when drastic changes in the way we organize and live our lives are forced on us. The amount of stress we experience, therefore, is largely dependent on how we adapt to circumstances.

One of the most prevalent causes of stress is our immediate environment. Urban living, in particular, with its associated problems of inadequate housing, noise, pollution, crowding, violence and poverty creates some of the most cumulative and pervasive forms of stress. These factors affect how we live, work and play, and much may depend on the infrastructure of the location, transport provision, and our ability to spend time away from our environment. If we feel unable to escape our surroundings, even for a brief time, then feelings of helplessness can grow to the point where they become very damaging to our self-image and the way we interact with other people.

There are ways of improving how we live and deal with stress that most of us recognize only subconsciously. For example, our home to most of us is more than a place to eat and sleep. In an increasingly hostile society we use our home as an oasis of calm. In our own homes we can shut the door on the outside world and surround ourselves with our personal possessions, family and friends. The 'feathering the nest' syndrome is well documented – it is an instinctive need to create a comfortable environment, one where we can relax and be ourselves.

In creating comfort, space is one of the most important factors. We all have invisible boundaries which outline our personal space. But these are difficult to maintain when our personal space is constantly being invaded. We should all be able to retreat inside ourselves and find peace, but many of us experience a physical lack of space that has an affect on our mental wellbeing as overcrowding and lack of privacy make personal calm all the more difficult to achieve. Also, advances in technology have led to increasing numbers of people working from home, and in many instances this has put a further strain on space allocation, as work space is carved out of resources already stretched between family members and various activities.

Our individual space requirements depend heavily on what we are used to. In Hong Kong, for example, where overcrowding has reached epidemic proportions, what most of us are used to in Britain would look positively luxurious. Building and space cost money, however, and in all societies those with lower incomes are usually restricted in their choice of accommodation or, increasingly, deprived of it altogether. Without privacy and space, quality of life undoubtedly suffers, as certain activities such as meditation, relaxation or making love need uninterrupted peace and quiet.

Light

Light is another important factor in determining the quality of our everyday lives. In the depths of winter most of us look forward to the long summer days ahead. This is because natural light is almost as vital for healthy living as the air we breath. It regulates levels of the hormone melanonin, which influences sleep, mood and the reproductive cycle. Our instinctive love of light and the sun explains our annual migration to hotter climates. A lack of daylight can influence the natural production of melanonin, creating lethargy and depression. SAD – seasonal affective disorder – is increasingly seen in the winter months. Sufferers feel antisocial, tired and depressed. In order to counter such feelings it is advisable to work beside windows and let as much daylight into the workplace or home as possible. Fluorescent lighting, the most unnatural from of light, should be avoided wherever possible. As artificial light is a necessary evil, it is best to use full spectrum lights, as they simulate daylight.

Natural light is as vital for healthy living as the air we breath. It regulates levels of the hormone melatonin, which influences sleep, mood and the reproductive cycle. Our instinctive love of light and the sun explains our annual migration to hotter climates.

Colour

Colour affects many aspects of our lives and can have a significant ffect on our moods and perceptions. We are all colour biased – e may chose colour as a response to their innate properties or e may just have a distinctive preference for it. Colours have physical as well as psychological effects. Research has shown that physilogical responses such as blood pressure and brain-wave patterns vary according to which colour we are being exposed to. For xample, exposure to red, the most stimulating colour, can lead o an increase of blood pressure while exposure to blue light has he opposite effect.

Colour can have a huge effect on our moods and ability to relax. Effective and intelligent use of colour is one of the easiest and cheapst ways to improve our surroundings. This is increasingly being ecognized by health and education authorities, and more thought ow goes into selecting the decor for classrooms, hospital wards nd waiting rooms. Scientific research has also shown that colours an have physical as well as psychological effects. It has been found, or example, that exposure to red light can often raise blood pressure, while exposure to blue light can actually lower it.

ife events and the pace of change

n the following table of stressful events, compiled by two American doctors, T. H. Holmes and R. H. Rahe (*Journal of Psychosomatic Research No. 11*, 1967), specific events are weighted on a scale from 0 to 100.

The chart suggests that it is *change itself* that is stressful – moving house, getting married, redundancy, etc – regardless of whether he change is regarded as favourable or unfavourable. Scores of bout 300 supposedly indicate a major life crisis, scores of 200 to 99 a moderate life crisis, and 100 to 199 a mild life crisis.

Event	Life Change Units
Death of a spouse	100
Divorce	73
Marital separation	65
Imprisonment	63
Death of a close relation	63

Personal relationships

The quality of personal relationships is traditionally regarded as one of the main sources of stress. The relationship between partners is the key factor, followed by the parent–child relation-ship. Factors that contribute to successful and relatively stress-free relationships include:

- communication
- realistic expectations
- honesty with yourself and partner
- quality time together
- listening
- quality time apart
- respect for yourself and partner

Home and family
Many sources of stress, such as bereavement, financial worries and relationship breakdowns, which feature prominently in the Holmes and Rahe scale, orginate within the family.

Increases in stress over the last 30 years can be partly explained by changing social factors. Within the context of a large extended family, and a close working and social environment, an individual benefits from contact and communication with others, receives feedback to establish realistic life goals and meaning, as well as useful information and practical help to overcome problems. The dissolution of these close social support networks makes the in-dividual more vulnerable to various stress-related chronic ill-nesses.

In the same period it has also become clear that, as well as being a source of support, affection and love, the home can also be the place where individuals, especially women and children, are most likely to suffer varying degrees of physical and emotional abuse.

Parenthood
Parenthood imposes heavy physical, emotional and financial bur-dens, which can crush the less resilient. Combining childcare and full-time employment is the most stressful of all, especially for the working mother, who is more likely to be responsible for a

bigger share of the housework and childcare than the father. In this situation, arguments, disagreements, misunderstandings, resentments and depression are more likely to surface. The following advice can help to reduce parental stress levels:

- care for yourself as well as the children
- keep a sense of self, apart from the role of parent
- plan, prepare and prioritize to exploit free time
- use free time in a creative and stimulating way
- partners should acknowledge and define shared responsibilities
- preserve healthy communication
- avoid self recrimination – no one is perfect
- be prepared to use family, friends and agencies for support

Occupational stress

Work provides an income and also fulfils a variety of other human needs – mental and physical exercise, social contact, a feeling of self-worth and competence. Work, however, is also a major source of stress, arising from the nature of the relations between management and employees, and that between colleagues in the workplace in general.

The modern world thrives on the work ethic, and we are taught at a very early age to equate personal adequacy with material success and professional status. Few of us are immune to the pressures placed on us by society to desire things – bigger televisions, faster cars, exotic holidays – that are symbols of status. Advertising and marketing strategies tap into this competitive urge we all have and create in us a need to go one better than people around us, in other words succumb to the 'keeping up with the Joneses' syndrome. This starts at an early age – basically in tandem with the learning process. The fear of failure and the challenge of peer pressure motivates us to work to achieve. In moderation, this can be healthy, as achievement goes hand in hand with self-esteem, but it also creates a cumulative stress that follows us from school to secondary education, through to our working lives.

For many of us, however, it is a struggle to keep up, and we often work unnaturally long hours in unfortunate working conditions just to keep our heads above water. It has become a truism nowadays to say that no job is for life. Temporary employment contracts and the threat of unemployment are now features of more and more peoples' working lives, and many feel lucky to have a job at all. Society, therefore, is forcing us to change our expectations of how we work, and this is taking its toll on our physical and emotional security.

In coping with the structural changes of our working lives, it is vital to try to embrace the positives among the negatives. Flexitime, job sharing and increased communication through technology and the 'information superhighway', offer new ways of working, which, if we are able to adapt to them, can offer us greater freedoms. More emphasis on leisure time and recreation should also mean more time to relax and relate to family and friends. We are starting to see worth in activities not necessarily related to the working environment. This control can be used to create a healthy, more relaxed style of living. Stress is a plague of current working practices, and even if we can't change our overall working situation, there are certain steps we can take to de-stress our days.

There is a lot of truth in the saying that a messy desk portrays a messy mind. Being chronically disorganized can be debilitating at work, where lack of planning is one of the most common causes of stress. Stressful environments are minimized when we impose a form of structure that can offer security against problems appearing 'out of the blue'. Too inflexible a pattern would be impractical, but keeping a diary, writing lists and prioritizing duties all help to stem stressful situations. Writing down objectives, duties and activities helps to make them seem more tangible and surmountable. Don't try to overload your mind with too much information – if you are already stressed there is more chance of you forgetting vital references and data – but if you take steps to keep control of things then you will work more efficiently.

People have different tolerances for routine and variety. Some personalities thrive under the security of a routine working day. In many ways it can be quite liberating, as adhering to a pattern means that you can fully concentrate on one task at a time and not get in a muddle attempting things that there may not be adequate time for. On the other hand, too much routine can be boring and demoralizing and eat away at your enthusiasm for the job. Variety at work holds interest and enthusiasm, but too little structure leads to overloading, confusion and stress.

Most of us need to strike a balance between routine and variety in order to enjoy work and maintain levels of efficiency. Monotony can be broken by looking ahead and planning when to switch from one job to another. Perhaps there is a way to inject some variety into your tasks – can you open up your job description? Those suffering under too great a workload should learn to say 'no', and not be afraid of the consequences. Pacing yourself is one of the most vital practices in achieving a relaxed lifestyle. Learn when to stop and stand back from your activity, the odd moment of calm will increase efficiency when you do return to your task.

Most people suffer from time deprivation, as it is perhaps one of life's most precious commodities. We have to juggle everything – work, family, friends, leisure, eating and sleeping – in only 24 hours. Every day most of us have to strip demands on our time down to the essentials, and usually it is the time spent working and commuting that dictates how much we can give to other activities.

Time deprivation leaves us feeling harassed, hurried and guilty. It may also damage relationships, as it can mean breaking arrangements because we 'just don't have the time'. Some people make the situation worse – as the saying goes, 'less haste, more speed'. They will procrastinate and waste time worrying about commitments in their social life and deadlines at work. Often they take on too much and end up fulfilling few or none of their aims. Work will pile up and relationships suffer as commitments are neglected, and the individual is left feeling panicked and chaotic.

It can be very difficult to change habits formed over a lifetime. Often the best way is to recognize weak points in time management and learn to deal with them. Prioritize and look at the steps mentioned earlier for dealing with organization. Also, don't punish yourself for not having the time to do everything or be everywhere – it is not humanly possible or desirable.

The drive for success

Western society is driven by the work ethic. We are taught at a very early age to equate personal adequacy with professional success, making us crave status and abhor failure. Our culture demands a monetary success together with professional identity, and it takes a strong personality to step off the ladder.

Changing work patterns

In our post-industrial society's climate of increasing unemployment and greater leisure time, many people feel lucky to have a job at all. Unemployment, redundancy, a shorter working week and the impact of new technology are affecting our physical and emotional security. Careers for life are no longer guaranteed, and more employers offer short-term contracts that preclude them from offering sickness or holiday pay. Financial and emotional burnout is therefore increasingly common among all levels of the workforce.

Working conditions

There can be little doubt that an individual's physical and mental health is adversely affected by unpleasant working conditions – such as high noise levels, too much or too little lighting, extremes of temperature, and unsocial or excessive hours.

Overwork

An individual may experience stress through an inability to cope with the technical or intellectual demands of a particular task. On the other hand, no matter how competent you are at your job, circumstances, such as long hours, unrealistic deadlines, and frequent interruptions, will all produce stress.

Underwork

An employee may experience boredom because there is not enough to do, or because a particular job is dull and repetitive.

Uncertainty

Uncertainty about an individual's work role – work objectives,

responsibilities, and colleagues' expectations – and a lack of communication and feedback can result in confusion, frustration,
helplessness, and stress.

Conflict
Stress may arise from work that an individual does not want to do
or that conflicts with their personal, social and family values.

Responsibility
The greater the level of responsibility the greater the level of stress.

Relationships at work
Good relationships at work with superiors, subordinates and colleagues are crucial. Within an organization, open discussion of
problems is essential to encourage positive relationships.

Change at work
Changes that alter psychological, physiological and behavioural
routines, such as promotion, retirement and redundancy, are extremely stressful.

Working conditions survey

Causes
3 points each
❑ company has been taken over recently
❑ staff reductions/lay-offs in the past year
❑ department/company had major reorganization
❑ staff expect company to be sold or relocated
❑ employee benefits significantly cut recently
❑ mandatory overtime frequently required
❑ employees have little control over their work
❑ consequences of making mistakes are severe
❑ workloads vary greatly
❑ most work is machine-paced or fast-paced
❑ staff must react quickly and accurately to change

2 points each

- ❏ few chances of opportunities for advancement
- ❏ red tape hinders getting things done
- ❏ inadequate staffing, money or technology
- ❏ pay is below the going rate
- ❏ sick and holiday benefits are below the norm
- ❏ employees are rotated between shifts
- ❏ new machines/work methods have been introduced
- ❏ noise/vibration levels are high or temperature keeps changing
- ❏ employees normally isolated from one another
- ❏ performance of work units normally below average

Remedies
3 points each

- ❏ staff recognized and rewarded for their contributions
- ❏ management takes firm action to reduce stress
- ❏ mental health benefits are provided
- ❏ company has formal employee communications programme
- ❏ staff given information on coping with stress
- ❏ staff given clear job descriptions
- ❏ management and staff talk openly with one another
- ❏ employees are free to talk with one another

2 points each

- ❏ work rules are published and are the same for everyone
- ❏ child care programmes are available
- ❏ employees can work flexible hours
- ❏ perks are granted fairly
- ❏ employees have access to necessary technology
- ❏ staff and management are trained in resolving conflicts
- ❏ staff receive training when assigned new tasks
- ❏ company encourages work and personal support groups
- ❏ staff have space and time for relaxation

1 point each

- ❏ staff assistance programme is available

❏ each employee's work space is not crowded
❏ staff can have personal items in their work areas
❏ management appreciates humour in the workplace
❏ programmes for care of the elderly are available

Subtract the total points for stress reducers from the total for stress producers. Results will range from minus 50 for excellent working conditions, to plus 60 points for a very stressful working environment.

Personality traits
Type-A and Type-B personalities
Two American cardiologists, Friedmann and Rosenman, noticed that many of their patients with heart disease shared similar personality characteristics and tended to find it difficult to adjust their lifestyle in a way that would aid recuperation. After detailed research they discovered a significant relationship between certain habitual behavioural patterns and stress-related illness. They reported that males with Type-A behaviour were six times as likely to suffer heart disease as men who exhibited Type-B behaviour. Type-A behaviour features four main patterns:

- *intense sense of time urgency* – always rushed, trying to achieve more in less time
- *inappropriate hostility and aggression* – excessively competitive, finds it difficult to relax and have fun; slight provocation may trigger hostility
- *multiple behaviour* – engages in two or more things simultaneously at improper times
- *lack of proper planning* – lack of planning to achieve required goals

Many studies of people who exhibit Type-A personalities in a wide range of contexts show that common characteristics include:

248

- work longer hours
- spend more time in classes (students)
- travel more for business
- get less sleep
- more involved in voluntary work, clubs, etc
- spend less time resting or relaxing
- work more around the home
- communicate less with their partners
- less marital sex
- derive little pleasure from socializing

Type-A behaviour places more stress on the cardiovascular system, stimulating high blood pressure, high heart rate and increased risk of heart attacks.

Type-B behaviour is the opposite: more relaxed, less hurried, less competitive. The main character traits include:

- *able to take the long view* – they don't try to meet unrealistic targets or to take on more than they can cope with; better at delegating
- *speed is not that important* – don't worry if not every task can be completed to deadline
- *sense of personal identity* – don't feel they have to earn respect and love; secure in who they are and what they do
- *sense of proportion* – no sense of constant struggle; always maintain a sense of balance at events in their lives

Classifying individuals as either Type-A or Type-B personalities helps to explain why some people are more prone to stress-related disease. It should be emphasized, however, that the distinction between these two personality types is not absolute; most people will fall between the two extreme types described.

Personality type questionnaire
In the list of attributes, circle the number that most closely represents your own behaviour.

#	Left	5	4	3	2	1	0	1	2	3	4	5	Right
1	Never Late	5	4	3	2	1	0	1	2	3	4	5	Casual about appointments
2	Not competetive	5	4	3	2	1	0	1	2	3	4	5	Very competetive
3	Anticipates what others are going to say (nods, interrupts, finishes for them)	5	4	3	2	1	0	1	2	3	4	5	Good listener
4	Always rushed	5	4	3	2	1	0	1	2	3	4	5	Never feels rushed
5	Can wait patiently	5	4	3	2	1	0	1	2	3	4	5	Impatient while waiting
6	Goes all out	5	4	3	2	1	0	1	2	3	4	5	Casual
7	Takes things one at a time	5	4	3	2	1	0	1	2	3	4	5	Tries to do too much
8	Emphatic in speech	5	4	3	2	1	0	1	2	3	4	5	Slow deliberate talker
9	Wants good job recognised by others	5	4	3	2	1	0	1	2	3	4	5	Seeks self-satisfaction regardless of others
10	Fast (eating, walking, etc.)	5	4	3	2	1	0	1	2	3	4	5	Slow doing things
11	Easy going	5	4	3	2	1	0	1	2	3	4	5	Hard-driving
12	Hides feelings	5	4	3	2	1	0	1	2	3	4	5	Expresses feelings
13	Many outside interests	5	4	3	2	1	0	1	2	3	4	5	Few outside interests
14	Satisfied with job	5	4	3	2	1	0	1	2	3	4	5	Ambitious

At one end of the scale is Type-A behaviour, the other is Type-B behaviour. High Type-A scores are obtained on the right side of the scale for questions 2, 5, 7, 11, 13, 14; High Type-A scores are obtained on the left side of the scale for questions 1, 3, 4, 6, 8, 9, 10, 12. Give yourself 10 points if you score at the end of the scale towards Type-A, working down to 0 points at the other end of the scale, which represents Type-B.

Childhood influences and upbringing

A traumatic childhood is likely to lead to greater levels of stress as an adult. A difficult childhood is also more likely to lead to low self-esteem, low self-assertiveness, difficulty expressing personal beliefs, attitudes and feelings, and a tendency to depend on others to provide a sense of emotional wellbeing and self-worth. Over-dependence upon others is likely to lead to frustration as expectations are inevitably dashed – leading to feelings of frustration, anger, depression and hopelessness in adulthood.

Unrealistic expectations

Unrealistic expectations are a common source of stress. People often become upset about something, not because it is innately stressful but because it does not concur with what they expected. Take, for example, the experience of driving in slow-moving traffic. If it happens at rush hour, you may not like it but it should not surprise or upset you. However, if it occurs on a Sunday afternoon, especially if it makes you late for something, you are more likely to be stressed by it.

When expectations are realistic, life feels more predictable and therefore more manageable. There is an increased feeling of control because you can plan and prepare yourself (physically and psychologically). For example, if you know in advance when you have to work overtime or stay late, you will take it more in your stride than when it is dropped on you at the last minute.

Attitudes and beliefs

A lot of stress results from our beliefs. We have literally thousands of premises and assumptions about all kinds of things that we hold to be the truth – everything from, 'You can't beat the system' and 'The customer is always right', to 'Men shouldn't show their emotions' and 'Children should tidy their rooms'. We have beliefs about how things are, how people should behave and about ourselves ('I can never remember people's names'). Most of our beliefs are held unconsciously so we are unaware of them. This gives them more power over us and allows them to run our lives.

Beliefs cause stress in two ways. The first is the behaviour that results from them. For example, if you believe that work should come before pleasure, you are likely to work harder and have less leisure time than you would otherwise. If you believe that people should meet the needs of others before they meet their own, you are likely to neglect yourself to some extent. These beliefs are expressions of a personal philosophy or value system, which results in increased effort and decreased relaxation – a formula for stress. There is no objective truth to begin with. These are really just opinions but they lead to stressful behaviour. Uncovering the unconscious assumptions behind actions can be helpful in changing one's lifestyle.

The second way in which beliefs cause stress is when they are in conflict with those of other people. However, it should always be remembered that personal assumptions are not the truth but rather opinions and, therefore, they can be challenged. In situations of conflict it is always helpful if the protagonists attempt to revise their beliefs, or at least admit that the beliefs held by the other person may be just as valid as their own. This mind-opening exercise usually helps to diminish stressful antagonism.

Relaxation response

Just as the body has an automatic process to prepare it for a 'fight or flight' situation, it can also go into what is called the 'relaxation response'. This stage of low arousal is less well known than the body's red-alert status, and it initially takes a concentrated effort in order to experience it. The symptoms of the 'fight or flight' response – increased metabolic rate, quickened heart rate and faster breathing – are the direct opposite of those experienced by the body while in a state of deep relaxation.

We need to be truly relaxed for the process to begin and for the body to feel the full benefits. Two branches of the automatic nervous system are responsible for most of the changes that take place. What is known as the 'sympathetic branch' slows down, allowing the 'parasympathetic branch' to assume a greater role, calming the body and mind and decreasing metabolism until it reaches a hypometabolic state – it was in a hypermetabolic state during the 'fight or flight' process.

During relaxation our bodies require very low maintenance, and the decrease in metabolism is similar only to that found in deep sleep. Our breathing becomes more regular and the heart rate decreases. In a sustained period of relaxation oxygen consumption actually falls below that measured during deep sleep. There is also a significant fall in blood lactate, a substance that enters the blood through the metabolism of skeletal muscles. This occurs three times faster during meditation than while sitting at rest.

Blood pressure is also lowered, but only to normal pre-stress levels. All these things allow the body to recover from the strains placed on it by everyday life.

The relaxation response also elicits a marked alteration in brain activity. The brain emits four types of waves, each with its own rhythm. Beta waves signify everyday conscious rhythms; delta waves are present during sleep; theta waves appear while in a dreamlike state; and alpha waves are more prominent when the mind is active, yet relaxed. Effective meditation manufactures a predominance of alpha and theta waves – signifying a state of restfulness and deep relaxation, where the mind is alert but not strained or confused. These waves appear almost as soon as the body starts to relax, increasing in frequency as the process intensifies, allowing clearer and more constructive thinking.

A prolonged period of relaxation will also increase the body's secretion of particular mood-altering chemicals, known as neurotransmitters. One of these, serotonin, is a powerful hormone that is associated with feelings of happiness and content-ment. Recent medical research suggests that a deficiency in this hormone is a contributory factor in cases of clinical depression.

Achieve relaxation and combat stress through self help

It would not be possible, or desirable, to eliminate all the effects of stress in our lives. The aim of stress management should be to harness and control the effects of stress to help to enrich our physical, mental and emotional well-being. Positive stress man-agement involves recognizing the existence and type of stress and then taking remedial action. By getting to the root causes of your stress, you can not only relieve current problems and symptoms, but you can also prevent recurrences.

Remedial action falls into three main categories:

- change your thinking
- change your behaviour
- change your lifestyle

Change your thinking
Reframing

Reframing is one of the most powerful and creative stress reduc-ers. It is a technique used to change the way you look at things in order to feel better about them. We all do this inadvertently at times. The key to reframing is to recognize that there are many ways to interpret the same situation. It is like the age-old ques-tion: Is the glass half empty or half full? The answer of course is that it is both or either, depending on your point of view. How-ever, if you see the glass as half full, it will feel different than seeing it as half empty because the way we feel almost always re-sults from the way we think. The message of reframing is this: there are many ways of seeing the same thing – so you might as well pick the one you like. Reframing does not change the exter-nal reality, but simply helps you to view things differently – and less stressfully.

Positive thinking

When faced with stressful situations try to avoid becoming pre-occupied with debilitating negative thoughts of powerlessness, dejection, failure and despair. Chronic stress can leave us vulner-able to negative suggestion, so try to focus on positives:

* focus on your strengths
* learn from the stress you are under
* look for opportunities in the stressful situation
* seek out the positive – make a change

Change your behaviour

Be assertive

Being assertive means taking control and advancing your own needs and aspirations whilst remaining aware of the wishes of others. Assertiveness helps to manage stressful situations, and will in time help to reduce their frequency. Lack of assertiveness is often a function of low self-esteem and low self-confidence, factors that aggravate stress levels and can turn even relatively benign situations and events into potential crises.

The key to assertiveness is verbal and non-verbal communica-tion. People who cannot adequately communicate their needs or wishes will create various problems for themselves. For example, the person who cannot say 'no' to others' requests is likely to be overwhelmed by external demands; the person who finds it diffi-cult to express personal feelings and thoughts will lack self-ful-filment and not be comfortable with his or her own identity; an overly aggressive style of communication will prevent an individual from forming close personal relationships.

We all display different degrees of passive, aggressive or asser-tive behaviour, at different times and in different situations. Prob-lems arise when a particular response is unhelpful for a particu-lar situation, and we find it difficult to change to a more appropri-ate style of response. Improving assertiveness is about learning how to extend the range of our communication style to allow a greater flexibility of responses in different situations.

It is important to acknowledge that we are all equal and have

the same basic rights (*see* Assert your rights below). Being too
passive means denying one's rights by failing to express honest
feelings, thoughts and beliefs, and allowing others to violate oneself. A passive person may express thoughts and feelings in such
an apologetic, self-effacing manner that others can easily disre-
gard them. Being non-assertive means allowing people to walk all
over you, denying the validity of your own needs, and surrender-
ing control over a situation to others. This leads to stressful feelings of anxiety, powerlessness, frustration and anger.

Being assertive involves standing up for your personal rights
and expressing your thoughts, feelings and beliefs directly, hon-
estly and spontaneously in ways that don't infringe the rights of
others. Assertive people respect themselves and others, and take
responsibility for their actions and choices. They recognize their
needs and ask openly and directly for what they want. If they fail
in these efforts, for whatever reason, they may feel disappointed
but their self-confidence remains intact. They are not reliant on
the approval of others.

Useful verbal and non-verbal assertive skills include the ability to

- Establish good eye contact, but do not stare.
- Stand or sit comfortably without fidgeting.
- Talk in a firm steady voice instead of rambling or shouting.
- Use gesture to emphasize points (hands, facial expressions,
  body posture).
- Use statements such as 'I think', 'I feel'.
- Use empathetic statements of interest such as 'What do you
  think', 'How do you feel?'
- Be concise and to the point. State clearly the message you
  want the other person to hear.

The more you stand up for yourself the higher your self-esteem. Your chances of getting what you want out of life improve
greatly when you let others know what you want and you stand up
for your own rights and needs. Expressing negative feelings at
the appropriate time avoids the build-up of resentment. Being

ess self-conscious and anxious, and less driven by the need for self-protection and control, you will be able to manage stress more successfully, and to love and appreciate yourself and others more easily.

Assert your rights

1 I have the right to express my feelings.
2 I have the right to express my opinions and beliefs.
3 I have the right to say 'yes' and 'no' for myself.
4 I have the right to change my mind.
5 I have the right to say 'I don't understand'.
6 I have the right simply to be myself, and not act for the benefit of others.
7 I have the right to decline responsibility for other people's problems.
8 I have the right to make reasonable requests of others.
9 I have the right to set my own priorities.
10 I have the right to be listened to, and taken seriously.

Any of the above can be personalized: if your boss asks you to work late at short notice, then by rights 3 and 7, your decision may be: 'I have the right to refuse this unreasonable request, I should have been given more warning.'

Get organized

Being chronically disorganized, either at work or in the home, is one of the most common causes of stress. Stressful environments are minimized when you impose a form of structure: this offers security against problems appearing 'out-of-the-blue'. Too inflexible a pattern would be impractical, but keeping a diary, writing lists and prioritizing duties all help to stem stressful situations. Writing down objectives, duties and activities helps to make them seem more tangible and surmountable. Don't try to overload your mind with too much information – if you are already stressed there is more chance of you forgetting vital references and data. If you keep control over what you are doing there is less chance of spiralling into professional and personal chaos.

Ventilation

There is an old saying that 'a problem shared is a problem halved'.
People who keep things to themselves carry a considerable and
unnecessary burden. Talking through a problem with others can
be the first step to eliminating it. It is worth developing a support
system – a few trusted relatives, colleagues or friends to talk to
when you are upset or worried. Often it's not events themselves
that are stressful but how we perceive them. Another form of communication that may be helpful is writing, for example in a private journal at home, or even letters to oneself, which should then
be destroyed. The value is in expressing the feelings and getting
them out. Rereading the letter just reinforces the upset and re-
awakens the anger.

Humour

Humour is a wonderful stress-reducer and antidote to upsets
both at home and at work; we often laugh hardest when we have
been feeling most tense. Laughter relieves muscular tension,
improves breathing, regulates the heart beat and pumps
endorphins – the body's natural painkillers – into the bloodstream.

Diversion and distraction

Take time out (anything from a short walk to a holiday) to get
away from the things that are bothering you. This will not resolve
the problem, but it gives you a break and a chance for your stress
levels to decrease. Then, you can return to deal with issues feeling more rested and in a better frame of mind.

Change your lifestyle through nutrition and exercise

Relaxation is virtually impossible if your body isn't maintained
properly. Nutrition and exercise are the cornerstones of a healthy
lifestyle, and so it is vital to achieve an equilibrium between the
two.

Food is the fuel we put into our bodies in order to survive, and
exercise creates the process that turns it into energy. In times
past, the equation was relatively easy to achieve – the balance

between energy input and output occurred naturally. We burnt up a lot of energy just keeping warm and doing a lot of physical work. Today's society, with its increased automation and sedentary jobs, makes it more difficult to maintain any equilibrium. Western society offers us abundant food and warmth with minimum physical outlay, so it has become all the more important consciously to monitor the balance of our diets.

Being overweight or underweight can create serious health problems. Obesity can cause diabetes, high blood pressure and heart problems. Being underweight is no more desirable in terms of health. An underweight body can lack the energy and strength to carry out effectively its functions, leaving the individual tired and listless. Add bad habits such as smoking or excessive alcohol consumption to either of these conditions and it often becomes very difficult for the body to cope.

Food management is important not just when it comes to checking weight, it can also improve your ability to relax and cope with stress. Food affects every organ of our bodies, including the heart, lungs and brain. The correct diet will encourage fitness and energy, nourish nerves, feed muscles, improve circulation and breathing, and support the immune system. It will promote a general feeling of positiveness and calm.

The eating process itself can create a feeling of wellbeing. What, and how, we eat says a lot about our emotional state – think of how a baby is calmed by the act of feeding, even if it is not hungry. We instinctively link eating to nurturing, comfort and security. At one extreme, anorexia nervosa and bulimia nervosa are examples of how emotional distress can affect our relationship with food. Yet all of us skip meals or overeat when we are feeling under pressure. As the digestive system shuts down during periods of stress, this is particularly dangerous and can lead to stomach problems and 'executive' ulcers.

To guard against ill-health it is vital to be aware of your body's needs. Often this means re-educating your body in terms of nutrition and taste – it can take a while for a 'junked-out' palate to become accustomed to unprocessed foods. But information has never been more accessible. Nutritional education is now seen as a step in preventive medicine, and the general principles are easy to follow.

Every food has its own nutritional make-up and has a unique effect on the mechanics of your body. What each food does for you depends on its core attributes and composition, and it can either enhance or aggravate your sense of wellbeing.

Most experts agree that a well-balanced diet is crucial in preserving health and helping to reduce stress. Certain foods and drinks act as quite powerful stimulants to the body and so are a direct cause of stress. This stimulation may be pleasurable in the short term, but more harmful with prolonged consumption.

Caffeine

In small doses caffeine can be a good thing. Its initial effects are increased alertness and activity in the muscles, nervous system and heart. Unfortunately, people often use caffeine to fuel an already overloaded system, thinking that it will improve their performance. Too much caffeine has the same effects on the system as prolonged stress – anxiety, over-stimulation, headache, migraine, emotional instability, palpitations – and should be avoided wherever possible.

Caffeine is a drug commonly found in food and drinks such as coffee, tea, chocolate and Coca-Cola. It is a strong stimulant that actually generates a stress reaction in the body by causing a rise in the relase of adrenaline. In small doses caffeine can have a positive effect on our health. People often use caffeine to fuel an already overloaded system. Some studies have also indicated a possible link between caffeine intake and high blood pressure and high cholesterol levels.

The best way to observe the effect of caffeine is to get it out of the system long enough to see if there is a difference in how you feel. After about three weeks many people notice a benefit. You feel more relaxed, less jittery or nervous, sleep better, have more energy (a paradox, since you are removing a stimulant), less heartburn and fewer muscle aches. To avoid withdrawal symptoms if is best to decrease intake by one drink per day until they you are down to zero, then abstain for three weeks.

Fats

There are some foods that, quite simply, are not good for you. It is important to cut back or drop these foods from your diet. Most people know that fat intake should be carefully monitored. Fats generally fall into two groups: saturated and unsaturated. Saturated fats are found in dairy produce, vegetable fats, palm oil, hard margarines, sauces and biscuits, and are the most dangerous. Polyunsaturated fats are a sub-group of unsaturated fats and are present in sunflower, corn and soya oil, nuts and soft margarines. Eating too much fat can lead to obesity, heart disease, strokes and cardiac arrest. Polyunsaturated fats do not raise cholesterol levels in the same way as saturated fats, and they can also help to restore everyday wear and tear.

It is important to limit the amount of fat in our diet. Too much fat causes obesity and puts unnecessary strain on the heart. There is also evidence that high-fat diets contribute to the growing incidence of breast, colon and prostate cancers in Western society.

- *saturated fats* – in milk, cheese, butter, animal fats, vegetable fats, biscuits, cakes and sweets
- *unsaturated fats* – which include *polyunsaturated fats* are found in sunflower oil, corn oil, soya oil, nuts, trout, mackerel and herring.

Nutritionists advise that we should substitute polyunsaturated fats for saturated fats wherever possible. This will help to avoid the tendency towards obesity and raised cholesterol levels in the blood, which can lead to cardiovascular disease and premature death.

Salt

Most of us eat much more salt than is healthy. Part of the reason our intake is so high is that salt is present in most foods as a preservative, making it difficult to avoid.

Salt should be minimized in your diet. Foods high in salt, such as refined convenience foods, bacon, ham, sausages and pickled items, should be avoided. The dangers of high salt intake are similar to our responses to stress. It can induce high blood pressure, irritate the menstrual cycle and have a stimulating and weakening effect on the adrenal glands, muscles and nervous system. Instead of salt use a salt substitute that is rich in potassium rather than in sodium.

Preservatives

Preservatives, antioxidants, colourings, raising agents, flavour enhancers and sweeteners, emulsifiers and stabilizers are all included in the 3,500 different additives frequently used by food manufacturers. Some are natural and some are completely synthetic, and most are silently injected into our diet. It is difficult to check the label on everything we buy in the supermarket, but it is well worth the effort to make ourselves aware of what we are taking home. Some of these additives have been found to have negative effects on our health and emotional wellbeing, and the only way to guard against them is through conscious awareness and nutritional education.

Sugar

Sugar is one of the most common food additives, and, unfortunately, it is also one of the most 'empty' of all foodstuffs. It induces a short-term boost of energy, but when we eat too much of it our adrenal glands are overloaded and become sluggish. This reduces our ability to relax and causes irritability and a lack of concentration. An overly high sugar intake will also strain our insulin-producing glands, perhaps inducing diabetes. More obvious problems include obesity, tooth decay and mood swings. These are particularly difficult problems for children to deal with, and parents must be aware of the dangers of placating a disruptive child with a bar of chocolate or a bag of sweets.

Sugar consumption can be reduced by eating fresh fruit for dessert instead of sugary puddings; drinking unsweetened fruit juices and sugar-free squashes and carbonated drinks; leaving out sugar in coffee and tea; looking for sugar-free labels on products in supermarkets; and avoiding junk foods.

Alcohol

The amount of alcohol we consume can also create health problems and contribute to stress levels. A limited intake can actually be very beneficial – red wine in particular contains things that are very good for us – but taken in excess, alcohol will destroy organs as well our emotional wellbeing. Dependency on alcohol is a disease in itself, which can create great distress not only for the alcoholic but for his or her family and friends as well.

Like caffeine, alcohol stimulates the secretion of adrenaline, producing the same problems of nervous tension, irritability and insomnia. Alcohol in excess will increase fat deposits in the heart and decrease immune function. Alcohol is also a toxin to the bone marrow, and has a severe impact on the liver, inhibiting that organ's ability to detoxify the body. These toxins include hormones released during stress, which will continue to circulate in the body if liver function is impaired.

Balance and nutrition

It should be clear by now that it is important to avoid too much salt, sugar and dairy products in our diet. These foods tend to promote adrenaline release, which decreases stress tolerance, and they also have a negative effect on cardiovascular health. As part of a balanced diet, the following foods will encourage fitness and energy, nourish nerves, feed muscles, improve circulation and breathing, support the immune system and promote a general feeling of positivity and calm:

- *whole grains* – wheat, rice, oats, barley, rye, corn – are a source of complex carbohydrates and essential vitamins and minerals and other nutrients that are of great value in improving stress tolerance
- *beans* – soybeans, kidney beans, broad beans, lentils, chick peas – are an excellent source of anti-stress B-vitamins

- *fresh fruit and vegetables* – are an excellent source of essential vitamins and dietary fibre

Nutrients

If you seek a more relaxed lifestyle, you should start by caring for yourself from the inside, and feed your body with only 'good' fuel. The general maxims of a healthy diet are to increase our intake of fruit, vegetables, carbohydrates and low fat proteins, such as fresh fish or lean meat. Fibre became a buzz word of the 1980's and it is still valued – but fortunately a healthy diet should preclude the need for endless bowls of bran. Fat is essential but, as discussed, only in restricted quantities.

Of course there are many foods that aid the mental and physical balance of our bodies. When we are under a lot of pressure and feel worn down by life, the body will benefit from supplements of substances that are devoured by a system under stress. Unfortunately, vitamins and nutrients can have a short shelf-life. Food has to be very fresh, as some vitamins are easily eroded by heat, light and storage. Overcooking can destroy the nutritional value of many foods, and it is always best to eat food raw or lightly cooked whenever possible. Buying organic food is another way of ensuring that our bodies get the nutrients they need.

Although nutrients are best taken in their most natural form, modern diets do not always allow this, and we often need to supplement our intake. It is now possible to obtain vitamins and minerals that are specifically targeted to help with stress. A deficiency of vitamin C is a common problem, as stress hampers our ability to create and absorb it. Such a deficiency can also damage our absorption of iron. Supplements of vitamin B6 are recommended when under stress, pregnant or during times of anxiety and worry. A lack of B6 can lead to physical and mental exhaustion. Zinc deficiency is a common sign of stress and can induce stomach problems, a breakdown of the immune system, poor healing, low appetite and fatigue. Iodine, linked to the thyroid gland, has a direct effect on the metabolic rate of the body, so a deficiency can cause exhaustion while supplements have a stimulant effect. For more information make time to visit your local health food shop or chemist – staff there will be glad to advise.

It is important to keep your diet and dietary behaviour as balanced as possible. The demands of modern-day life sometimes make it difficult to adhere to a well-balanced diet. There will always be times when the processed, overcooked oven meal is just too convenient, or when you really don't have time to sit down for a bite. Given this inevitability, it is all the more important to monitor what you eat and try to make up for the days when you do not have the time or inclination to prepare something more wholesome. This is the only way to let your body cope and to lessen any anxiety you may have about not eating properly.

Vitamins and minerals

Vitamins are a group of chemically unrelated, organic nutrients that are essential in small quantities for normal metabolism, growth, and physical wellbeing. These nutrients must be obtained through diet, since they are not synthesized in the body. In general, all the vitamins required by the average person can be obtained from a natural, well-balanced diet. However, stress increases cellular activity, which leads to increased nutrient usage, and under chronic stress certain vitamin deficiencies may occur.

The following vitamins and supplements are available from most chemists and health shops. For more information contact your doctor, local health shop, pharmacist or alternative health practitioner.

Vitamin C

Vitamin C deficiency is a common problem caused by stress, which hampers the body's ability to create and absorb the vitamin. Vitamin C deficiency has been linked to a range of illnesses and disorders, including scurvy, lethargy and fatigue, a weakened immune system and degenerative diseases such as arthritis and arteriosclerosis. Alcohol and cigarettes are also thought to inhibit the action of vitamin C. Foods rich in vitamin C include fresh fruit and vegetables.

Vitamin B6

Vitamin B6 is essential to the health of the nervous system. It is important in maintaining a healthy immune system, and there is evidence that B6 plays a role in limiting the growth of certain tumours and skin cancers. B6 relieves a wide variety of PMS symptoms, such as breast tenderness, weight gain (water retention) and irritability. This very important vitamin has also been shown to be helpful in reducing or eliminating symptoms of nervous tremors and epileptic seizures. A lack of B6 can lead to physical and mental exhaustion, and has been linked to anaemia.

Supplements of vitamin B6 are recommended when under stress, for morning sickness during pregnancy, and for anxiety. Foods rich in vitamin B6 are fish, fresh vegetables, pulses and whole grain cereals.

Vitamin B12

Vitamin B12 is vital for blood formation and a healthy nervous system. Living with persistent and unmanaged stress can and will eventually result in symptoms of physical deterioration and mental and emotional breakdown. B12 helps you to fight disease, recover more quickly from viral infections and helps to restore a sluggish appetite. Foods rich in B12 are red meats, fish and dairy products.

Vitamin B5 (pantothenic acid)

Pantothenic acid is essential for the proper functioning of the adrenal glands, the health of which is so important to the management of stress. Most experts agree that pantothenic acid supplements are recommended to help to alleviate the symptoms of chronic stress.

Selenium

This trace element is essential for normal growth and development. It acts as an anti-oxidant, an anti-polluting agent and helps to strengthen the immune system. Research indicates a possible link between heart disease and selenium deficiency. Nutritionists advise that selenium supplements are best taken together with vitamin E.

Iron

Iron deficiency leads to tiredness and exhaustion, anaemia and moods of depression. A deficiency in iron can result from vitamin C deficiency, which limits the absorption of iron in the body. Symptoms of iron deficiency include brittle nails, paleness and mouth ulcers. Foods rich in iron include pulses, grains, fish, poultry, meat, spinach, potatoes and peas.

Zinc

Zinc deficiency is a common sign of stress, and can cause stomach problems, a breakdown of the immune system, poor healing, low appetite and fatigue. Foods rich in zinc include seafood, dairy products, meat, ginger root and soya beans.

Iodine

The body's supply of iodine is dependent on a healthy thyroid gland, which determines the metabolic rate of the body – so a deficiency can cause exhaustion, whilst iodine supplements have a stimulant effect. Foods rich in iodine include seafoods, spinach and green peppers.

Calcium

Calcium is essential for healthy bones, joints, teeth, nerves, muscles and for efficient blood clotting. Foods rich in calcium include dairy products, pulses, apples and cabbage. Some foods, such as bread and milk, have added calcium and are advertised as calcium-fortified.

Super health foods

There are certain foods that are super foods – packed full of nutritional value in such beautifully balanced forms that they are easy to assimilate. Much richer in specific nutrients than ordinary or processed food, if you incorporate these super foods into your diet, you will boost your energy levels and achieve a personal equilibrium that is one of the most basic – and long-lasting – aspects of relaxation in the truest sense of the word.

Almonds

Almonds are an important source of the minerals zinc, magnesium, potassium and iron, so that a small handful of the nuts can transform a light salad into a well-balanced meal. You should eat vitamin C-rich foods at the same time, because almonds also contain oxalic and phytic acid, which can prevent your absorption of this vitamin.

Apricots

The brighter the fruit, the more beta-carotene it contains, and apricots are very high in vitamin A. Dried apricots are a wonderful source of beta-carotene during the winter months.

Avocado pears

Avocados are an almost complete food – so much so, that in some parts of the world babies are weaned using mashed avocado. They are rich in potassium and vitamin A.

Barley

This grain has a very high mineral content. It has lots of calcium, potassium and B-complex vitamins, making it especially useful for anyone suffering from stress or fatigue. Add a handful of barley to home-made chicken soup ('Jewish penicillin') for a soothing and nourishing meal. It also lowers the level of cholesterol in the body.

Beetroot

For hundreds of years, beetroot has been used as a folk remedy for anaemia and liver problems. It helps the digestive system – especially when grated raw, perhaps served with grated apple and carrot and dressed with lemon juice and olive oil. It is much better eaten in this way rather than drowned in vinegar.

Broccoli

Like other members of the crucifer family – cabbage, cauliflower, Brussels sprouts, etc – broccoli has a protective effect against disease. It is rich in vitamin C, iron, beta-carotene and folic acid. Like all green vegetables, it should be lightly cooked (steaming is ideal) to preserve most of its nutrients.

Carrots

A single carrot will supply all your vitamin A needs for a whole day. Nibbling carrot sticks is a much healthier pastime than grazing on salted peanuts and crisps. Research has shown that carrots have a protective effect against ultraviolet rays, so they can help you to look younger for longer as well.

Celery

According to Hippocrates, celery calms the nerves – perhaps because of its high calcium content. It helps eliminate waste via the urine, due to the effect it has on the kidneys.

Cider vinegar

Made by fermenting the juice of whole, fresh apples, cider vinegar's beneficial effects come from the high mineral content of apples. It is unusually high in potassium, calcium, phosphorus, sodium and trace elements. It increases blood oxygenation, improves metabolism, strengthens digestion and increases blood clotting ability. Two teaspoonfuls of cider vinegar in a glass of water on an empty stomach first thing in the morning is helpful to people with weight problems.

Garlic

Like sprouts, garlic has been used as a cure-all for millennia. Inscriptions on the Great Pyramid at Gizeh in Egypt mention garlic as one of the foods eaten by its builders.

Some naturopaths believe that common infectious diseases, like flu and bronchitis, are caused by an accumulation of toxins in the body that gradually undermines the functions of internal organs.

Garlic has been shown to be an excellent antiseptic. It was used with amazing success in treating soldiers with infected wounds during both World Wars. In the Second World War, the wounds of British soldiers were treated with garlic. Some of the wounds were already gangrenous, but garlic checked the spread of the gangrene and resulted in the shedding of gangrenous tissue. As recently as 1965 the Russians flew 500 tons of garlic to Moscow to fight a flu epidemic, and some people still call garlic 'Russian penicillin'.

Garlic also helps clear fat accumulations from the blood vessels, lower cholesterol, and protect against bacterial and viral infections.

Grapes

Grapes are very cleansing and regenerating. Grape fasts – eating nothing but grapes and drinking water for a day or two – are a well-known method of detoxifying the body. They are an ideal food, not only for convalescents, but for anyone suffering from fatigue or depression,

Kelp

Kelp – or seaweed – is a wonderful source of iodine, which helps protect the body against the radioactivity in the atmosphere that contributes to early ageing. It is rich in B-complex vitamins, vitamins D, E and K, magnesium and calcium. It is particularly good for hair and nails.

Kelp tablets are not concentrated; they are simply dehydrated seaweed, so six or eight of them should be taken after each meal for good results.

Lecithin

Lecithin is important in maintaining a healthy nervous system and is vital in helping the body resist stress. Daily lecithin consumption means that body fats are converted into energy more quickly, and existing fat deposits will slowly disperse. It breaks up cholesterol so that it can pass through artery walls, and has been shown to increase immunity to virus infections and help prevent gallstones. It also helps to cleanse the liver and purify the kidneys and, because of its choline and unsaturated fatty acid content, it is very good indeed for the condition of the skin.

Lecithin can be bought in granule form from health food shops.

Mixed three seeds

Pumpkin, sunflower and sesame seeds, ground in a blender or coffee grinder in equal proportions, make a wonderful complete protein to sprinkle on salads or fruits. They are extremely rich in vitamins, and are excellent for hair and skin as well as general health. Pumpkin seeds are rich in B vitamins, phosphorus, iron and zinc. Sesame seeds are rich in magnesium and potassium and have been used for generations to treat fatigue, insomnia and sexual dysfunctions. They also contain more calcium than milk, cheese or nuts and are a good source of vitamin E. Sunflower seeds are rich in iron, the B-complex vitamins, magnesium and zinc.

Molasses

A tablespoonful of black-strap molasses supplies as much calcium as a glass of milk, as much iron as nine eggs, more potassium than any other food, and the B-complex vitamins in good balance. It is also rich in magnesium, vitamin E and copper, and is a very valuable food for women who tend to be anaemic. It is an alkali-forming food, beneficial for maintaining a proper acid-alkaline balance in the body. A tablespoon of molasses and the juice of half a lemon in a mug of hot water is a good way to start the day. It is also very good for the condition of your skin and hair.

Warning: Diabetics must not use molasses.

Oats

Oats are a uniquely soothing food for the nerves. They are amazingly high in calcium, potassium and magnesium, together with lots of B-complex vitamins, which are all vital to a healthy nervous system. They also help lower cholesterol levels. A bowl of porridge, perhaps with a spoonful of honey or molasses, makes a uniquely calming breakfast for a child on the morning of an exam.

Potatoes

Potatoes have a well-known soporific effect: they contain a substance very like chloroform. Research suggests that certain foods cause contentment and lifting of depression by altering brain chemistry in a similar way to drug therapy. To prevent downward mood swings, a chemical called serotonin must be present in the brain in proper amounts. The body makes serotonin from the amino acid tryptophan. Under ordinary circumstances, tryptophan has to compete with other amino acids to get into the brain. But when more carbohydrate than protein is eaten, tryptophan has much less trouble getting in. A potato is not only an ideal carbohydrate: a medium potato contains only about 90 fat-free calories, as well as vitamins A, C, B₁, B₆, niacin, iron, potassium and fibre. What could be more comforting or soothing than a creamy mass of freshly whipped up potato with a swirl of olive oil or a knob of fresh, cold butter melting on top?

Rabbit

Much lower in fat than beef or lamb, rabbit – especially wild rabbit, if you can get it – makes delicious slow-cooked dishes to warm and soothe on a cold winter's evening. Rabbit with prunes and Guinness is bursting with nutrients. Serve with barley instead of rice or potatoes for the ultimate nourishing and relaxing treat.

Sprouted grains

Sprouted grains and seeds have been used in diets for thousands of years, especially by the Chinese. They are amazing powerhouses of live food nourishment. They are rich in vitamins A, C, D, E, K and B complex, in calcium, phosphorus, potassium, magnesium, iron, high quality protein and enzymes. Sprouts are rich in vitality factors because, unlike most vegetables, they are eaten at the peak of their freshness – when they are still growing.

Sprouts contain an amazing quantity of enzymes. As we age, our bodies become less efficient at producing enzymes from food, which often leads to indigestion or flatulence. Sprouts, by giving us lots of enzymes, produce more efficient digestion and improved metabolism of food into energy. As well as being highly nutritious, sprouts are extremely low in calories.

How to grow sprouts:

Seeds to sprout include alfalfa (considered to be the richest in minerals), wheat, mung beans, buckwheat, lentils, sesame seeds, soya beans and chickpeas.

Put a heaped tablespoonful of seeds or grains into a jar, cover it with lukewarm water and leave it overnight. In the morning, covering the jar with a piece of muslin or cheesecloth held in place with a rubber band, pour off the water and rinse the seeds in fresh lukewarm water (not hot – or you will kill them). Pour off the excess water through the cloth and put the jar on the windowsill. In the evening, rinse again and pour off excess. Repeat the rinsing twice a day, and, in three to six days – depending on the kind of seeds used – you will have sprouts to sprinkle on your salads or steam lightly and enjoy with a sprinkling of olive oil and lemon juice. Patent plastic sprouters are now available that make sprouting even easier.

Spirulina

Spirulina is a blue-green, single-celled alga, microscopic in size and spiral in shape – hence its name. It thrives in warm alkaline lakes such as Lake Texcoco in Mexico. It was so highly valued by the Aztecs that it was used as currency.

The B_{12}, folic acid and chlorophyll content of spirulina makes it useful in the treatment of anaemia and liver disorders.

Spirulina is helpful in weight control. Its protein contains a high proportion of the amino acid phenylalanine, which is transformed into brain neurotransmitter substances that control appetite, energy level and mood. The appetite is curbed and a state of wellbeing is maintained. The usual dose is three tablets taken half an hour before each meal.

Wheat germ

Wheat germ is the richest known source of vitamin E. It is also rich in magnesium, copper, manganese, calcium and phosphorus. Sprinkled on yoghurt or cereal, it a superb source of protein But it is rich in fat – a tablespoonful a day is enough.

Hypoglycaemia

If you are suffering from hypoglycaemia – often called 'the great imitator' because it mimics so many mental and emotional disorders – you will find it almost impossible to relax completely. A large proportion of patients receiving psychotherapy – more than half, it is thought – are in fact hypoglycaemic. Symptoms include: irritability, exhaustion, nervousness, depression, faintness and dizziness, cold sweats, headaches, confusion, heart palpitations lack of sex drive, lack of concentration, blurred vision, phobias and allergies.

Hypoglycaemia, or low sugar levels in the blood, was discovered in 1924 by Dr Seale Harris. At that time it was called hyperinsulinism because it was thought to be caused by excessive insulin secretion due to an overactive pancreas. The excess insulin causes rapid uptake of glucose by the cells and tissues of the body, leaving the blood depleted of glucose. When glucose is in short supply, cell function is impaired, leading to physical and mental problems.

Low blood sugar may impair mental health even more than physical health because it deprives the brain and nervous system of oxygen.

During digestion, all ingested carbohydrates (sugars and starches) are converted to glucose, which is the only carbohydrate the body can use. After a meal, particularly one with a high sugar content, surges of glucose enter the blood, causing the pancreas to secrete insulin. Insulin causes rapid uptake of glucose by almost all of the tissues of the body and also promotes the conversion of excess glucose to glycogen, a more compact form of glucose that can be stored in the liver for future use. The pancreas, however, is only part of the mechanism that controls blood sugar. The whole process originates in glucoreceptor (glucose-sensitive) nerve cells in the brain from which impulses travel to the pituitary gland, adrenal glands, liver and finally the pancreas. In this sophisticated sugar-control chain, there are also hormones that convert glycogen back to glucose to raise the blood glucose level. The hormones that do this are glucagon, also secreted by the pancreas, and adrenaline, secreted by the adrenal glands. In this way, opposing forces are constantly at work, balancing each other, so that blood sugar levels are kept within fairly narrow limits. But they do not always succeed and, if the blood sugar level gets too low, hypoglycaemia occurs.

Some people inherit or develop an overactive pancreas, which secretes excessive amounts of insulin even when only small amounts of sugar enter the blood. Sometimes, the pancreas may react slowly and insulin does not enter the blood until the sugar level has already fallen – this is retarded hypoglycaemia. On the other hand, secretion of glucagon and adrenaline, the hormones that balance the action of insulin, may be too low. Hypoglycaemia can also be caused by allergies or an imbalance in the autonomic nervous system. Other causes are excessive consumption of alcohol, tobacco, coffee, overeating and emotional stress. Whatever the reason, hypoglycaemia develops when the delicate balance of the systems and substances that control blood sugar is upset.

Theoretically, sugar would appear to be the ideal food to raise blood sugar levels. But sugar is the one food that hypoglycaemics should avoid. In fact, sugar will eventually contribute to lower blood sugar levels.

When we eat sugar, it is readily absorbed into the blood, where it raises blood sugar levels, triggering the pancreas to secrete insulin, which will cause glucose to be absorbed into the tissues. Insulin, because it breaks down much more slowly than sugar, remains circulating in the blood for several hours, lowering blood sugar level even lower than the original level. It triggers the hypoglycaemic symptoms again, creating a craving for more sugar. So the hypoglycaemic eats more sugar, which deepens the vicious circle. The high consumption of refined sugar is thought to be the main cause for the higher rates of hypoglycaemia.

When we start consuming huge amounts of white sugar, our pancreas becomes highly stressed. The occasional binge can be dealt with, but when large intakes of refined carbohydrates are the norm, the strain on the sugar-regulating mechanism becomes intolerable and it breaks down. The pancreas may develop an over-sensitivity to sugar and produce more insulin than is really needed to keep a normal sugar level. This results in a consistently low blood sugar level, which deprives the brain and the nervous system of vital oxygen and produces all the symptoms of hypoglycaemia.

Coffee (especially when taken with sugar) and soft drinks that are high in caffeine contribute to hypoglycaemia by acting on the adrenal glands, brain and liver while sugar is flooding the blood stream. Too much salt in the diet depletes potassium and stress and allergies overtax the adrenal glands. Vitamin deficiencies – particularly zinc, chromium, B vitamins, magnesium, potassium and vitamin E – also contribute to hypoglycaemia. So it is easy to see that the condition, which has such a devastating effect on so many people's equilibrium, is mainly a nutritional disorder.

The influence of sugar in the body goes far beyond carbohydrate metabolism. Fatty acid synthesis and oxidation, cholesterol synthesis and the accumulation of ketone bodies, are all in part controlled by the rate at which glucose is broken down within cells.

Refined sugar causes more build-up of fat than any other carbohydrate except alcohol. This, in turn, means a greater susceptibility to heart attacks and high blood pressure.

Changes in Western eating habits over the last couple of generations have been in the direction of fewer complex carbohydrates (cereals, potatoes etc) and more simple sugars.

Life stresses are also an important factor. Under conditions of stress, more adrenaline is secreted, releasing more sugar from the liver. Repeated stress can impair the function of the adrenal glands, reducing the body's ability to cope with stress. When this happens we get depressed easily, and also develop hypoglycaemic symptoms. Persistent stress is a major cause of depression.

Like diabetes, hypoglycaemia is diagnosed by means of a glucose tolerance test, which can be arranged through your doctor.

A healthy diet, which means only rarely consuming simple sugars or junk food, can keep hypoglycaemia at bay. Plenty of complex carbohydrates and vegetables, together with a good multivitamin and multimineral supplement will go a long way towards this.

There are some simple rules that will improve your diet. These are not to be followed slavishly of course, the occasional sweet treat will do little harm if the mainstay of your diet is good, fresh food.

1 Eat good quality food

If we are what we eat, we do not want to put substandard materials into our bodies. Stick to good, natural foods that have nourished people for generations: fresh vegetables and fruit; fresh fish; poultry, game, beef and lamb – reared organically, if possible; wholegrains; nuts; seeds; pulses, free-range eggs; cold-pressed oils; cheeses, butter and milk.

2 Eat regularly

It is better to eat four or five small meals spread throughout the day, rather than starving all day and bingeing on a large dinner at night. This is also very important for keeping your blood sugar level constant.

3 Eat fresh foods in season

It is sensible to eat a really fresh, locally grown carrot, rather than some green beans that have been flown from Kenya and will have lost some nutrients in transit. It is also cheaper. Local produce is also more likely to have been harvested at its peak. Exotic fruits and vegetables are often chemically treated to ripen them artificially in transit.

4 Avoid over-processed and refined foods

Use wholemeal rather than white flour and eat brown rice rather than white. Try not to eat mass-produced cakes and pastries and sugary cereals. It is easy to munch your way through a packet of high-fat, high-salt crisps merely out of habit, without enjoying them. If you change your diet for a healthier one, after a while the artificial cream gateau will lose its appeal.

5 Eat in moderation

Exercise a little self control. It is not necessary to weigh every wedge of cheese or count out the strands of spaghetti. Listen to your body. A glass of wine occasionally is fine – but not if you go on to down the entire bottle.

6 Eat slowly and calmly

Take time to sit down and enjoy your meal. Grabbing some food and bolting it, when short of time, will play havoc with your digestion.

It is a good idea to begin meals with a salad; this will encourage your digestion to work efficiently, as well as curbing your appetite. Base your meals as much as possible around fresh fruit and vegetables.

Exercise

But getting the diet right is only part of the picture. It is impossible to overestimate the significance of exercise in a healthy and relaxed lifestyle. If a body is never pushed beyond its regular pace, relaxation periods will invariably have less benefit. Exercise doesn't just promote an increase in physical fitness; people who exercise regularly can enjoy a range of secondary benefits.

Regular exercise improves sleep, reduces headaches, improves concentration and increases stamina. Endorphins are released into the brain during exercise and these chemicals promote a sense of positiveness and happiness that will last for some time after the actual activity. This is an effective tool in the fight against depression and a vital move in the preparation for a relaxed life.

People are often accused of putting too much time into their careers or families, and strenuous physical activity is a great antidote to that. In today's society there is a general emphasis on sedentary lifestyles, and it is trend that shows little sign of slowing down. This makes it difficult to find an appropriate outlet for mental negativity and accumulated physical frustration. Physical exertion is great for releasing the toxic emotions that threaten a relaxed sense of wellbeing. You can thrash out tension, anger, frustration and aggression, exercising your mental muscles along with your physical ones.

Exercise, like relaxation, is a personal thing. Just as you will prefer one relaxation method over another, you probably won't like all forms of activity. Your preferences will be affected by your individual personality, physical capabilities and the time you have available. Realistically tailoring your activity to your lifestyle is the best way to ensure that the exercise is kept up.

Skilled sports such as skiing or golf are obviously more appealing if you have the time to invest in learning the game and developing your ability to a certain level. Highly competitive sports such as squash should be viewed with caution if you already have an exceptionally stressful lifestyle. Most experts would advise some form of noncompetitive exercise, like swimming, weight-training or walking, for those with limited time and resources. Even as little as twenty minutes a day put aside for such activities will be of great benefit.

Aerobic exercises

Aerobic activities include swimming, long-distance running, bicycling, rowing, cross-country skiing and even walking – if it is brisk enough. These differ from the other sorts of exercise because they demand your body's efficient use of oxygen throughout the whole time you are doing them.

Oxygen is the ignition factor in the burning of energy from the foods you eat. A good supply is always necessary for your body's metabolic processes to take place efficiently. When your cells – particularly your brain cells – have a good supply, you have stamina, feel well and don't tire easily. If you often feel tired, become depressed easily and have trouble concentrating, it is likely that your body is not getting enough exercise. Taking aerobic exercise will change all that. Any movement of sustained rhythm that puts a constant demand on your heart – raising your pulse rate to between 120 and 160 beats a minute – will bring about several important changes in your body:

It will tone your muscles and improve your circulation. It will increase the number and the size of the blood vessels that carry blood from your heart all over your body so you will have better transport of oxygen. It will increase your body's capacity to take in oxygen by strengthening the chest wall and making you breathe more easily. This oxygen will generate energy. It will make your bones, joints and ligaments stronger so they are more resistant to injury. It will increase the level of energy-rich compounds and enzymes in your body, making it easier for you to use the nutrients in your food. As the efficiency of your heart increases, pumping more blood with each beat, your basic pulse rate will decline.

Walking
Walking is often overlooked as an aerobic activity. A brisk, purposeful walk will improve your muscle condition, your circulation and your posture.

All you need is a good pair of strong shoes and a lightweight, waterproof jacket. Start off by walking for thirty minutes a day. Walk fast enough to make yourself a little out of breath and vary your route so you are not walking on flat ground all the time.

After a week or two, you can increase the time you walk to about forty-five minutes. By now you should be seeing the benefits: you will probably be sleeping better, your concentration will be sharper and you will feel better balanced emotionally.

Walking is an ideal aerobic exercise because you can do it wherever you are – in the country or the city. You need no equipment to measure your progress – you do not need to stop and take your pulse. Get into the habit of walking briskly every day and you will be rewarded with a fit body, glowing skin and a new sense of wellbeing.

Running
Running is the most satisfying form of aerobic exercise for many

people. No special training is needed and it can be done anywhere – at home or on holiday. All you need is a good pair of running shoes and the self-discipline to get started. You may be surprised to find that before long you too are hooked and can't imagine life without this liberating activity.

Before you start on a programme of running, it is important to check your fitness. If you are over thirty-five, suffer from high blood pressure, have a family history of heart disease or have recently been ill, it is a good idea to have a check-up with your doctor to make sure that running is safe for you.

There is a simple way to check your own fitness level. Simply walk two miles in thirty minutes at a brisk pace and ask yourself how you feel afterwards. If you feel no nausea or dizziness you are fit enough to start a graded programme of running. If, however, you find the two-mile walk difficult, persevere until you can do it comfortably in half an hour. You may be surprised how quickly this happens – walking for half an hour each day can have a marked effect on your condition. Here is a programme that you can follow:

First week:

Take a brisk walk of one mile, breaking into a jog of roughly 50–100 metres whenever you feel like it. In between these jogs, walk at a steady pace but do not force yourself. Pushing yourself too hard in the beginning is counter-productive and you could end up with strains or injuries that set you back. You should feel relaxed enough that you are able to appreciate your surroundings.

Second week:

Walk/jog for a mile, alternating about 100 strides of each at a stretch.

Third week:

Walk/jog for one and a half miles, increasing your jogging intervals to 150 strides with 100 strides of walking in between.

Fourth week:

Jog for a while at the speed that you find most comfortable. Don't worry if you have to stop from time to time to walk, although by now you should be finding that minor discomforts are fleeting and that you can run through them.

Fifth week:

Run a mile in less than nine minutes.

Sixth week:

Jog/run for one and a half miles or more. By now you should have passed through the initial barrier and be beginning to reap all the rewards of your perseverance. You will be more aware of your body and able to listen to what it is telling you. Your stamina will be increased and you can vary your running by pushing yourself more on the days when you feel in top condition and ready for a challenge.

By the end of six months, you should be able to run easily and steadily for between half an hour and an hour, covering a distance between three and nine miles. This programme leads on to a flexible regime of running. Enjoy running and don't get fixated with rigid training schedules. To reap the true benefits of running, aim to run for thirty minutes at least three times a week. This is more effective at building fitness than one running session of one and a half hours. If you want to run every day, it is a good idea to take one day off each week to give your muscles a chance to restore themselves and build up their store of glucose again. This day of rest will only improve the quality of your running.

Running has knock-on effects for health and relaxation. The more you run, the more you will feel in touch with your body. You will find yourself naturally drawn towards healthier foods, your skin will be clearer, and health problems like constipation and insomnia will disappear. As you look better and feel better, you may feel that running is addictive in the best sense of the word.

What to wear

Clothes made from fabrics that breathe, like cotton, are much better than those made from man-made fibres. In summer a pair of shorts and a T-shirt are ideal: running in bare legs increases the sense of freedom. In winter a cotton tracksuit with a fleecy lining is fine, perhaps with a lightweight waterproof jacket when it's raining. If it is very cold outside a wool cap will protect your ears.

Proper running shoes are not cheap, but they are an excellent investment. They should be not too flexible, without studs and with a high-density sole. Some excellent soles are made of microcellular rubber. Some soles on running shoes extend up the toe and heel to take account of the rocking movement from heel to toe that comes with running. The padded instep helps to absorb shock from running on hard ground. These special design features make you far less likely to risk the sort of injury to tendons or muscles that can come if you run in an old pair of tennis shoes. There should be plenty of room inside for your toes to move about and the heel should be slightly raised to help prevent injury to your Achilles tendon that comes with overstretching. It should have at least five set of holes for laces, so the shoe hugs your foot: in fact, the shoes should feel, when you are out and running, as if they are part of your feet. Plastic shoes are not a good idea because they make your feet sweat: light leather or nylon is a much better bet.

Cotton socks help absorb shock and, because you can change them every time you run, they keep your shoes fresh.

Warm up

It is not a good idea to jump straight out of bed and go running. You need to warm up your muscles and get your metabolic rate up first. If you run when your muscles are stiff or cold after a long period of inactivity, you are much more likely to pull a muscle or injure a joint. Simply moving about the house briskly for ten minutes will ease your body into action but, if you have time, it is a good idea to do some warm-up exercises. These will also limber the back of your legs, tighten your tummy muscles and strengthen your ankles – covering the muscle areas that running leaves out. Here are six stretching and firming exercises that many regular runners rely on:

1 For your calf muscles and Achilles tendons: stand a little under a metre from a tree or wall. With your feet flat on the ground, lean into it until the backs of your legs hurt a little. Hold the position for ten seconds and then relax. Repeat six times.

2 For tight hamstrings at the back of your legs: keeping your legs straight, put one heel up on a table at waist level (lower, if you cannot reach that high). Now lower your head down to your knee until you feel the strain. Hold the position for ten seconds, holding on to your leg or foot to steady yourself if you need to. Repeat (with each leg) six times.

3 For lower back and hamstrings: lie on your back, arms at your sides. Keeping your legs straight, bring them up over your head. Now lower them as far as possible above your head – touching the floor if you can. Hold for ten seconds and relax. Repeat six times.

4 For your shin muscles: sit on the edge of a table and hold a weight of about two kilograms on the front part of your foot just behind the toes (a small bucket or old paint tin filled with stones is ideal). Keep them there for a few seconds and then lower. Repeat a few times with each foot.

5 For your quadriceps: sit on the table and hang the weight over the toes of one foot so the bucket or tin is resting on the floor and you are not stretching the knee ligaments. Now straighten your knee, raising the weight. Hold for a few seconds and then lower. Repeat six times with each leg.

6 For tummy muscles: do twenty sit-ups with your knees bent and your feet tucked under a heavy piece of furniture if this helps you keep your balance. Clasp your hands behind your head and keep your chin in, curling your body up from the floor.

If you don't have time to go through this routine before you run, start running very slowly and keep to a slow, steady jog for the first five minutes or so until your muscles start to warm up. This is very important if you want to protect yourself from injury.

Never run after a meal, a hot bath, or when you are feeling really cold.

Cool down

It is just as important to cool off properly after a run, and your muscles should cool off gradually. A good way of achieving this is by walking for five or ten minutes after every run. This keeps extra blood flowing through the muscles and helps your body to eliminate the waste products of exercise such as lactic acid, which can otherwise make you stiff or sore.

If you like, do some stretching exercises, such as bending over from the hips. You should find that any muscular aches and pains vanish quickly as your body responds to your new regime and works itself into condition.

Problems

Don't worry if you get a stitch while you are running. Stop and walk or jog slowly through it until it passes. As you become fitter, stitches will become fewer. If you find areas of skin becoming irritated where they rub together – between the thighs, for example – apply a little petroleum jelly to the spot.

If you experience a sharp pain in a muscle, you should stop running. You may have torn some fibres and the muscle may harden and swell, which is a sign that it is bleeding inside. Place a cold compress – like a bag of frozen peas – on the area and, if the pain doesn't go away in a couple of days, it is a good idea to see your doctor. Of course, if you experience a sharp pain in your chest, you must stop running at once and seek medical advice.

Progress

When you first start running you will find yourself breathing deeper and faster as your body seeks more oxygen to meet the new demands being made on it. You may feel some stiffness in your chest as your muscles expand to help you to breathe more fully. After some minutes of running, you will probably experience the 'oxygen debt', when your body demands more oxygen than it is able to process efficiently at that moment. It is quite common at this point to feel that you want to stop. Walk slowly for a while, breathing deeply.

You may also find that your joints feel stiff, with your legs as heavy as lead. They are merely letting you know that they are being used in a way that is unusual for them. This is perfectly normal and will pass.

You will find, however, that when you are able to run for between six and ten minutes without having to stop and walk, you will come into your second wind. Suddenly your running is easier and you find yourself breathing more freely, coursing forward in a fresh and unrestricted way. If you are new to running, it will take time to reach this phase but, as you persevere, eventually it will come every time you run.

After several weeks running, when you can run for half an hour or so without stopping, you may experience your 'third wind'. You run until your legs are beginning to feel heavy and you are breathing hard. You are just thinking that you should stop, when your running suddenly changes gear, becoming almost automatic. Your body feels lighter and you feel as if you could run on and on. This kind of euphoria is known as 'runner's high' and is one of the reasons that running is such a good tool for anyone seeking relaxation in the deepest sense of the word. Perceptions are heightened and, as your mind clears, problems are seen in their proper perspective. It doesn't happen during every run, but it is an experience well worth working towards.

If you make running part of your routine, you will find that you gain energy in every area of your life – mental and physical.

It is important not to push yourself too hard in the beginning, especially if you are not used to regular exercise. It is always a good idea to seek advice on which form of sport to take up and to consult your doctor before you begin. Ease yourself into an exercise programme, as doing too much too soon could lead to physical exhaustion or injury. Also remember that the body benefits more from short periods of regular exercise than from infrequent bursts.

It is impossible to overestimate the importance of exercise in managing stress. The stress reaction encourages a state of high energy but there is usually no place for that energy to go; therefore, our bodies can stay in a state of arousal for hours at a time. Exercise is the most logical way to dissipate this excess energy. It is what our bodies are trying to do when we pace around or tap our legs and fingers. It is much better to channel it into a more complete form of exercise like a brisk walk, a run, a bike ride or a game of squash. During times of high stress, we could benefit from an immediate physical outlet – but this often is not possible. However, regular exercise can drain off ongoing stress and keep things under control: it improves sleep, reduces headaches, creates a feeling of wellbeing, helps concentration and increases stamina. Chemicals called endorphins are released into the brain during exercise. Morphine-like in their effect, these substances promote a sense of positivity and happiness, which will last for some time after exercising.

At the very least, it is important to exercise three times per week for a minimum of 30 minutes each time. Aerobic activities like walking, jogging, swimming, cycling, squash, skiing, aerobics classes and dancing are suitable. Choose things you like to do or they will feel like a chore and you will begin to avoid them. It is important not to push yourself too hard in the beginning, and to seek medical advice on which form of sport to take up. The body benefits more from short periods of regular exercise rather than infrequent bursts. Ease yourself into an exercise programme, as doing too much too soon could lead to physical exhaustion or injury.

Sleep

As mundane as it sounds, sleep is an important way of reducing stress. Fatigue is a common component of chronic stress (in some cases resulting from stress-induced insomnia), and when tired it is more difficult to cope with stressful situations. These dynamics can create a vicious cycle. When distressed individuals get more sleep, they feel better and are more resilient and adaptable in dealing with day-to-day events.

Most people know what their usual sleep requirement is (the range is five to ten hours per night; the average being seven to eight), but a surprisingly large percentage of the population is chronically sleep-deprived. If you do feel constantly tired, go to bed 30 to 60 minutes earlier and monitor the results after a few days or a week. If you are still tired, go to bed 30 minutes earlier than this. Eventually, there will be a pattern which does help to reduce stress. The three criteria of success are:

- waking refreshed
- plenty of daytime energy
- waking naturally before the alarm goes off

Sleeping-in is fine, but if you sleep too long, it throws off your body rhythms during the following day. It is better to go to bed earlier.

Daytime naps are an interesting phenomenon. They can be valuable if they are short and timed properly (i.e. not in the evening). The catnap is a short sleep (five to 20 minutes) that can be rejuvenating. A nap lasting more than 30 minutes can make you feel groggy. If you suffer with insomnia daytime naps are not a good idea. Beyond these cautionary notes, getting more sleep can be important in reducing stress and helping you to cope and function better.

Leisure

No one would expect a tennis player to complete an entire match without taking breaks. Surprisingly though, many otherwise rational people think nothing of working from dawn to dusk without taking a break and then wonder why they become distressed.

Stop smoking

Many people use cigarettes as a coping mechanism in times of stress, and it seems that smoking can help to reduce stress in the short term. The long-term hazards of smoking, however, far out-weigh its palliative properties. Smoking is one of the major causes of illness and death worldwide. Cigarettes unquestionably cause a variety of cancers, especially of the lung and bladder, and also contribute to the development of hypertension, respiratory ill-ness and heart disease.

Pacing

It is important to learn to monitor stress and energy levels, and then pace ourselves accordingly. Pacing is about awareness and vigilance – knowing when to extend ourselves and when to ease up. It is also about acting on the information supplied by our bod-ies. The graph below illustrates the relationship between stress and performance, and leads to the following important conclu-sions:

- Increased stress produces increased performance, initially.
- Once you pass a certain point (the hump), any more stress results in decreased performance. Trying harder at this point is unproductive or even counterproductive. The only sensible option is to take a break.
- We need a certain amount of stress to function well. However, stress becomes harmful when there is too much, when it lasts too long, or when it occurs too often.
- One of the first symptoms of distress is fatigue, which we tend to ignore. It is a good idea to take steps to reduce stress levels at this point, before fatigue becomes exhaustion.

The other key to pacing is taking periodic rest. Too many peo-ple go far too long without breaks. Just as we all have cycles of deep sleep and dream sleep throughout the night (at roughly 90- to 120-minute intervals), we also have cycles through the day (peaks of energy and concentration interspersed with troughs of low energy and inefficiency). These cycles are called ultradian rhythms because they happen many times per day (as opposed to the 25-hour circadian rhythm). We need to watch for these troughs and take 20-minute breaks when they occur, as opposed to working through them and building up stress.

It is not always convenient for us to take breaks when nature tells us to, but we can all become better at this. A mid-morning break, lunch, a mid-afternoon break and supper divide the day into roughly two hour segments. These time-outs can include catnaps, meditation, daydreaming, a social interlude, a short walk, a refreshment break, a change to low-concentration tasks, or listening to music. Like the catnap, it is simply a good investment of time that pays itself back quickly in increased productivity and reduced stress.

Work/leisure balance

Optimizing the balance between work and leisure is an important means to eliminating unwanted stress in our lives. Despite all our labour-saving devices, leisure is still an elusive commodity for most people. Statistics show that we are working an extra three hours per week compared with 20 years ago. That translates into an extra month of work each year. Add to that the phenomenon of the two career family (which makes family and leisure time even more scarce) and you start to get a picture of society on an accelerating treadmill.

Leisure time and levels of distress are inversely proportional – the less leisure, the more stress. It may be useful to divide your life (excluding sleep time) into four compartments (work, family, community and self) and then to assess what percentage of your time and energy in an average week goes into each part. There is no normal range, but when work is over 60 per cent and/or when self is less than 10 per cent this indicates there may be a problem with stress. We all require time to meet our own needs (self-care, self-nurturing, etc) and when that is neglected, trouble usually follows. Self-directed activities can include exercise or recreation, relaxation, socializing, entertainment and hobbies.

The word leisure is derived from the Latin word *licere,* which means 'permission'. The main reason so many people do not have enough leisure is that they are not giving themselves permission to make the time to enjoy it. Leisure is one of the most pleasant stress relievers ever invented, and it is strange that people resist it so much.

Conventional treatment for stress

It may not always be possible to alleviate all the causes and symptoms of stress without professional help. In addition to the family doctor, there is a great variety of various alternative therapies and medicines available, many of which provide excellent stress relief.

Tranquillizers

There are a variety of tranquillizing drugs that act to suppress the central nervous system, thereby reducing anxiety and other stress-related symptoms. Benzodiazepines, such as Valium, Librium or Ativan, are the most commonly prescribed minor tranquillizers. Because these products have few side effects and are relatively safe in overdose, they have come to replace barbiturates as prescribed sedatives and sleeping pills.

Benzodiazepines depress mental activity and alertness, but do not generally make you drowsy or clumsy as do barbiturates, but they do affect driving and similar skills. Alone, benzodiazepines cannot produce the 'high' that alcohol or barbiturates produce, and after up to two weeks' continuous use, they may become ineffective as sleeping pills, and after four months may become ineffective against anxiety. Long-term dependence is more likely to be psychological; the pills become a means of coping with stressful events, and there may be severe anxiety if the drug is unavailable. Withdrawal symptoms appear in many users if they suddenly stop taking such drugs after about eight years' treatment with normal doses. Symptoms include insomnia, anxiety, tremor, irritability, nausea and vomiting. Such symptoms are more noticeable with shorter-acting benzodiazepines such as lorazepam and temazepam.

In the 1950s and 1960s doctors would prescribe minor tranquillizers almost indiscriminately and for indefinite periods. Nowadays the medical profession is more aware that the short-term benefits of these drugs can be outweighed by long-term problems of dependency and withdrawal. In Britain in 1988, the Committee on Safety of Medicines recommended that minor tranquillizers should be prescribed for a period of no longer than two to four weeks.

Counselling and psychotherapy

There are various support organizations and counselling services available to help with stress management. These range from expensive specialist stress-management experts to free stress clinics run by local doctors. Counselling is especially good for short-term problems: trained experts help you to examine the causes of problems and devise strategies to avoid negative behaviour patterns and restore a sense of physical and emotional wellbeing.

Psychotherapy is used for resolving deeper, long-term emotional and psychological problems. Psychotherapy is usually offered by psychiatrists, clinical psychologists, and psychiatric social workers. Psychiatric social workers are trained in treatment methods and often work as part of a treatment team in hospitals or clinics. Today psychotherapy is being practised more and more by paraprofessionals, who have less training but may be supervised by a professional or may be trained to work with specific problems using specific methods.

Psychotherapy is conducted in several formats. Individual therapy refers to a therapist's work with one person on his or her unique problem; the relationship between client and therapist may be particularly important in producing change. In group therapy, therapists meet with a group of patients, and the interactions between patients become an important part of the therapy process.

Many different theories or schools of psychotherapy exist. Two of the more common are psychodynamic therapy and behavioural therapy.

Psychodynamic therapy

Psychodynamic therapy makes the fundamental assumption that emotional disorders are merely symptoms of internal, unobservable and unconscious conflicts between personality components. These conflicts result from unresolved family conflicts, experienced in early stages of childhood, that become reactivated in problem situations in adulthood. The aim of psychodynamic therapies is to revive the early conflict and to transfer it to the relationship with the therapist. The symptoms are removed when the therapist helps the patient to resolve the conflict in the transference relationship. The therapist interprets the transference to the patient and helps him or her overcome resistances to accepting the interpretation. Additional methods, such as dream interpretation or word-association techniques, are used to aid in uncovering unconscious material. Sigmund Freud's psychoanalysis is the primary example of a psychodynamic therapy.

Behavioural therapy

Behavioural approaches assume that all behaviour is learned. Emotional disorders are considered to be conditioned responses or habits that can be modified by the same principles of learning that govern all behaviour. From this perspective psychotherapy means providing corrective learning or conditioning experiences. Different therapy techniques are employed for remedying specific disordered behaviours. In social–skills training, for instance, patients practise handling difficult interpersonal situations via role playing.

Natural methods of therapy – relaxation techniques

An effective way to reduce stress in the body is through certain disciplines that fall under the heading of relaxation techniques.

Just as we are all capable of mounting and sustaining a stress reaction, we have also inherited the ability to put our bodies into a state of deep relaxation, called the 'relaxation response'. In this state, all the physiological events in the stress reaction are reversed: the pulse slows down, blood pressure falls, breathing becomes slower, and the muscles relax. But whereas the stress reaction is automatic, the relaxation response has to be deliberately induced. Fortunately, there are many ways of doing this. Sitting quietly in a park or beside the fireplace, gently petting the family cat, reclining on the sofa and other restful activities can generate this state. There also are specific skills that can be learned that are efficient and beneficial.

A state of deep relaxation achieved through meditation or self-hypnosis is actually more physiologically restful than sleep. These techniques are best learned through formal training courses, which are taught in a variety of places. Books and relaxation tapes can be used when courses are not available or are beyond your budget. On days when exercise is not possible, relaxation techniques are an excellent way to bring down the body's stress level. Whereas exercise dissipates stress energy, relaxation techniques neutralize it, producing a calming effect. As little as 20 minutes once or twice per day confers significant benefit.

Planning ahead

Making time in a busy schedule is probably the hardest of all the relaxation criteria to satisfy. You may need to obtain the cooperation of your friends, family or colleagues. If people close to you see you disappearing behind a locked door for twenty minutes or so, they may start wondering – so explain to them what you are doing. You may have to endure a bit of leg-pulling until other people come to appreciate the importance of it to you. If you fail to get support, then you will have to change your itinerary (or your friends).

Choose a time when you are least likely to be disturbed: early morning or late at night, if necessary. You should prepare yourself for relaxation by exercising moderately for five to ten minutes beforehand. You should also exercise moderately for up to three minutes afterwards to help you reorientate. Twenty minutes is the minimum time to spend on this three-part routine.

Get comfortable

It is up to you to ensure that you relax in a completely disturbance-free atmosphere. There must be no radio, no TV, no background music, no incense. Turn on the telephone answering machine and turn down the ringer if it is in the same room. It is best to avoid meals just before relaxation.

Find a comfortable chair in which to sit. Your back and neck should be straight, your shoulders not hunched forward. Your hands should rest comfortably in your lap half open. Your feet should be on the floor and your legs should not be crossed, just sit naturally. Next make sure there is nothing in the room to distract you, such as insects, draughts, direct sunlight. If you're relaxing in a group do so with experienced people – there's nothing less conducive to relaxation than an outburst of giggles from your flatmate or the person who shares your office.

Loosen off tight clothing like belts, ties and shoe laces. If you must lie down to get comfortable, rest your hands about an inch away from your body either side and don't cross your legs. Physical discomfort of any sort will provoke the secretion of adrenaline to spur you into remedial action, creating a sense of restlessness. Listen to what your body is trying to tell you about avoidable discomfort in your posture and remove the source before you go on.

Correct breathing

Breathing for relaxation should be moderate, slow and rhythmic. Don't hold your breath, and conversely, don't take short gasping breaths. Your whole chest should be involved in breathing – not just the top half – so use both chest and diaphragm muscles. Don't fully inhale or exhale and above all, don't force your breathing, make it natural. Sigh or take deep breaths if you need to – but do try to make it moderate, slow and rhythmic.

'Don't hold your breath' is an often heard expression, and one that suggests that we are always in full control of our breathing. Usually, of course, we are, but that is not always the case. During a normal day we take between 16,000 and 21,000 breaths. This automatic action is one of the first things to go when we become stressed. Our breathing gets shallower and accelerates erratically. Erratic breathing patterns lead to disorientation and emotional wavering, which can create even more stress – thus a vicious cycle begins. Investigating the breathing pattern and learning to control it is an important step in learning to control stress.

The brain controls our breathing by checking the ratio between oxygen and carbon dioxide in the blood. We exhale when the carbon dioxide makes the blood too acidic. Hyperventilation (fast, deep breathing) makes us expend too much carbon dioxide, leaving the blood in an alkaline state. This induces dizziness and disorientation, as the brain is starved of carbon dioxide.

Habitual hyperventilation causes fainting, numbness, palpitations, sweating and chest aches – all symptoms of carbon dioxide deficiency. These create a cause and effect cycle – erratic breathing induces other unpleasant symptoms, which in turn make our breathing worse.

Obviously, these symptoms occur when we are very stressed. But there are more subtle signs that breathing patterns could be better – gulping, holding the breath, moving the upper chest when talking and breathing, and frequent yawning.

Try a simple test to find out if you are breathing correctly. Lay a hand on the upper section of your chest and the other hand on the lower part of your rib-cage. If only your chest moves when you breathe, then you are breathing ineffectively. If the lower edge of the rib cage expands and the stomach rises at the start of each breath, then you are breathing correctly.

When stress hits, regular breathing is the first thing to go. To enable you to maintain easy breathing under stress, it is important to practise breathing exercises. It can sometimes seem difficult to slow down and become conscious about such an automatic act, but regular controlled breathing exercises are a very good way of getting your whole body to relax and to work out stress. Just a few minutes each day given over to fully concentrating on these exercises will bring great relief from stress.

Bad posture can effect the flow of air in and out of the body. Try lying down on your back to give the lungs and diaphragm freedom to move and leave the body relaxed and flexible. By removing the upright strain on your body and lungs there is more chance of developing an easy breathing pattern.

While breathing, focus on raising the abdomen, and filling lower, mid and upper sections with air. Be aware of the expansion of your ribs as you hold your breath – concentrate on that feeling. To exhale, pull in your diaphragm towards the back of your spine, slowly and smoothly. Try to ensure that you fully empty your lungs before inhaling again. This is commonly overlooked when breathing, which means that the lungs are never used to their full potential.

Correct attitude

The human mind is a highly complex, mostly automatic processing machine. If you have expectations that are not met, your mind will unconsciously generate a stress response as the first stage in remedying the situation. That stress response will initiate a host of subliminal physiological reactions that make you feel like doing something – the heart rate increases, muscles tense, and a lowering of the body's surface temperature makes you feel uncomfortable. Your attitude, your expectations and your intent are the foundation of your thoughts and your actions. If this foundation is not in keeping with your reality your relaxation will not be complete. Therefore, set your intent on relaxing without expectations and when you get it right it will be a very peaceful, restful and invigorating twenty minutes.

Thought control

Thinking is a form of internalized action, a visualization of consequences. Through thought we are distinguished from animals who act on instinct alone. However, the mind is an imperfect mirror, and every thought carries with it a kind of charge capable of setting off a stress response before rational decision making can take its turn. For relaxation this is a problem because that thought charge is just as potent as any external stimulus, as anxiety sufferers know only too well.

In order to relax effectively, that is, to reduce the stress response to a minimum for a meaningful period of time, thought has got to be put on hold – you have to stop the internal dialogue.

In the mind there are preconscious entities that float around, dragging you into self-dialogue. Recognizing these entities and avoiding their lure is a skill arrived at only with practice, and you must practise this skill every time you relax.

Perseverance

It may look easy to start with, but the benefits of this exercise are mainly long term. Other than noticing an improvement in your ability to sleep at night (or catnap during the day) you may spend many sessions doubting that benefit until you have grown stronger mentally and physically. It is important to persevere – 20 minutes minimum – every day.

Meditation

Meditation is central to the Hindu way of life, and is also an integral part of the other great oriental religions, Buddhism and its close cousin, Zen. It also has its place in Sufism, Christianity and Judaism. (That said, meditation does not require adherence to any of the faiths and religions that advocate it.)

Many people view meditation as peaceful but ineffectual self-centredness. They are wrong: the benefits to be gained from meditation in any of its various forms are many. Those who meditate regularly believe that it leads to a significant lowering of mental tension and negative emotions, while at the same time increasing efficiency at work and deepening the sense of inner calm. This feeling of wellbeing brings physical benefits: regular meditation eliminates or reduces stress; can ease migraine and tension headaches; reduces blood pressure; benefits the heart; and reduces the pain of menstrual cramps.

In its simplest form, meditation is nothing more than allowing the mind to be lulled by a simple repetitive sensation – waves lapping on the beach, the tinkling of a fountain, repeating a word or sound over and over again, even something as mundane as the sound of machinery, any of these, and countless others, can be used as something on to which the mind focuses so strongly that problems and anxieties are crowded out. In its more refined, mystical guise, it is a means to total self-fulfilment, being completely at one with the universe.

Meditation is neither a time-consuming process – 20 minutes a day are all that is needed – nor is it, as many suspect, a form of self-hypnosis. Practised properly, it is a life-enhancing voyage during which preconceived opinions and ideas fade, the senses and the intellect are refined and the ability to concentrate is increased.

A simple meditation technique

Sit in a comfortable chair, with your feet flat on the floor, your legs and arms uncrossed. (This can also be done lying down, but you might fall asleep). Rest your hands on your upper legs, with your palms down. Close your eyes, so your mind won't be distracted by what is going on around you.

Direct your focus of awareness to a place six inches (about 20 centimetres) directly above the centre of the top of your head. Here is a location in consciousness which is always calm and radiant, no matter what is going on elsewhere in your mind or body, or around you. It is called the 'upper room'. Think of a point of pure, crystal-white light here. Don't 'try' to visualize it. If you see it, fine, but if you don't, it doesn't matter. As you think of the point of white light, it grows brighter, expanding into a little star, three inches (about 10 centimetres) in diameter.

Think and let the star burn away the veils that have kept it hidden all these years. Direct the star to open, releasing a downpour of cleansing and purifying life energy. This energy is crystal-clear, like fresh spring water.

Let the energy flow through your hair, scalp, into the bones of your head and face, into your brain, eyes, ears, nose, mouth, down the neck, through your shoulders, arms and hands. Experience it flowing through your chest and back, abdomen, hips, pelvic area, upper legs, knees, lower legs, ankles and feet. Think and let the soles of your feet open, releasing the energy into the earth beneath your feet. Now it is flowing through your whole body.

Think of the bottoms of your feet closing, so the energy begins to reflow up through the areas you have cleared out. Experience it in your legs, hips, torso, shoulders, arms, hands, neck and head. Let it overflow out of the top of your head, surrounding your body with an aura of crystal-clear white light.

Bring your hands together, almost but not quite touching, palms facing each other, out in front of your body. Experience the energy flowing through your hands. You could use this energy to heal others, by laying your lighted hands on the person's head, heart, or wherever they have discomfort. Whatever you touch with your hands lighted this way will be filled with inner light-fire-energy.

If you experience discomfort anywhere in your body as you are working with the inner light, think of the 'consuming fire' aspect of the energy. Hold the focus of it in the area of discomfort to burn through the obstructions to the flow of your pure life energy. Afterwards, take a few minutes to assimilate the radiant essence of the light into any area that you have cleared out with the consuming fire aspect.

In addition to your focusing of the energy during meditation, as described above, you can work with the downpour anytime and anywhere, day or night, with your eyes open or closed, as appropriate to the situation. You can use it as an inner shower while you take your outer shower in the morning. Every time you think of the star and the white light downpouring, it continues for about 30 minutes. So you can literally fill your day with inner light. It's also a great way to go to sleep at night. For stress-reduction it is best to practice the technique for at least a few minutes every day.

Autogenic training

Autogenic training is a form of therapy that seeks to teach the patient to relax, thereby relieving stress. This is achieved by the patient learning a series of six basic exercises that can be undertaken either lying flat on the back, sitting in an armchair or sitting wards the edge of a chair with the head bent forwards and the chin on the chest. The six exercises concentrate on (a) breathing and respiration (b) heartbeat (c) the forehead to induce a feeling of coolness (d) the lower abdomen and stomach to induce a feeling of warmth (e) the arms and legs to induce a feeling of warmth (f) the neck, shoulders, arms and legs to induce a feeling of heaviness.

It is now well established that a number of illnesses and disorders are related to, or made worse by, stress. By learning the techniques and exercises of autogenic training, the person is able to achieve a state of relaxation and tranquillity, sleeps better and generally has more energy and a greater feeling of wellbeing. Autogenic training is taught at group sessions involving a small number of people (about six is usual).

Patients with a variety of disorders may benefit from autogenic training, which can also help people who feel under stress without particular physical symptoms. Illnesses that may be helped include irritable bowel syndrome, digestive disorders, muscular aches and cramps, ulcers, headaches and high blood pressure. Also, anxieties, fears and phobias, insomnia and some other psychological illnesses. This form of therapy can benefit people of all age groups, although it is considered that children under the age of six may not be able to understand the training. Therapists in autogenic training usually hold medical or nursing qualifications and expect to obtain a full picture of the patient's state of health before treatment begins. Therapy is both available privately and through the National Health Service in some areas of Great Britain.

Massage

Inactive lifestyles and sedentary occupations have created a society of people with cramped, stooped, and neglected postures. By realigning our bodies, massage can help to repair damaged postures. Not only does massage help to coax the spine and corresponding physiology back into position, it also makes us more aware of our bodies. Relieved of muscle tension, the body feels lighter and can therefore be borne more naturally and with mor poise. Used in conjunction with postural therapies such as th Alexander technique (*see* page 18), massage is a valuable contri bution towards a relaxed yet controlled posture.

Many of the benefits of massage come through the healer–pa tient contact. Our hands are one of the most sensitive parts of ou body – we experience much of our sense of touch through ou hands. Hand healers are believed to help people through thei hands, often without even touching the body. There is a certai element of this in massage techniques. The masseur is commu nicating feelings of harmony and relaxation through their hands allowing a benign force to flow into the client. Many practitioner therefore believe that it is important for the masseur to be in positive state of mind.

During a massage the patient is coaxed from emotional an occupational stresses and brought into the intense arena of th here and now. Such one-on-one non-verbal communication is valuable element in our overstressed lifestyles.

For more on the benefits and techniques of massage *see* pag 42.

Yoga

Yoga is a technique of self-awareness that has been practised i the East as a physical, psychological and philosophical disciplin for over 5,000 years. The word 'yoga' derives from the Sanskr *yuk,* meaning 'to bind together', and the aim of yoga is to inte grate the mind and the body and commune with the universa process of being.

Yoga is not a religion and does not require adherence to an particular dogma; it is basically a technique for personal develop ment, enabling people to explore and fulfil their physical and spir itual needs. Over the last quarter of the twentieth century yog has become increasingly popular in the West, and its effective ness in relieving stress is widely acknowledged within the medi cal profession. Practised regularly, yoga creates mental clarit emotional stability, deep relaxation and body awareness.

See page 75 for a fuller explanation of the benefits and positions of Yoga.

Traditional Chinese medicine

About 2,500 years ago, deep in the mountains of Northern China, Taoist priests practiced Ki Gong – meditative movement revealing and cultivating the vital life force. They believed this force, ki (pronounced 'chi' in China, 'ki' in Japan), was inseparable from life itself. They discovered that ki animated not only body and earth, but was the energetic force of the entire universe. Traditional Chinese medicine is a philosophy of preserving health, and is based first and foremost on an understanding of the ultimate power of ki. In contrast to much of Western medicine, traditional Chinese medicine is a preventative practice, strengthening the immune system to ward off disease.

In traditional Chinese medicine, ki is manifested both as *yin* (cold, dark, and 'interior'), and *yang* (warm, light, and 'exterior'). In fact, ki is present in all the opposites we experience, such as night and day, hot and cold, growth and decay. And although yin and yang may be perceived as opposites, they are actually inseparable. The recognition of one is essential to the recognition of the other. The balance between them is like the motion of night and day; at the instant darkness reaches its zenith at midnight, the cycle has begun to flow steadily towards dawn. At noon, the zenith of light, the day begins slowly to turn towards the darkness of night. All the internal organs of the body are subject to this nocturnal–diurnal swing of the universe.

This world view further holds that ki, manifesting as yin/yang, makes up the universe in the form of five elements: wood, fire, earth, metal, and water. These five elements also represent our bodily constitution as human beings, making us one with the universe. Ki flows into our bodies, up from the earth in its yin form and down from the heavens in its yang form. The energy channels in our bodies through which it moves are called 'meridians'.

These meridians do not directly correspond to any anatomical component recognized by Western medicine. The best way to understand the flow of ki through the meridians is to compare to the flow of blood in our veins and arteries. If our blood does not reach our toes, they become dead. If our blood does not flow freely we have high or low blood pressure. If our blood clots, we have an embolism or a stroke. Similarly, unbalanced or stagnant ki can cause many diseases and ailments. In fact, traditional Chinese medicine is based on the principle that every illness, ailment, and discomfort in the body can be explained in terms of an imbalance of ki.

Each meridian is related to one of the five elements. For example, the heart meridian is related to the element fire, the kidney and bladder to water. Along the meridians are pressure points, or 'gateways', special places where ki can become blocked. With the help of a trained practitioner, its flow can be freed and balance restored.

Out of the belief system of traditional Chinese medicine arose many healing methods, all directed to the balancing of ki. These include acupuncture, shiatsu, Tai Chi Ch'uan and herbalism.

Acupuncture

This is a form of traditional Chinese medicine that uses the gentle insertion of hair-fine needles into specific points on the body to stimulate the flow of one's ki, or natural healing energy. As we have already seen, according to ancient Chinese medicine Ki flows through the body in channels, called meridians, and illness is the result of an imbalance of ki.

Most people are surprised to learn that acupuncture needles are very thin (from ten to fifteen acupuncture needles can fit into one conventional hypodermic needle). Acupuncturists can attain a high level of skill in gently placing these tiny needles into the skin with a minimum of discomfort.

Acupuncture excels in those areas in which conventional medicine offers limited relief – chronic disease, pain control, and stress-related disorders. Acupuncture treatments are drug-free; you avoid side effects or dependency. However, you should always inform ny practitioner about all pre-existing conditions, the names of ll medicines you are taking, whether you are, or could be, pregant, and if you have a cardiac pacemaker or cosmetic implants. our acupuncturist will be able to evaluate your specific situation ith this information to ensure the best form of treatment.

See also Acupuncture page 11.

hiatsu

hiatsu is a Japanese healing art combining the principles of traitional Chinese medicine with practices similar to those of acuuncture but performed without needles. Shiatsu is a balance – a ance – between practitioner and receiver, in which the healing ower of both build upon each other to clear and balance the vital fe force known as ki.

Shiatsu is a Japanese word: *shi* meaning 'finger', and *atsu* meanng 'pressure'. But shiatsu is more than acupressure. It is a comination of many different techniques, including pressing, hookng, sweeping, shaking, rotating, grasping, vibrating, patting, lucking, lifting, pinching, rolling, brushing, and, in one variaion – barefoot shiatsu – it includes walking on the person's back, egs, and feet.

But these are merely the physical techniques. With an awareess of psychological and spiritual implications, shiatsu has beome, indeed, a kind of dance between giver and receiver. A unique apport develops between the practitioner and client, because hiatsu relies on the simple but powerful experience of touch to waken the client's own self-healing powers. This 'touch comunication' between practitioner and client is fundamental to all ealing methods.

See page 154 for more on Shiatsu.

romatherapy

n the past the human sense of smell was crucial to our survival – e could smell intruders, sense which plants were poisonous and rack game through their odour. Obviously, the need for this abil-ty has lessened, and we are now more likely to appreciate the

smell of the latest perfumery sensation, or suffer under the stenc
of cigarettes or cigars. However, we are still extremely suscepti
ble to smell – both personal and environmental. We all have ou
own unique smell (pherones), apart from body odour, and whil
our recognition may be subconscious, it has more effect on ou
responses and behaviour than we may realize. Our emotions an
physical harmony can be effected through our sense of smell. Th
effect of pleasant or unpleasant smells on the harmony of ou
bodies is well documented, and utilized through the art c
aromatherapy.

Aromatherapy uses essential oils, which are extracted from aro
matic plants and trees. A holistic medicine, it shares the sam
principles as acupuncture, reflexology and herbal medicine, t
name a few. These arts are complementary and work on the prin
ciple of promoting mental serenity and bodily health – treatin
the person as one entity.

The therapy works from the principle that life itself is utterl
intangible, that its core or essence cannot be seen, felt or ana
lysed. When we talk about life, we talk about our souls and emo
tions, as well as our physical and physiological presence. Th
Chinese call it ki, and it represents the energy that propels u
through each day of our lives and creates the world around us
This force is present in every plant and tree, and aromatherap
deals with extracting this organic 'essence' and using it to enhance
cure and protect. Essential oils can affect mood, alleviate fatigue
reduce anxiety and promote relaxation. When inhaled they wor
on the nervous system and brain through stimulation of th
olfactory nerves. When absorbed through the skin, stronger com
ponents are released into the bloodstream.

See page 312 on Aromatherapy.

Biofeedback

This refers to the use of monitoring equipment to measure an
control levels of relaxation. Training can be given after the scien
tific data is examined.

Although great feats of body and mind control have bee

eported in Eastern medicine for centuries, it has only been in he past two decades that Western medicine has accepted the fact hat humans can, indeed, regulate their own heart rate, circulaion, temperature, muscle tension, and other body functions that vere mostly thought to operate only automatically. That acceptance came largely through the development of the biofeedback machine, which teaches people to become aware of various body unctions and to control them with conscious intent, using reaxation and mental imagery techniques.

Today biofeedback is widely used for the treatment of chronic pain and stress-related disorders. Even astronauts have used bioeedback to control the nausea of space sickness.

If you go for biofeedback therapy, you will be asked to sit in a comfortable chair in front of a machine that looks like a TV set. Electrode sensors (wires) from the biofeedback machine will be taped to your body, usually on your forehead, neck, back, or orefinger. With the help of relaxing music or a taped voice that uggests relaxation techniques, you will be asked to reduce the muscle tension throughout your body. Later you way also be asked to slow your heart rate, even warm your hands by increasing their blood flow. While you're trying to accomplish these eats, the machine measures your muscle tension, heart rate and blood flow, and 'feeds back' how well you are doing. This feedback can be in the form of audible beeps, pictures, or graphic ines.

After learning what the correct response feels like by working with the machine and practising at home, you should eventually be able to achieve the same response without the machine.

Hydrotherapy

Floatation

A form of sensory deprivation, floatation involves lying face up in an enclosed, dark tank of warm, heavily salted water. There is no ound, except perhaps some natural music to bring the client into dream-like state. It is exceptionally refreshing and induces a deep, relaxing sleep.

Neutral bath

Before the development of tranquillizers, the most dependable and effective method of calming an agitated patient was the use of a neutral bath. The patient was placed in a tub of water, the temperature of which was maintained at between 33.5°C and 35.6°C (92°F to 96°F), often for over three hours, and sometimes for as long as twenty-four hours. Obviously, this is not a practical proposition for the average tense person.

As a self-help measure, the neutral bath does, however, offer a means of sedating the nervous system if used for relatively short periods. It is important to maintain the water temperature at the above level, and for this a bath thermometer should be used. The bathroom itself should be kept warm to prevent any chill in the air.

Half an hour of immersion in a bath like this will have a sedative, or even soporific, effect. It places no strain on the heart, circulation or nervous system, and achieves muscular relaxation as well as a relaxation and expansion of the blood vessels: all of these effects promote relaxation. This bath can be used in conjunction with other methods of relaxation, such as breathing techniques and meditation, to make it an even more efficient way of wiping out stress. It can be used daily if necessary.

Hot bath

Most people know the relaxing benefits of a hot bath. A bath with the temperature between 36.5°C and 40°C (98°F and 104 F) is very useful as a means of muscle relaxation. To begin with, five minutes immersion in a bath of this temperature is enough. This can be stepped up to ten minutes a day, as long as no feelings of weakness or dizziness arise. It is important to realize that a brief hot bath has quite a different effect from a long one.

For other methods of hydrotherapy *see* page 30.

Herbalism

The use of medicinal herbs to alleviate illness is based on ancient techniques. When used properly, traditional herbs are non-addictive, have no side effects and can have impressive results. Herbs are particularly useful in treating nervous tension, depression, insomnia, PMS, nervous headaches and migraines. Herbal remedies are also extremely important in helping to reduce stress by their effects on the immune, circulatory and neuromuscular systems.

See page 344 for Herbal Remedies.

Homeopathy

Put most simply, homeopathy is based on the belief that substances which are poisonous in large doses can be beneficial in small doses. Various substances can be taken in the form of pills, capsules, sachets of powder, sachets of granules or liquids. These homeopathic remedies can be bought in chemists and health shops, or obtained from a practitioner. *See* page 485 for Homeopathy .

Hypnotherapy

Because it can be used to treat conditions where psychological aspects are important, hypnotherapy is a valuable means of treating stress-related illnesses; although it is not clear how hypnosis works, and the links between hypnosis and entertainment have contributed to prejudice against its use as a therapeutic tool.

See page 180 for more information on Hypnotherapy.

Pet therapy

The evidence is clear that owning and caring for a family pet can help to reduce stress levels. Pets provide their owners with unconditional love and loyalty. In return, the experience of caring for the animal imparts a sense of belonging and opportunities for play and amusement. Relationships with animals are largely free of the threats and responsibilities inherent in human intercourse. The rewards may not be so great, but for many animal lovers there can be no substitute for the emotional rewards of owning a pet.

Physiological tests have shown that stroking and petting animals can improve general health, lower blood pressure, reduce anxiety and produce a reduction in stress levels.

Certain institutions, such as hospitals, old people's homes, and even prisons, have noticed an improvement in their inmates' mental, physical and emotional health and behaviour when given access to animals.

Reflexology

Reflexology is a method for activating the natural healing resources of the body. Forms of reflexology have been in use for at least 3000 years (paintings depicting the art have been discovered in an Egyptian doctor's tomb dating back to 2330 BC). The science of reflexology as it is practised today was developed fairly recently, and its use as a complementary therapy has been on the increase ever since.

Reflexology works on the principle that the body is divided into ten zones that run lengthwise from head to toe, where the reflex areas for all the organs, glands and body parts are found. Energy runs through these zones. Reflexologists believe that if this constant flow of energy is impeded by a blockage or congestion, illness sets in. A reflexologist, by using constant, rhythmic pressure on the reflexes of the patient's feet, breaks down the blockage, allowing the return of free-flowing energy and deep relaxation to occur, thus enabling the body's own healing mechanisms to take effect.

See also page 89 for more on reflexology.

Tai Chi Ch'uan

The aim of Tai Chi (the ch'uan is usually dropped) is to combine motion, unity and dance so that those who practise its art surrender to the natural flow of the universe and become one with it – exactly the aim of more passive meditation.

Tai Chi is a means of exploring the processes of mind and body through creative movement and reflects the I Ching belief that nature is always in motion. It is said to have originated with the meditation of a Taoist monk, Chang San-feng, who one day saw a magpie trying to attack a snake. The reptile teased the bird by writhing and curling in a spiral motion, always remaining just out of the bird's reach. Similar movements are now an integral part of Tai Chi.

In Tai Chi, the image of water symbolizes the flow of energy and the way it yields to the form of its container. Earth is seen as a link between person and planet. The use of circular forms of expression shows unity and containment.

It is not possible to learn Tai Chi from the pages of a book. Traditionally, the practise was handed down from master to pupil. Today most large towns offer Tai Chi classes, and anyone wishing to learn its ways and mysteries should join a group.

The classes always begin with a period of meditative stillness, and then the pupils step forward on the right foot – an energy step with fire being visualised shooting from the palms of the hands. The energy is pulled back into the body and the weight transferred to the left foot, everyone now visualizing water cascading over them. With the body turning to the left, the palms are rotated and curved back to the right. The body continues to turn to the right with both feet firmly fixed to the floor, then the left foot is brought round, returning the body to the centre.

Tai Chi is a processs of self-discovery and, like yoga, demonstrates the link between body movement and posture and contemplative states of being. In the words of one expert, Al Huang, who wrote the classic *Embrace Tiger, Return to Mountain*, 'Tai Chi is to help you get aquainted with your own sense of personal growth, the creative process of just being you.'

Aromatherapy

Healing through aromatherapy

Aromatherapy is a method of healing using very concentrated essential oils that are often highly aromatic and are extracted from plants. Constituents of the oils confer the characteristic perfume or odour given off by a particular plant. Essential oils help the plant in some way to complete its cycle of growth and reproduction. For example, some oils may attract insects for the purpose of pollination; others may render it distasteful as a source of food. Any part of a plant – the stems, leaves, flowers, fruits, seeds, roots or bark – may produce essential oils or essences but often only in minute amounts. Different parts of the same plant may produce their own form of oil. An example of this is the orange, which produces oils with different properties in the flowers, fruits and leaves.

Art and writings from the ancient civilizations of Egypt, China and Persia show that plant essences were used and valued by priests, physicians and healers. Plant essences have been used throughout the ages for healing – in incense for religious rituals, in perfumes and embalming ointments and for culinary purposes. There are many Biblical references that give an insight into the uses of plant oils and the high value that was attached to them. Throughout the course of human history the healing properties of plants and their essential oils has been recognized and most people probably had some knowledge about their use. It was only in more recent times, with the great developments in science and orthodox medicine, particularly the manufacture of antibiotics and synthetic drugs, that knowledge and interest in the older methods f healing declined. However, in the last few years there has been a great rekindling of interest in the practice of aromatherapy with many people turning to this form of treatment.

Extraction of essential oils

Steam distillation, solvent extraction, maceration, defleurage, enfleurage

Since any part of a plant may produce essential oils, the method of extraction depends upon the site and accessibility of the essence in each particular case. The oils are produced by special minute cells or glands and are released naturally by the plant in small amounts over a prolonged period of time when needed. In order to harvest the oils in appreciable amounts, it is usually necessary to collect a large quantity of the part of the plant needed and to subject the material to a process that causes the oil glands to burst. One of the most common methods is *steam distillation*. The plant material is paced tightly into a press or still and steamed at a high temperature. This causes the oil glands to burst and the essential oil vaporises into the steam. This is then cooled to separate the oil from the water. Sometimes water is used for distillation rather than steam. Another method involved dissolving the plant material in a solvent or alcohol and is called *solvent extraction*.

This involves placing the material in a centrifuge, which rotates at high speed, and then extracting the essential oils by means of a low temperature distillation process. Substances obtained in this way may be called *resins* or *absolutes*. A further method is called *maceration* in which the plant is soaked in hot oil. The plant cells collapse and release their essential oils, and the whole mixture is then separated and purified by a process called *defleurage*. If fat is used instead of oil, the process is called *enfleurage*. These methods produce a purer oil that is usually more expensive than one obtained by distillation. The essential oils used in aromatherapy tend to be costly as vast quantities of plant material are required to produce them and the methods used are complex and costly.

Storage and use of essential oils

Essential oils are highly concentrated, volatile and aromatic. They readily evaporate and change and deteriorate if exposed to light, heat and air. Hence pure oils need to be stored carefully in brown glass bottles at a moderate temperature away from direct light. They can be stored for one or two years in this way. For most purposes in aromatherapy, essential oils are used in a dilute form, being added either to water or to another oil, called the *base* or *carrier*. The base is often a vegetable oil such as olive or safflower which both have nutrient and beneficial properties. An essential/carrier oil mixture has a short useful life of two or three months and so they are usually mixed at the time of use and in small amounts.

Techniques used in aromatherapy
Massage

Massage is the most familiar method of treatment associated with aromatherapy. Essential oils are able to penetrate through the skin and are taken into the body, exerting healing and beneficial influences on internal tissues and organs. The oils used for massage are first diluted by being mixed with a base and should never be applied directly to the skin in their pure form in case of an adverse allergic reaction.

An aromatherapist will 'design' an individual whole body massage based on an accurate history taken from the patient and much experience in the use of essential oils. The oils will be chosen specifically to match the temperament of the patient and also to deal with any particular medical or emotional problems which may be troubling him or her.

Although there is no substitute for a long soothing aromatherapy massage given by an expert, the techniques are not difficult to learn and can be carried out satisfactorily at home.

Bathing

Bathing most people have experienced the benefits of relaxing in a hot bath to which a proprietary perfumed preparation has been dded. Most of these preparations contain essential oils used in romatherapy. The addition of a number of drops of an essential il to the bath water is soothing and relaxing, easing aches and ains, and can also have a stimulating effect, banishing tiredness nd restoring energy. In addition, there is the added benefit of nhaling the vapours of the oil as they evaporate from the hot wa- er.

nhalation

nhalation is thought to be the most direct and rapid means of reatment. This is because the molecules of the volatile essential il act directly on the olfactory organs and are immediately per- eived by the brain. A popular method is the time-honoured one f *steam inhalation,* in which a few drops of essential oil are added o hot water in a bowl. The person sits with his or her face above he mixture and covers the head, face and bowl with a towel so hat the vapours do not escape. This can be repeated up to three mes a day but should not be undertaken by people suffering rom asthma. Some essential oils can be applied directly to a hand- erchief or onto a pillow and the vapours inhaled in this way.

Steam inhalation with essential oils constitutes a wonderful, ime-honoured way of alleviating the symptoms of colds and flu, nd can also be beneficial to greasy skins. Steam inhalations hould, however, be avoided by asthmatics unless under direc- ion from a medical practitioner, as the steam can occasionally rritate the lungs.

ompresses

ompresses are effective in the treatment of a variety of muscu- ar and rheumatic aches and pains as well as bruises and head- ches. To prepare a compress, add 5 drops of oil to a small bowl of vater. Soak a piece of flannel or other absorbent material in the olution. Squeeze out excess moisture (although the compress hould remain fairly wet) and secure in position with a bandage r cling film. For acute pain, the compress should be renewed vhen it has reached blood temperature, otherwise it should be left in position for a minimum of two hours and preferably over night. Cold water should be used wherever fever or acute pain or hot swelling require treatment, whereas the water should be ho if the pain is chronic. If fever is present, the compress should be changed frequently.

Hair treatments/scalp tonics

Many hair conditions such as dryness, excessive grease, or dan druff will respond to aromatherapy using specific recipes of es sential oils diluted in a nourishing base oil. For instance, 60 drops of an essential oil diluted in 100 mls of base oil (such as olive or sweet almond) will make a wonderful conditioning treatment Simply rub the oils thoroughly into the scalp, then wrap the hai in warm towels and allow the oil to penetrate the hair and the scalp for an hour or two. The choice of oil depends of cours upon the desired effect: chamomile and rosemary, for instance will condition and promote healthy hair growth, bergamot an tea tree are helpful in dandruff control whilst lavender has repel lent qualities which will deter lice and fleas.

Face creams, oils and lotions

For the face, essential oils should be mixed with base oils in much the same way as for massage, the main difference being that more nourishing oils such as apricot kernel and avocado should be used in preference to ordinary vegetable oils. (It should be noted that avocado is a fairly heavy oil and its use is best reserved for dry skin.) Essential oils can also be added to a non-perfumed col cream or lotion and used for problem complexions.

Most essential oils have antiseptic properties and can be used to treat infective skin conditions. Certain oils (such as rose and neroli) are anti-inflammatory and have a soothing effect, whereas sandalwood is useful in the treatment of superficial broken veins Rose and neroli are also excellent for care of mature skins. For dry cracked skin, the addition of wheatgerm and avocado oil (with their high vitamin E content) to preparations will relieve the con dition. In general, aromatherapy can improve the skin by ncouraging toxin removal, stimulating cell growth and renewal and mproving circulation. A gentle circular massage with the tips of he fingers should be used on the face, and special care must be aken not to stretch or drag the delicate skin around the eye area.

lower waters

`lower waters constitute a refreshing and soothing aid in the treatnent and prevention of skin conditions such as eczema and acne, nd can be easily prepared at home. Simply add around 20 drops f essential oil to an amber glass bottle containing 100 mls of pring water, then leave it to stand in a dark place for a few days. `ilter the water through some coffee or similar filter paper, then pply to the skin as required using a cotton wool pad.

athing and showering

.dd a few drops (5–10) of essential oil to the bath water after the vater has been drawn, then close the door to retain the aromatic apours. The choice of oils is entirely up to the individual, depend-1g on the desired effect, although those with sensitive skins are dvised to have the oils ready diluted in a base oil prior to bathing.

Bathing in essential oils can stimulate and revive or relax and edate depending on the oils selected: rosemary and pine can have soothing effect on tired or aching limbs, chamomile and laven-er are popular for relieving insomnia and anxiety, etc. A similar ffect (although obviously not quite as relaxing) can be achieved vhilst showering by soaking a wet sponge in essential oil mix, 1en rubbing it over the body under the warm spray.

itz bath

, sitz, or shallow, bath in the appropriate essential oil can bring normous relief in conditions such as haemorrhoids, thrush and ystitis.

oot bath

`ired, swollen feet can be refreshed by bathing in a basin of hot water ontaining 4–5 drops of lavender, peppermint, rosemary or thyme.

Hands

Dry, chapped hands may be soothed by soaking in a bowl of warm water containing a few drops of essential oil such as patchouli or rose.

Mouthwash and gargles

Used strictly in the correct dilutions, essential oils provide a natural, gentle way to help clear up mouth ulcers, oral thrush and infected gums, but it cannot be stressed too much that essential oils should never be swallowed.

Neat application and internal use

Generally, the application of undiluted essential oils directly to the skin should be avoided as many are highly irritant. However there are one or two exceptions which have been safely applied to the skin undiluted for centuries. These include lemon oil, which can be applied neat to warts (Vaseline can be applied around the wart to protect the surrounding skin); lavender, which can be safely applied directly to burns, cuts, bites and stings; and tea tree, which may be dabbed on spots. Any other oils must be used in dilution unless under careful direction from a trained aromatherapist.

Many essential oils are highly toxic when taken orally and there are **no circumstances** in which they may safely be taken at home in this way.

Mode of action of essential oils

Although the subject of a great deal of research, there is a lack of knowledge about how essential oils work in the body to produce their therapeutic effects. It is known that individual essential oils possess antiseptic, antibiotic, sedative, tonic and stimulating properties, and it is believed that they act in harmony with the natural defences of the body such as the immune system. Some oils, such as eucalyptus and rosemary, act as natural decongestants whereas others, such as sage, have a beneficial effect upon the circulation.

Conditions that may benefit from aromatherapy

A wide range of conditions and disorders may benefit from aromatherapy and it is considered to be a gentle treatment suitable for all age groups. It is especially beneficial for long-term chronic conditions, and the use of essential oils is believed by therapists to prevent the development of some illnesses. Conditions that may be relieved by aromatherapy include painful limbs, muscles and joints due to arthritic or rheumatic disorders, respiratory complaints, digestive disorders, skin conditions, throat and mouth infections, urinary tract infections and problems affecting the hair and scalp. Also, period pains, burns, insect bites and stings, headaches, high blood pressure, feverishness, menopausal symptoms, poor circulation and gout can benefit from aromatherapy. Aromatherapy is of great benefit in relieving stress and stress-related symptoms such as anxiety, insomnia and depression.

Many of the essential oils can be safely used at home and the basic techniques of use can soon be mastered. However, some should only be used by a trained aromatherapist and others must be avoided in certain conditions such as pregnancy. In some circumstances, massage is not considered to be advisable. It is wise to seek medical advice in the event of doubt or if the ailment is more than a minor one.

Consulting a professional aromatherapist

Aromatherapy is a holistic approach to healing hence the practitioner endeavours to build up a complete picture of the patient and his or her lifestyle, nature and family circumstances, as well as noting the symptoms which need to be to be treated. Depending upon the picture that is obtained, the aromatherapist decides upon the essential oil or oils that are most suitable and likely to prove most helpful in the circumstances that prevail. The aromatherapist has a wide ranging knowledge and experience upon which to draw. Many oils can be blended together for an enhanced effect and this is called a 'synergistic blend'. Many aromatherapists offer a massage and/or instruction on the use of the selected oils at home.

Base oils

Because essential oils are extremely concentrated and also because of their tendency to evaporate rapidly, they need to be diluted with carrier or base oils. Generally it is not advised that essential oils should be applied undiluted to the skin, although there are one or two specific exceptions. It is very important to use a high quality base oil, as oils such as baby or mineral oil have very poor penetrating qualities which will hamper the passage of the essential oil through the skin. Indeed, it would be better to use a good quality vegetable or nut oil for babies in preference to proprietary baby oils as the vegetable oil is more easily absorbed and contains more nutrients.

Although the choice of base oil is largely a matter of personal preference, it is useful to note that many vegetable oils possess therapeutic properties of their own. Any of sweet almond, soya bean, sunflower, jojoba, olive, grapeseed, hazelnut, avocado, corn or safflower will provide a suitable base for essential oils, although these should preferably be of the cold-pressed variety that have higher nutrient levels.

Pure essential oils should retain their potency for one to two years but once diluted in a base oil will only last for three months or so before spoiling. They should also be stored at a fairly constant room temperature in corked dark glass bottles or flip-top containers as they will deteriorate quickly when subjected to extremes of light and temperature. Adding some vitamin E or wheatgerm oil to the mixture can help prolong its usefulness. For massage oils, it is best to make up a very small quantity of essential oil in base oil for each application because of its poor keeping qualities.

Below is a very rough guide to the dilution of essential oils. However, you will find many variations and differing opinions on this depending on the preference of individual therapists, and their recipes will differ accordingly.

Base Oil	Essential Oil
100 ml	20–60 drops
25 ml	7–25 drops
1 teaspoon (5 ml)	3–5 drops

Blending essential oils

Essences can be blended to treat specific ailments, and some aromatherapy books contain precise recipes for blends. When two or more essential oils are working together in harmony, this is known as a synergistic blend. Obviously, it takes many years of experience to know which combinations of plant essences will work most effectively together, but as a rough guide, oils extracted from plants of the same botanical family will usually blend and work well together, although it is by no means necessary to stick rigidly to this rule as other combinations may be just as successful. Really, a number of factors need to be taken into account when preparing a blend of oils for a patient, such as the nature of his/her complaint, his personality or frame of mind. For home use, it is not usually beneficial to blend more than three oils for any one preparation.

Around the home

There are a variety of ways in which your home can be enhanced by the use of essential oils. Fragrances, pomanders, ring burners and diffusers can all be used in conjunction with essential oils to impart a wonderful scent to a room. (Essential oils should be put into water and vapourized and not burned as they are inflammable. Follow the instructions on ring burners carefully and never put essential oils directly onto a hot light bulb.) Most essential oils also have antimicrobial properties which make them extremely useful when the occupants of the room are suffering from colds and flu. Oils such as myrtle and eucalyptus also seem to have a soothing effect on coughs and can be used in the bedroom where they will release their aroma throughout the night.

Fragrancers, pomanders, and ring burners can all be purchased quite cheaply from shops and indeed make very welcome gifts, but it is not neccessary to use any extra equipment to benefit from essential oils in the home. By adding a few drops of essential oil to a bowl of water or soaking a cotton ball in the oil and placing it in a warm place the same effect can be achieved. You can also sprinkle logs and twigs before placing them on the fire or barbecue to create a soothing aroma.

In case of colds or flu, a bowl of water is actually preferable as it has a humidifying effect on the air. Three or four drops of an appropriate essential oil such as eucalyptus or cypress sprinkled on a handkerchief can also be inhaled periodically to alleviate the worst symptoms of sinusitis, colds and headaches. Similarly, 2–drops of a relaxing essential oil on the pillow at night can help to alleviate insomnia.

How essential oils work

Inhalation, application and bathing are the three main methods used to encourage the entry of essential oils into the body. When inhaled, the extremely volatile oils may enter via the olfactory system, and permeation of the skin occurs when they are diluted and applied externally. By bathing in essential oils, we can inhale and absorb the oils through the skin simultaneously.

Little is known about how essential oils actually affect the mind and the body, although research is currently ongoing in the USA and the UK. However, the effectiveness of aromatherapy has been supported by recent research in central Europe, the USA, the UK and Australia. It appears that most essential oils are antiseptic and bactericidal to some degree, whilst some even seem to be effective in fighting viral infections.

On inhalation, essential oil molecules are received by receptor cells in the lining of the nose, which will transmit signals to the brain. Electrochemical messages received by the olfactory centre in the brain then stimulate the release of powerful neurochemicals into the blood which will then be transported around the body. Molecules inhaled into the lungs may pass into the bloodstream and be disseminated in the same way.

When rubbed or massaged into the skin, essential oils will permeate the pores and hair follicles. From here, they can readily pass into the tiny blood vessels (known as capillaries) by virtue of their molecular structure, and then travel around the body.

Once absorbed, the action of the oil depends upon its chemical constituents. Most essential oils are high in alcohols and esters, although a few contain a high concentration of phenols, aldehydes

322

and ketones. The latter are powerful chemicals and their use should be avoided by all save the skilled professional.

Special care

You may find that your professional aromatherapist will use some of the following oils, but these are generally unsafe for use by the lay person.

Generally

Aniseed, cinnamon bark, cinnamon leaf, clove bud, clove leaf, clove stem, fennel (bitter), pine, parsley, nutmeg.

During pregnancy

Basil, cedarwood, clary sage, fennel, juniper, marjoram, myrrh, rosemary, sage,
thyme, parsley, nutmeg.

Prior to exposure to sun

Bergamot, lemon, mandarin, orange, fennel.

Hypertension

Sage, thyme, cypress.

Aromatherapy massage at home

Before beginning an aromatherapy massage, there are a number of steps that should be taken in order for the subject of the massage to derive full benefit from the treatment.

1. It is important to take a brief history from the patient in order to be able to select the correct oils. This will involve an assessment of his/her emotional state as well as any physical complaints.
2. At least an hour should have elapsed since the last meal prior to receiving or giving a massage.
3. Make sure your clothing is loose and will not obstruct your movements.

4 Ensure that hands are clean and nails short.
5 Have some tissues ready, and make sure your oil is easily accessible.
6 Make sure your hands are warm before touching your subject

The room should be warm so that your subject will be comfortable even though only partly dressed. Lighting should be subdued, and the telephone should be disconnected to avoid interruption. Perhaps music could be played softly in the background but this is a matter of preference and convenience. It is a good idea to have a compatible essence evaporating in the room prior to commencement. The massage surface needs to be firm, therefore a normal sprung bed is unsuitable – instead, pad the floor or use a futon or similar firm mattress.

First of all the subject may have a warm bath or shower in order that the pores are open and receptive to the essential oil. This however, is a matter of personal preference on the part of the therapist. The subject should be positioned comfortably and should be covered with towels, exposing only the area that is to be massaged at any one time in order to avoid embarrassment and cold. Hair should be tied out of the way.

Basic techniques

The following constitutes only a very basic guide to massage movements and is no substitute for a comprehensive aromamassage course. However, massage can be used to great benefit at home using the following simple movements and suggestions:

Effleurage

This is the most often used therapy movement, and constitutes a simple, gentle stroking movement. Note that deep pressure should *never* be used by an untrained person. The strokes may be long or short, gentle or firm, but the whole hand should be used, always pushing the blood towards the heart, thus promoting venous return. This stroke promotes muscle relaxation and soothes the nerve endings.

Petrissage

In petrissage, the flesh is gently rolled between the thumbs and fingers in a movement not unlike kneading dough. This technique is best used on the back and on fatty areas. The idea is to stimulate the circulation and lymphatic flow and thereby increase the rate of toxin expulsion.

Head massage

Put a little of the essential massage oil on the fingertips and massage in circular movements over the scalp and temples.

Massage for tension headaches and migraine

Work from the base of the neck and scalp for a few moments, using effleurage strokes firmly, again with the chosen oil(s) on the fingertips

Neck massage

Neck massage should be carried out with the patient sitting on a chair with some support in front. Working around the base of the neck and scalp, use small upward and outward circular movements. Move slowly up, down and around the sides of the neck, alternating firm and gentle movements.

Shoulder massage

Using gentle anticlockwise effleurage movements, stroke firmly from the shoulders to the neck.

Arm massage

Use effleurage and petrissage movements upwards in the direction of the armpit, concentrating on muscular and fatty areas. Avoid bony areas.

Back massage

Avoiding the vertebrae, use gentle or firm petrissage or effleurage movements. Stroke all the way from the lumbar to the shoulders, move the hands outwards across the shoulders and return slowly down the outer area of the back. Repeat this movement to induce deep relaxation.

Abdominal massage

Use a clockwise effleurage stroke, taking care not to apply too much pressure.

Leg massage

Always massage the legs in an upward direction. Avoid bony area and *never* massage varicose veins.

Massage for menstrual or gynaecological problems

Always use gentle effleurage movements and do not exert any pressure on the lower abdomen. Begin at the lower back and slide forwards and downwards across the hips. Repeat several times.

Feet massage

Work in the direction of toe to heel, using the fingers uppermos and the thumb under the foot.

Common ailments

Stress-related disorders

Anxiety	basil, bergamot, geranium, lavender marjoram(sweet), melissa, neroli, sandalwood vetiver.
Mild shock	basil, chamomile, melissa, peppermint, rosemary
Depression	bergamot, chamomile, geranium, jasmine lavender, neroli, patchouli, rose, rosemary, sage*
Fatigue	clary sage, eucalyptus, juniper berry, peppermint rosemary.

Skin complaints/disorders

Dry skin	bergamot, chamomile, geranium, jasmine lavendar, melissa, neroli, patchouli, sandalwood ylang ylang.
Oily skin	cypress, lemon, tea tree.

Acne	bergamot, cedarwood, chamomile, cypress, eucalyptus, fennel, geranium, juniper berry, lavender, lemon, myrrh, parsley*, patchouli, petitgrain, rose, rosemary, sandalwood, tea tree.
Eczema	chamomile, geranium, juniper berry, lavender, melissa.
Psoriasis	bergamot, chamomile, eucalyptus, lavender, peppermint.

Feminine/gynaeological disorders

Amenorrhoea	chamomile, clary sage, fennel, geranium, sage*.
Dysmenorrhoea	cypress, geranium, rose.
Hot flushes	chamomile, clary sage, jasmine, lavender, neroli, petitgrain, sandalwood, ylang ylang.
Mastitis	chamomile, clary sage, geranium, lavender, rose.
Period pain	clary sage, lavender, marjoram
PMT	geranium, lavender, neroli, petitgrain, rose.

* oils marked with an asterisk can have adverse effects and are normally recommended to be used under the guidance of a professional aromatherapist

Select A – Z of Essential Oils

The following section is by no means an exhaustive one, but aims to include the most popular oils readily available today. Similarly whilst therapeutic uses have been suggested, therapists will differ in the choice of oils for particular complaints, just as a general practitioner may prescribe one remedy for a specific complaint, whereas his partner in the same practice may favour another treatment for the same complaint.

Aniseed
Pimpinella anisum
Aniseed seems to have a carminative (flatulence-expelling) effect on the alimentary canal and is therefore useful in the treatment of flatulence and indigestion. It has a strong antiseptic effect, and its antispasmodic properties can be effective against period pains. It also seems to stimulate lactation postnatally and is used in lozenges and cough sweets for its decongestant effect. Its anti-parasitic effect makes it useful in the treatment of lice and scabies.

CAUTION: Can be irritant to sensitive skins and narcotic in large doses. It is not suitable for home use and should only be used by a qualified aromatherapist.

Basil
Ociymum basilicum
Basil is now grown in many countries of the world although it originates from Africa. The herb has a long history of medicinal and culinary use, and was familiar to the Ancient Egyptian and Greek civilizations. Basil is sacred in the Hindu religion and has many medicinal uses in India and other Eastern countries. The whole plant is subjected to a process of steam distillation to obtain the essential oil used in aromatherapy. Basil is valued for its soothing

and uplifting effects – its sweet, liquorice-like fragrance alleviates fatigue and depression and has a general tonic effect. Basil has a refreshing, invigorating effect and also has antiseptic properties. It can be effective in treating respiratory infections such as colds, bronchitis, asthma and sinusitis. It can also alleviate the symptoms of fever, gout and indigestion. It seems to be equally effective in relieving tired and over-worked muscles and is widely used in baths, inhalation and massage. Its strongly antiseptic effect sooths skin abrasions and assists the healing process. It also has insect repellent qualities. As a digestive aid, basil's antispasmodic effect has made it a favoured herb in cookery throughout the ages.

CAUTION: Basil should be avoided during pregnancy. It can also have a depressant effect, so it should be used in moderation. It is relatively non-toxic, but should be well diluted to avoid possible skin irritation.

Bay
Laurus nobilis

Both *Laurus nobilis* and its West Indian cousin *Pimenta racemosa* are valuable in the treatment of colds, flu and bronchitis. As discovered by the ancients, it also promotes digestion, and combats dyspepsia and flatulence. The West Indian oil is favoured in the treatment of rheumatic pain because of its anti-inflammatory properties and is widely used as a general tonic. Both can be used in inhalation, baths and massage.

CAUTION: Avoid application to sensitive skins.

Benzoin
Styrax benzoin

For skin complaints, benzoin is indicated in the treatment of chapped, inflamed or irritated skin. Its antiseptic properties make it a popular choice for urinary, respiratory and throat infections. Benzoin also has uplifting qualities which can relieve stress and nervous tension when used in a massage oil. As an expectorant, many therapists recommend a few drops of benzoin in a pint of hot water as an inhalation.

CAUTION: Compound tincture of benzoin (which contains other substances including aloe, tolu balsam and storax) occasionally causes sensitivity, but benzoin itself is generally non-toxic and non-irritant.

Bergamot
Citrus bergamia

Oil of bergamot is obtained from a plant that is a native species of some Asian and Eastern countries. The oil was first used and traded in Italy and derives its name from the northern city of Bergamo. In Italian medicine, it was popular as a remedy for feverish illnesses and to expel intestinal worms. It has also been used in cosmetics and perfumes, as the flavouring of Earl Grey tea, and in other foods. Recent research carried out in Italy indicates a wide variety of therapeutic applications for bergamot, including urinary tract and respiratory infections.

Its strong antiseptic effect makes it a good choice for the treatment of skin, throat and mouth infections.

In particular, scalp and skin conditions such as psoriasis, acne and ulcers will often respond to treatment with bergamot, especially where stress and depression may have played a part in lowering resistance to infection. When combined with eucalyptus, its soothing effect will afford relief to sufferers of cold sores and shingles. Insomnia, anxiety and depression can be alleviated by the uplifting and refreshing nature of this oil. It also has a natural deodorizing effect and can be used both as a breath freshener and as a personal deodorant.

CAUTION: Bergamot can irritate the skin if used in concentrations in excess of one per cent. It is phototoxic and should not be used in home-made suntan oil.

Cajeput
Melaleuca cajeputi

In addition to the above, therapists have found cajeput helpful for relief of a wide variety of complaints. Used in baths, diffusers, inhalation and massage, cajeput can bring relief from asthma, bronchitis, sinusitis and throat infections. Occasionally it has been used to treat diarrhoea and indigestion.

CAUTION: It may be irritant to the skin if used in high concentrations.

330

Cedarwood
Juniperus virginiana

Cedarwood seems to be beneficial in skin and scalp conditions such as alopecia, acne, dandruff and eczema. It also helps the body to fight respiratory infections and problems and has a mild diuretic effect which can be useful in the treatment of urinary tract infections. Cedarwood has been credited with aphrodisiac qualities.

CAUTION: High concentrations may irritate the skin, and on **no account** must cedarwood be used during pregnancy as it is a powerful abortifacient.

Camomile, Chamomile (Roman)
Chamaemelum nobile

There are several varieties, but Roman chamomile is the essential oil of choice for home use. It is used by therapists to treat many skin complaints and promotes the healing of burns, cuts, bites and inflammations. It is also effective in allergic conditions and can have a beneficial effect on menstrual problems when used regularly in the bath. It seems to be effective in reducing stress and anxiety and problems such as headache, migraine and insomnia. As an analgesic, it is used in the treatment of earache, toothache, neuralgia and abscesses, and is popular for treating childhood illnesses.

CAUTION: Chamomile is generally non-toxic and non-irritant, but may cause dermatitis in very sensitive individuals.

Cinnamon
Cinnamomum zeylanicum

This oil possesses a warm, spicy aroma and has been favoured in the treatment of nausea, dyspepsia, flatulence and other digestive disturbances. Its warm, soothing qualities can be beneficial to rheumatism when used in massage oil on the affected parts.

These soothing, relaxing qualities also impart a strong stress-relieving effect.

CAUTION: Cinnamon can be irritant to the mucous membranes in large doses. Oil distilled from the bark is especially irritant to skin and mucous membranes and should never be directly applied. It is unsafe for home use and must only be used by a trained aromatherapist.

Clary Sage
Salvia sclarea

Clary sage is possessed of antispasmodic, antidepressant, balsamic, carminative, tonic, aperitive, astringent, anti-inflammatory, bactericidal and antiseptic qualities. It is valuable in stress-related conditions and has an anti-hypertensive effect. A thick mucilage can be made from the seeds, which was traditionally used for removing particles of dust from the eyes. Clary sage is also indicated in the treatment of colds and throat infections. It is also good for regulating menstrual problems and for soothing problem skin, particularly if dry or sensitive.

CAUTION: It should be avoided during pregnancy and also in conjunction with alcohol consumption. However, in general, clary sage has very low toxicity levels and is therefore preferable to garden sage for use in aromatherapy.

Clove
Eugenia aromatica

Clove is a useful antiemetic and should also be used for dyspepsia. It has a powerful antiseptic and a mild analgesic action which make it popular in the relief of gum infections and aching teeth. Its expectorant effect is valuable in the treatment of bronchitis and catarrh. It is widely used as an antihistamine and an antirheumatic and to treat skin conditions such as scabies and athlete's foot. It is also good for treating infections, especially colds and flu, and is often an ingredient of commercially available digestive tonics and mouthwashes.

CAUTION: It can cause mucous membrane irritation and is therefore best used in small doses. It can be dangerous and is best used only by a trained aromatherapist.

Cypress
Cupressus sempervirens

Cypress is thought to be beneficial to the urinary system and seems to help in conditions involving a loss of fluid. These include excessive perspiration, diarrhoea and menorrhagia. Used in the bath, cypress brings great relief to tired aching legs and feet. On the skin, or in a massage oil, its antiseptic and astringent actions can have a balancing effect on oily skin and provide an aid to healing. Cypress is often used by therapists to reduce swellings and nasal congestion, and it is useful in the treatment of colds and flu.

CAUTION: Not to be used by those suffering from hypertension, otherwise non-irritant and non-toxic.

ucalyptus

ucalyptus globulus

Eucalyptus is a native species of Australia and Tasmania but is now grown in many countries throughout the world. The plant has a characteristic pungent odour, and the oil obtained from it has disinfectant and antiseptic properties, clears the nasal passages and acts as a painkiller. The leaves and twigs are subjected to a process of steam distillation in order to obtain the essential oil used in aromatherapy. The diluted oil is used for muscular and rheumatic aches and pains, skin disorders such as ringworm, insect bites, headaches and neuralgia, shingles, respiratory and bronchitic infections and fevers. Eucalyptus is used in many household products and in remedies for coughs and colds. Its analgesic properties are often used to ease the discomfort of shingles, chicken pox and herpes as well as to soothe muscular aches and sprains.

CAUTION: When diluted, eucalyptus is safe to use externally, but can be fatal if taken internally.

ennel (Sweet)

oeniculum vulgare

Fennel has properties similar to those of aniseed, so that it is frequently used to treat colic and flatulence. It is also a mild natural laxative. It is credited with an action similar to oestrogen and is thought to stimulate milk production in nursing mothers. This action also indicates fennel in the treatment of menopausal symptoms. As a mild diuretic, it slows the build-up of toxic waste,

which is a causative factor in gout and liver problems. Fennel
also suitable for children's complaints.

CAUTION: Avoid use on sensitive skin or prior to exposure
sun. It should not be used by epileptics or pregnant wome
Bitter fennel oil can be dangerous and is best used only by
trained aromatherapist.

Frankincense
Boswellia carteri

The inhalation of frankincense is used to relieve the sympton
of bronchitis and laryngitis, and its soothing effect is useful i
the treatment of asthma, attacks of which may be brought o
by anxiety or emotional stress. It is also indicated in urinar
tract problems such as cystitis and is sometimes used as a ute
ine tonic. Its healing properties have long been valued in th
treatment of wounds, and it is often used in skin preparatio
for mature skins. It has an extremely relaxing aroma and is ide
in the bath for soothing away the day's stress.

Geranium
Pelargonium graveolens

Geranium is an excellent 'all-round' oil, with a wide range
uses, particularly for menopausal problems and pre-menstru
tension. Its diuretic quality makes it a wise choice for fluid r
tention, and cellulitis and mastitis often respond well to it. F
skin conditions and emotional disorders, it is a popular choic
in the bath and in massage oil. Serious skin conditions ofte
respond to its antiseptic and anti-fungal qualities.

CAUTION: Generally non-toxic and non-irritant, it may caus
contact dermatitis in hypersensitive individuals.

Jasmine
Jasminum officinalis

Because jasmine is so costly, it is not much used in hon
aromatherapy, but like all essential oils it does have therapeut
uses. Its heady, uplifting scent makes it useful in the treatme
of stress-related illnesses. It also has a smoothing effect on sk
and is a valuable component in skin care preparations. It al
seems to have a regulating effect on the menstrual cycle, an

has been successfully used for throat problems, coughs and catarrh. However, as there are many less expensive oils that will perform these functions, jasmine's main use is as a fragrance ingredient in perfumes.

CAUTION: Although non-toxic and non-irritant, it has, on occasion, caused an allergic reaction

Juniper Berry

Juniperus communis

Juniper is a native species of many northern countries and has a long history of medicinal use. It has stimulant, tonic and antiseptic properties. It is beneficial in the treatment of stress and sleeplessness. In cases of debility, it helps by acting as a tonic for the digestion and boosting the appetite.

Juniper seems to be beneficial to the digestive system, the female reproductive system and the menstrual cycle. It also helps regulate problem skin and is favoured by therapists in the treatment of acne, eczema, dermatitis and haemorrhoids. It helps disperse uric acid build-up and is therefore useful in the treatment of gout and other joint problems. It is a good stress-reliever, especially when used in the bath, and has a mild diuretic action which indicates its use in cystitis. Juniper also acts as an appetite stimulant, and is often used to get rid of intestinal parasites. It can be used in massage and baths.

CAUTION: Juniper stimulates uterine contractions and therefore should not be used in pregnancy. It should also be avoided by those with kidney disease. Generally non-toxic, but it may be slightly irritant.

Lavender

Lavendula vera

The highly perfumed lavender is a native species of the Mediterranean but has long been popular as a garden plant in Britain and many other countries. It has antiseptic, tonic and relaxing properties, and the essential oil used in aromatherapy is obtained by subjecting the flowers to a process of steam distillation. It is considered to be one of the safest preparations and is used in the treatment of a wide range of disorders.

Lavender is an appetite stimulant, a tonic and an antispasmodic. It is particularly effective in the treatment of minor burns and scalds, wounds, sores and varicose ulcers, and is generally one of the most versatile and widely used oils for healing. It also has a strong antiseptic effect and is employed in many cosmetic preparations and as an insect repellent. It is also used in the treatment of muscular aches and pains, respiratory problems, influenza, digestive problems, and genito-urinary problems such as cystitis and dysmenorrhoea. Its soothing effect is recommended for headaches and pre-menstrual tension. Lavender is a very safe oil and can even be applied undiluted to the skin.

Lemon
Citrus limonium

As a massage oil lemon can have a very stimulating effect on the circulation, and seems to have the ability to stimulate the body's own immune system. Therefore, it is frequently used to treat circulatory problems and respiratory ailments such as asthma, bronchitis and catarrh. As a digestive aid, lemon can have a calming effect on dyspepsia. As a natural cosmetic, lemon has an astringent and toning effect.

CAUTION: It is generally safe but should not be used prior to exposure to sunlight.

Lemongrass
Cymbopogon citratus

Combined with neroli in a massage oil, lemongrass brings relief to muscular aches and pains. It also has a sedative effect on the central nervous system, inducing a deep sense of relaxation when used in the bath. Lemongrass has an extremely strong bactericidal and fungicidal effect, which indicates its use in a variety of infections such as athlete's foot and thrush. It is also helpful in digestive disturbances such as colitis and indigestion, especially where stress or anxiety is a factor.

CAUTION: It is generally non-toxic, but occasionally dermatitis has been reported in sensitive individuals. Use under the guidance of a trained therapist.

Mandarin
Citrus nobilis

Mandarin is still a popular oil in the treatment of digestive weaknesses and liver disturbances and is especially preferred for children and the elderly because of its gentle nature. For stress, anxiety, insomnia and nervousness, its use is recommended in conjunction with other citrus oils. Like neroli, it is also a wonderful skin tonic, particularly for acne and oily skins. It is also indicated in the treatment of fluid retention.

CAUTION: Generally very safe, although its use on the skin is not recommended prior to exposure to sunlight.

Marjoram (Sweet)
Origanum marjorana

Marjoram can be extremely effective in reducing the pain and swelling of muscular damage, bruises and sprains, and arthritis. It has an extremely hypnotic effect, which is useful in inducing sleep and calming emotions, especially when used in the bath. It can also be effective in menstrual problems. Marjoram is also a popular treatment for colds and coughs, bronchitis and asthma, and has a carminative and antispasmodic action on colic, constipation and flatulence.

CAUTION: It should be avoided by pregnant women as it has a strong emmenagogic effect.

Melissa True
Melissa officinalis

Melissa is used in the treatment of respiratory disorders, nausea, indigestion and skin disorders. It is said to regulate menstruation and fertility, and is helpful in the treatment of anxiety and depression because of its revitalising properties. It also relieves wasp and bee stings and aids their healing. *The British Herbal Pharmacopoeia* recommends it for flatulent dyspepsia, neurasthenia and depressive illness.

CAUTION: It has caused occasional sensitization and dermal irritations and is therefore best used in low concentrations. Rarely stocked commercially, most melissa oils are blends and should be labelled so.

Myrrh
Commiphora myrrha

Myrrh has a stimulant effect on the mucous membranes and therefore a useful expectorant. It is still used in Chinese medicine to treat menstrual disturbances and complaints, haemorrhoids and sores. It is also indicated for dental problems and an effective antiseptic gargle for throat infections. It has long been known as an appetite stimulant and is a valuable ingredient in beauty treatments for mature skin.

CAUTION: Myrrh has an emmenagogic action and therefore should not be used by pregnant women.

Niaouli
Melaleuca viridiflora

Niaouli has a sweet, fresh fragrance and is strongly antiseptic and non-irritant, making it popular in the treatment of acne, boils and other skin irritations. It also makes a very stimulating chest rub and is good when vaporized.

Neroli
Citrus aurantium

Neroli is an extremely expensive oil to produce because of the volume of flowers required, but it is very much in demand because of its wonderful aroma. This is frequently harnessed in massage oil because of its power to uplift, calm and relax. It is also believed to have qualities that are beneficial to the skin and is widely used to prevent stretch marks and scarring, to reduce thread veins and as an aid for dry, sensitive skin. Neroli's stress-relieving qualities indicate its use in a wide variety of complaints, ranging from colitis and diarrhoea to palpitation, insomnia and pre-menstrual tension.

Nutmeg
Myristica fragrans

Nutmeg is recommended in *The British Herbal Pharmacopoeia* for a variety of digestive complaints such as dysentery, nausea, dyspepsia, flatulence and diarrhoea. It has powerful stimulant properties that lend it to the treatment of poor circulation, poor appetite and menstrual irregularities. It can also be applied locally in massage to soothe aches and pains and to relieve rheumatism. Its warming effects are particularly welcome in the winter, and it has strong stimulant properties that lend it to the treatment of poor circulation.

CAUTION: It must not be used in high doses or for extended periods of time, as essential oil of nutmeg can induce hallucinations and hypnosis. Avoid its use during pregnancy. Nutmeg should always be well diluted, even for bathing purposes, as it can cause skin irritation. It can be dangerous and should be used only under the supervision of a trained aromatherapist.

Orange (Sweet)
Citrus sinensis

Sweet orange essential oil is very useful in the treatment of respiratory infections such as colds, bronchitis and influenza, and is thought to increase bronchial secretions. It can also help oily and dull complexions when used as part of a skin care routine. Having similar stress-relieving qualities to neroli, it is also helpful in the alleviation of stress-related complaints. As a gentle aid to digestion, it is often used to ease dyspepsia and constipation.

CAUTION: It is generally safe but should not be applied to the skin prior to exposure to sunlight.

Parsley
Petroselinum Crispum

Parsley has a diuretic and emmenagogic effect, which makes it useful for menstrual problems. It also has the power to reduce fever and has a soothing effect on colic, flatulence and indigestion. It is used for treating bladder and kidney problems, and is also indicated in the treatment of arthritis, rheumatism and sciatica, cystitis and urinary tract infections.

CAUTION: Oil of parsley is moderately toxic, therefore it is wise to use it in moderation and to avoid it completely in pregnancy. It should be used only under the supervision of a trained aromatherapist.

Patchouli
Pogostemon patchouli

Patchouli possesses a soothing, calming, earthy scent. It is a good antiseptic with anti-inflammatory properties, which makes it a sensible choice in the treatment of minor burns. Patchouli has also been credited with aphrodisiac powers, and is excellent for relieving a variety of skin disorders including acne, athlete's foot, eczema and dry and cracked skin. It is also used for treating poisonous snakebites in Japan and Malaysia.

Peppermint
Mentha piperita

Peppermint is a native plant of Europe with a long history of medicinal use dating back to the ancient civilizations of Egypt, Greece and Rome. Oil of peppermint is obtained by subjecting the flowering parts of the plant to a process of steam distillation. The essential oil of peppermint has a calming effect on the digestive tract and is excellent for the relief of indigestion, colic-type pains, nausea, travel and morning sickness. It is also an extremely gentle inhalation for asthma. It is cooling and refreshing, and useful in the treatment of colds, respiratory symptoms and headaches.

Peppermint is widely used in remedies for colds and indigestion, as a food flavouring, especially in confectionery, and in toothpaste.

CAUTION: Possibly irritant to sensitive skin – use in moderation.

Petitgrain
Citrus bigordia

Petitgrain can be used as a mild antidepressant substitute for neroli, and is effective in the alleviation of anxiety and insomnia. It is also valuable in skin care, having a balancing and toning effect on greasy skin conditions. In the digestive system, it reduces the symptoms of dyspepsia and flatulence.

Pine
Pinus sylvestris

Pine has a strong antiseptic quality, valued for its effectiveness in treating respiratory conditions and relieving asthma, blocked sinuses and catarrh when used as an inhalation. Its stimulating effect also makes it a good choice as a warming massage oil for muscular pains and strains. It has a multitude of other applications for cuts and sores, arthritis and rheumatism, cystitis and urinary tract infections, fatigue, stress, anxiety and neuralgia.

CAUTION: Those with a tendency towards sensitive skin should avoid bathing in pine oil. Pine oil should only be used under the direction of a trained aromatherapist and is unsafe for home use.

Rose
Rosa centifola

Rose has a supremely feminine and deeply sensual aroma, which is the traditional mainstay of the perfume industry. Rose oil has a wonderful antidepressant effect that may be harnessed in body and face massages, baths or vaporizers to treat anxiety, stress and depression. It also has a gentle balancing effect on gynaecological disorders and is said to have aphrodisiac properties.

Rosemary
Rosemarinus officinalis

Rosemary has a wide application and is effective in the treatment of numerous complaints. Possessing a powerful aroma, rosemary is favoured as a decongestant in inhalation and an invigorating muscle-strengthening massage oil. Skin and hair problems can respond well to rosemary, and gargling with it will freshen the breath. Above all, rosemary seems to possess remarkable memory and concentration-enhancing properties. Other therapeutic uses are in digestive disorders, headaches and stress.

CAUTION: It should be avoided during pregnancy and should not be used by epileptics.

Sage
Salvia officinalis

Sage is a native plant of the northern coastal regions of the Mediterranean and has a long history of medicinal and culinary use dating back to the ancient civilizations of Greece and Rome. The essential oil used in aromatherapy is obtained by subjecting the dried leaves to a process of steam distillation. Sage has an expectorant effect when used in inhalations, and its astringent and cooling properties make it a popular choice as a tonic, an appetite stimulant and as a fever reducer. Its antiseptic effects are beneficial to sore throats and mouth problems if used in a gargle or mouthwash. It is also used to improve poor circulation, sore throats, colds and viral infections, bronchitic and catarrhal complaints, rheumatism, arthritic pains, joint sprains and strains, mouth infections and headaches. Sage is widely used as a flavouring in foods and in some household preparations and toiletries.

CAUTION: It should be avoided during pregnancy and if epileptic. Sage is toxic if ingested and is best substituted with clary sage for home use.

Sandalwood
Santalum album

Its preservative powers are often employed to lengthen the life of creams and potions. Sandalwood is a wonderful facial oil, with a soothing emollient effect on dry or sensitive skin. This oil also has a powerful relaxing effect and can alleviate upset stomachs, especially where nervous tension or stress has been a causative factor. Sandalwood also seems to have a powerful antiseptic effect that is particularly useful in the treatment of cystitis and urinary tract infections. It is also favoured for menstrual problems, as a sedative and for catarrh.

Tea Tree
Melaleuca alternifolia

Tea tree contains four substances that do not occur anywhere else in nature and, next to thyme, is the most antiseptic of all oils. It is also strongly disinfectant, antibacterial, anti-fungal, and antiviral – all qualities that make tea tree an invaluable weapon in the treatment of a multitude of infections. Similarly, it also seems to offer a boost to the body's own immune system whenever threat of infection occurs. Tea tree should be considered when treating any of the following problems: colds, influenza, bronchitis and asthma, warts and verrucas, burns and inflammation, thrush and similar fungal infections, mild shock and hysteria. It can be used undiluted on facial spots and, in a cream, on sunburn.

CAUTION: It is generally very safe, but may cause sensitization in some people.

Thyme (Sweet)
Thymus vulgaris

Thyme is a strong antiseptic, perhaps the strongest of any oil, and is also a powerful stimulant to the appetite, the immune system, and the central nervous system. Respiratory infections, coughs and asthma all seem to respond well to thyme oil, especially if used in inhalations and gargles. Note, however, that gargles must not be swallowed and care must be taken to use the thyme in low dilutions. Its use is indicated in a wide variety of fungal, bacterial and viral infections, in the treatment of wounds and sores and as an aid to the immune system.

CAUTION: It should not be applied undiluted to the skin or used during pregnancy, or on children's skin. Always dilute prior to use in the bath. In fact, generally it is best used in low concentrations. There are several types of thyme, some of which can be dangerous. Only sweet thyme is safe for home use.

Ylang ylang
Cananga odorata

Ylang ylang is a native species of the Far Eastern islands of Indonesia, the Philippines, Java and Madagascar. To obtain the essential oil used in aromatherapy, the flowers are subjected to a process of steam distillation. Like most essential oils ylang ylang has a strong antiseptic effect, but it is best known for its euphoric and aphrodisiac properties. The nervous system can also benefit greatly from its relaxing powers, and its antidepressant powers can also be harnessed to treat mild shock, anger and stress. It has a calming effect on the heart-beat rate and can be used to relieve palpitations, tachycardia, hypertension (raised blood pressure), depression and shock.

It is used widely as an ingredient in skin care, having a wonderful tonic effect and gentle action.

CAUTION: It is generally very safe, although sensitization has been reported in a small number of cases. Used excessively, it can cause nausea or headache.

Herbal Remedies

History of the use of herbal remedies

Herbalism is sometimes maligned as a collection of home-made remedies to be applied in a placebo fashion to one symptom or another, provided the ailment is not too serious and provided there is a powerful chemical wonder-drug at the ready to suppress any 'real' symptoms. We often forget, however, that botanical medicine provides a complete system of healing and disease prevention. It is the oldest and most natural form of medicine. Its record of efficacy and safety spans centuries and covers every country worldwide. Because herbal medicine is holistic medicine, it is, in fact, able to look beyond the symptoms to the underlying systemic imbalance; when skillfully applied by a trained practitioner, herbal medicine offers very real and permanent solutions to concrete problems, many of them seemingly intractable to pharmaceutical intervention.

Early civilizations

The medicinal use of herbs is said to be as old as mankind itself. In early civilizations, food and medicine were linked and many plants were eaten for their health-giving properties. In ancient Egypt, the slave workers were given a daily ration of garlic to help fight off the many fevers and infections that were common at that time. The first written records of herbs and their beneficial properties were compiled by the ancient Egyptians. Most of our knowledge and use of herbs can be traced back to the Egyptian priests who also practised herbal medicine. Records dating back to 1500 BC listed medicinal herbs, including caraway and cinnamon.

The ancient Greeks and Romans also carried out herbal medicine, and as they invaded new lands their doctors encountered new herbs and introduced herbs such as rosemary or lavender into new areas. Other cultures with a history of herbal medicine are the Chinese and the Indians. In Britain, the use of herbs developed along with the establishment of monasteries around the country, each of which had its own herb garden for use in treating both the monks and the local people. In some areas, particularly Wales and Scotland, Druids and other Celtic healers are thought to have had an oral tradition of herbalism, where medicine was mixed with religion and ritual.

The first publications

Over time, these healers and their knowledge led to the writing of the first 'herbals', which rapidly rose in importance and distribution upon the advent of the printing press in the 15th century. John Parkinson of London wrote a herbal around 1630, listing useful plants. Many herbalists set up their own apothecary shops, including the famous Nicholas Culpepper (1616–1654) whose most famous work is *The Complete Herbal and English Physician, Enlarged,* published in 1649. Then in 1812, Henry Potter started a business supplying herbs and dealing in leeches. By this time a huge amount of traditional knowledge and folklore on medicinal herbs was available from Britain, Europe, the Middle East, Asia and the Americas. This promoted Potter to write *Potter's Encyclopaedia of Botanical Drugs and Preparations*, which is still published today.

The decline of herbal medicine

It was in this period that scientifically inspired conventional medicine rose in popularity, sending herbal medicine into a decline. In rural areas, herbal medicine continued to thrive in local folklore, traditions and practices. In 1864 the National Association (later Institute) of Medical Herbalists was established, to organize training of herbal medicine practitioners and to maintain standards of practice. From 1864 until the early part of this century, the Institute fought attempts to ban herbal medicine and over time public interest in herbal medicine has increased, particularly over the last 20 years. This move away from synthetic drugs is partly due to possible side effects, bad publicity, and, in some instances, a mistrust of the medical and pharmacological industries. The more natural appearance of herbal remedies has led to its growing support and popularity. Herbs from America have been incorporated with common remedies and scientific research into herbs and their active ingredients has confirmed their healing power and enlarged the range of medicinal herbs used today.

Its rise and relevance today

Herbal medicine can be viewed as the precursor of modern pharmacology, but today it continues as an effective and more natural method of treating and preventing illness. Globally, herbal medicine is three to four times more commonly practised than conventional medicine.

Nowhere is the efficacy of herbalism more evident than in problems related to the nervous system. Stress, anxiety, tension and depression are intimately connected with most illness. Few health practitioners would argue with the influence of nervous anxiety in pathology. Nervous tension is generally acknowledged by doctors to contribute to duodenal and gastric ulceration, ulcerative colitis, irritable bowel syndrome and many other gut-related pathologies.

We know also, from physiology, that when a person is depressed, the secretion of hydrochloric acid – one of the main digestive juices – is also reduced so that digestion and absorption are rendered less efficient. Anxiety, on the other hand, can lead to the release of adrenaline and stimulate the over-production of hydrochloric acid and result in a state of acidity that may exacerbate the pain of an inflamed ulcer. In fact, whenever the voluntary nervous system (our conscious anxiety) interferes with the autonomic processes (the automatic nervous regulation that in health is never made conscious), illness is the result.

Herbalists rely on their knowledge of botanical remedies to rectify this type of human malfunction. The medical herbalist will treat a stubborn dermatological problem using 'alternatives' specific to the skin problem, and then apply circulatory stimulants to aid in the removal of toxins from the area, with remedies to reinforce other organs of elimination, such as the liver and kidneys. Under such natural treatment, free of any discomforting side effects, the patient can feel confident and relaxed – perhaps for the first time in many months.

Curiously, this is an approach that has never been taken up by orthodox medicine. There, the usual treatment of skin problems involves suppression of symptoms with steroids. However, the use of conventional antihistamines or benzodiazepines often achieves less lasting benefit to the patient because of the additional burden of side effects, such as drowsiness, increased toxicity, and long-term drug dependence.

Herbs, on the other hand, are free from toxicity and habituation. Because they are organic substances and not manmade synthetic molecules, they possess an affinity for the human organism. They are extremely efficient in balancing the nervous system. Restoring a sense of wellbeing and relaxation is necessary for optimum health and for the process of self-healing.

Naturally, the choice of a treatment should be based upon a thorough health assessment and the experience and training of a qualified herbal practitioner. The herbalist will then prepare and prescribe herbal remedies in a variety of different forms, such as infusions, loose teas, suppositories, inhalants, lotions, tinctures, tablets and pills. Many of these preparations are available for home use from chemists, health shops and mail-order suppliers.

Herbs for stress management

Chamomile

This has a relaxing effect on the mind and body. It is an excellent sedative for anxiety and muscle tenseness. Many people enjoy its benefits in the form of chamomile tea.

Valerian

This is the ideal tranquillizer. The rhizomes of this plant contain a volatile oil (which includes valerianic acid), volatile alkaloids (including chatinine), and iridoids (valepotriates), which have been shown to reduce anxiety and aggression. So effective is Valerian in relieving anxiety while maintaining normal mental awareness, that it enables us to continue the most complicated mental exercise without drowsiness, loss of consciousness or depression. Valerian has been usefully taken before an examination or a driving test!

Peppermint

This is effective for treating digestive discomfort: it relieves indigestion, flatulence, constipation and nausea. Peppermint is also a good mind tonic, helping to clarify ideas and focus concentration. It is also helpful in alleviating the symptoms of colds and influenza. peppermint and chamomile tea is thought to be effective in reducing the pain of tension headaches and migraines.

Vervain

This is not only effective against depression but also strongly supports the detoxifying function of the liver. Its French name is still 'Herbe Sacre'; an old English name is 'Holy Wort' – it was one of the seven sacred herbs of the Druids. Today we know that the antispasmodic qualities of Verbena are largely due to the glycoside verbenalin. Recent Chinese research has linked the plant with dilation of arteries in the brain: a likely explanation of its usefulness in treating migraine, especially when this problem is accompanied by liver congestion. It is certainly of use to treat exhaustion and depression.

St John's Wort

Also called *Hypericum perforatum*, St John's wort has analgesic and anti-inflammatory properties, with important local applications to neuralgia and sciatica. Systemically, its sedative properties are based on the glycoside hypericin (a red pigment), which makes it applicable to neurosis and irritability. Many herbalist use it extensively as a background remedy.

Lemon balm

This herb is both carminative and antispasmodic, and is active specifically on that part of the vagus nerve that may interfere with the harmonious functioning of the heart and the stomach. Recent research has indicated that the action of the volatile oil begins within the limbic system of the brain and subsequently operates directly upon the vagus nerve and all the organs that are innervated by it. Accordingly, neurasthenia (complete nervous prostration), migraine, and nervous gastropathy are amenable to its healing power.

Lime flowers

These are thought to be helpful in controlling anxiety and hyperactivity. They are also effective for treating insomnia, high blood pressure and for soothing muscles and nerves.

Borage

This is an effective mind tonic, which helps to alleviate headaches, migraine and depression.

Oats

Oats is one of the great herbal restoratives of the nervous system. The plant contains a nervine alkaloid that is helpful in angina and in cardiac insufficiency. It has also been used in the treatment of addiction to morphine, narcotics, tobacco and alcohol.

Soothing herbal drinks

Warm milk and honey

Perhaps with a dash of cinnamon, this is an ideal drink to take at bedtime. It will help you relax and ward off insomnia.

Hop tea

Three hop cones, or heads, infused in a cup of boiling water whenever you begin to feel excessively tense, is a marvellous remedy for anxiety and insomnia.

A soothing herb tea to sustain a feeling of equilibrium

> 25g (1 oz) each dried chamomile flowers,
> lime flowers, hibiscus blossoms and
> marigold flowers
> 15g (½ oz) each dried peppermint leaves
> and vervain
> 1 teaspoon whole fenugreek seeds
> 100g (4 oz) Lapsang Souchong tea

Mix all the ingredients together and store in a dark airtight container. Use 1 teaspoon to 300 ml (½ pint) of boiling water in a te pot and leave to infuse for five minutes before straining and serv ing with a slice of lemon and a teaspoon of honey if desired. Thi is a very calming tea that soothes feelings of anxiety. It also help to clear your head and settle an upset tummy. One cup take morning and night will promote a feeling of wellbeing.

Another calming tea, especially good for the nerves

> 1 teaspoon each grated valerian root and
> dried mint
> ½ teaspoon each dried chamomile and lav-
> ender flowers
> 600 ml (1 pint) boiling water

Infuse the dry ingredients in the water for 15 minutes then strai and take a glass three times a day for one week only.

Two tonic teas to sip when feeling depressed

Sip either 2 teaspoons of dandelion and 1 of basil infused in 60 ml (1 pint) of boiling water, or 2 teaspoons each of nettle, bas and melissa infused in 600 ml (1 pint) of boiling water.

A tonic tea to relieve stress and anxiety

> 1 tablespoon each fresh dandelion and
> nettle tops
> 1 teaspoon each fresh blackcurrant and
> borage leaves
> 600 ml (1 pint) boiling water

steep the greenery in the water for five minutes. Strain and drink with lemon and honey.

dock wine

Dock is one of the great tonic herbs because it is extremely high in iron. Here is a recipe for an old-fashioned dock wine.

> 175g (7 oz) dock root
> 15g (½ oz) liquorice wood
> 7g (¼ oz) juniper berries
> 100g (4 oz) raw cane sugar
> 2 litres (3½ pints) organic red wine

Put all the ingredients together in a china container, cover and place either in a very slow oven or in a bain marie. Continue to heat gently until the mixture is reduced by half. Strain, bottle and seal tightly. Drink a sherry glass of the dock wine every morning for two weeks.

rosemary in wine

Steep 6 sprigs of rosemary in a well-sealed bottle of sweet white wine for 14 days. Take 1 wineglass as a daily tonic.

sage tonic

Take 100g (4 oz) of fresh sage leaves and put them in a bottle of organic white wine for two weeks. Sweeten to taste with honey and leave for another day. Press and strain through muslin. Bottle, and take 1 sherry glass before lunch and dinner.

You can also infuse sage leaves in boiling water, strain and sweeten with honey for an uplifting sage tea.

A–Z of Herbal Remedies

Aconite *Aconitum napellus*. COMMON NAME: Monkshood, blu
rocket, friar's cap, wolfsbane.

OCCURRENCE: indigenous to mountain slopes in the Alps an
Pyrenees. Introduced into England very early, before 900 AD.

PARTS USED: the leaves used fresh and the root when dried.
contains alkaloidal material – aconitine, benzaconine an
aconine amongst other compounds.

MEDICINAL USES: the plant is poisonous and should not be use
except under medical advice. It is an anodyne, diaphoretic, feb
rifuge and sedative. Used for reducing fever and inflammatio
in the treatment of catarrh, tonsillitis and croup. It may be use
in controlling heart spasm.

ADMINISTERED AS: tincture, liniment and occasionally as injectio

Agrimony *Agrimonia eupatoria*. COMMON NAME: Church steeple
cockeburr, sticklewort.

OCCURRENCE: field borders, ditches and hedges throughou
England. Found locally in Scotland.

PARTS USED: the herb. Contains a particular volatile oil, tanni
and a bitter principle.

MEDICINAL USES: mild astringent, tonic, diuretic, deobstruent.
has a reputation for curing liver complaints and is very goo
for skin eruptions and blood diseases. Also recommended
treat the sting and bite of snakes.

ADMINISTERED AS: liquid extract.

Alder *Alnus glutinosa*. COMMON NAME: Betula alnus.

OCCURRENCE: commonly found throughout Britain, usually i
moist woods or by streams.

PARTS USED: the bark, wood, shoots, catkins and leaves have a
been used as dyes. The bark and leaves contain tannic acid.

MEDICINAL USES: tonic and astringent. Used as a decoction to bathe swelling and inflammation, particularly of the throat.
ADMINISTERED AS: decoction.

Aloes *Aloe perryi, Aloe vera.*

OCCURRENCE: indigenous to East and South Africa and introduced into the West Indies.
PARTS USED: the drug aloes is described as 'the liquid evaporated to dryness which drains from the leaves.' It contains two aloin compounds, barbaloin and isobarbaloin, as well as amorphous aloin, resin and aloe-emodin in differing proportions.
MEDICINAL USES: emmenagogue, purgative, vermifuge, anthelmintic. It is generally administered along with carminative and anodyne drugs, and acts on the lower bowel. The liquid form may be used externally to ease skin irritation.
ADMINISTERED AS: fluid extract, powdered extract, decoction, tincture.

Allspice *Pimento officinalis.* COMMON NAME: Pimento, jamaica pepper, clove pepper.

OCCURRENCE: indigenous to the West Indies and South America; cultivated in jamaica and central America.
PARTS USED: the fruit, which contains a volatile oil made up of eugenol, a sesquiterpene and other unknown chemicals.
MEDICINAL USES: aromatic, stimulant, carminative. Allspice acts on the gastro-intestinal tract and is usually added to drinks tonics and purgatives for flavouring. The spice may also be used for flatulent indigestion and hysteria. Allspice is frequently used as a spice and condiment in food or drinks.
ADMINISTERED AS: essential oil, distilled water, powdered fruit, fluid extract.

Almond, Sweet *Amygdalus communis* var. *dulais.* **Almond, Bitter** *Amygdalus commis* var. *amara.*

OCCURRENCE: native trees of western Asia and North Africa and cultivated in most Mediterranean countries and Great Britain.
PARTS USED: the nut and the oil expressed from it.
MEDICINAL USES: sweet almonds have demulcent and nutritive properties, but since the outer skin can cause irritation of the

alimentary canal, almonds are normally blanched and the skin removed before being used as food. The oil produced is emollient, demulcent, nutritive and slightly laxative, and is mainly used in cosmetics but is also taken internally as a medicine. is of benefit in allaying acrid juices, softening and relaxing solid materials, bronchial diseases, tickling coughs, hoarseness and nephritic pains. Sweet almonds are made into emulsions with barley water or gum arabic to treat gravel, stone, kidney disorders and bladder and biliary duct problems, with more success than almond oil.

Bitter almonds yield a volatile oil upon distillation with water which is used as a flavouring agent. These almonds contain the glucoside amygdalin and the chemical emulsin that acts on the glucoside to produce glucose, prussic acid and benzaldehyde in the presence of water. Prussic acid is poisonous and use of bitter almond oil must be carefully monitored. In the Middle Ages, the oil was used for intermittent fevers, hydrophobia and as an aperient, diuretic and vermifuge drug, but is seldom administered medicinally now. The cake left after expressing the oil has a special dietary value and is often made into flour for cakes and biscuits for diabetic patients. Almond oil is used in trade as a lubricant for watches, and in soaps and toiletries.

ADMINISTERED AS: expressed oil, bitter almond oil (with prussic acid removed).

Anemone, Pulsatilla *Anemone pulsatilla*. COMMON NAME: Pasqueflower, meadow anemone, wind flower.

OCCURRENCE: found locally in chalk downs and limestone areas of England.

PARTS USED: the whole herb. It produces oil of anemone upon distillation with water.

MEDICINAL USES: nervine, antispasmodic, alterative and diaphoretic. It is beneficial in disorders of mucous membranes and of the respiratory and digestive passages. Can be used to treat asthma, whooping cough and bronchitis.

ADMINISTERED AS: fluid extract.

Anemone, Wood *Anemone nemorosa*. COMMON NAME: crowfoot, windflower, smell fox.

OCCURRENCE: found in woods and thickets across Great Britain.

PARTS USED: the root, leaves and juice.

MEDICINAL USES: this species of plant is much less widely used than it has been previously. It used to be good for leprosy, lethargy, eye inflammation and headaches. An ointment made of the leaves is said to be effective in cleansing malignant ulcers.

ADMINISTERED AS: decoction, fresh leaves and root, ointment.

Angelica *Angelica archangelica*. COMMON NAME: Garden Angelica, *Archangelica officinalis*.

OCCURRENCE: found native to some sites in Scotland although more abundant in Lapland and is a common garden plant in England.

PARTS USED: the root, leaves and seeds. The leaves contain volatile oil, valeric acid, angelic acid, a bitter principle and a resin called angelicin. The roots contain terebangelene and other terpenes while the seeds also yield two acid compounds.

MEDICINAL USES: Angelica has carminative, stimulant, diaphoretic, diuretic, aromatic, stomachic, tonic and expectorant properties and is good for colds, coughs, pleurisy, wind, colic and rheumatism. It is used as a stimulating expectorant and is good for digestion.

ADMINISTERED AS: powdered root, liquid extract, infusion or as a poultice.

Angostura *Galipea officinalis*. COMMON NAME: Cusparia bark, *Cusparia febrifuga, Bonplandia trifoliata, Galipea cusparia*.

OCCURRENCE: a small tree native to tropical South America.

PARTS USED: the dried bark, which has the active ingredients angosturin, the alkaloids galipine, cusparine, galipidine, cusparidine and cuspareine, as well as a volatile oil and an unidentified glucoside.

MEDICINAL USES: aromatic, bitter, tonic, stimulant, purgative. There is a long history of usage by native South Americans as a stimulant tonic. It is useful in bilious diarrhoea and dysentery, but in large doses it has a purgative and cathartic effect on the body.

ADMINISTERED AS: infusion, powdered bark, tincture, fluid extract.

Anise *Pimpinella anisum.* COMMON NAME: Aniseed.

OCCURRENCE: native to Egypt, Greece, Crete and western Asia; its cultivation spread to central Europe and North Africa.

PARTS USED: the fruit. Upon distillation, the fruit yields a fragrant volatile oil that is made up of anethol, choline, a fixed oil, sugar and mucilage.

MEDICINAL USES: carminative and pectoral. It is very useful against coughs and chest infections and is made into lozenges or smoked to clear the chest. Aniseed tea is good for infant catarrh, and aids digestion in adults. Anise seed is an ingredient of cathartic and aperient pills, to relieve flatulence and lessen the griping caused by purgative herbs. It can also be given in convulsions quite safely.

ADMINISTERED AS: essence, essential oil, tincture, powdered seeds, tea and pills.

Apple *Pyrus malus.* COMMON NAME: Wild Apple, *Malus communis,* crab-tree.

OCCURRENCE: native to Great Britain and found throughout the temperate regions of the northern hemisphere.

PARTS USED: the fruit and bark. Apples contain water, protein material, carbonaceous matter, vitamins, organic acids, salts of potassium, sodium, carbon and magnesium.

MEDICINAL USES: diuretic, slightly astringent. The organic acids in the fruit benefit sedentary people and ease liver problems, gout and indigestion. Apple juice or cider is drunk frequently in some areas e.g. Normandy, where problems of stone or calculus are unknown because of the diuretic effects of apples. Apples can also help cure constipation, scurvy, sleeplessness or bilious complaints. They act as an excellent dentifrice (tooth cleanser) and are applied as a poultice to sore eyes when rotten. A decoction of the bark is used against intermittent and bilious fevers, while cooked apples are used in sore throats, eye problems, and in skin and tissue infected with the *Streptococcus pyogenes* bacterium. Dropsy is helped by drinking cider in which horseradish was steeped.

ADMINISTERED AS: fresh fruit, expressed juice, fermented drink, infusion, decoction, poultice.

Apricot *Prunus armeniaca*. COMMON NAME: Apricock, *Armeniaca vulgaris*.

OCCURRENCE: originally found in northern China, the Himalaya region and temperate Asia. Now cultivated across temperate regions of Europe and introduced into England in the sixteenth century.

PARTS USED: the kernels and the oil expressed from them. The oil contains olein and the glyceride of linolic acid. The cake left after oil removal produces an essential oil upon distillation that contains the glucoside amygdalin and is chemically identical to the essential oil from the almond. It is used in confectionery and as a food flavouring.

MEDICINAL USES: apricot oil is substituted for oil of almonds in cosmetics, because of its lower cost. It has a softening action on the skin.

ADMINISTERED AS: expressed oil, essential oil.

Areca Nut *Areca catechu*. COMMON NAME: Betel nut, pinang.

OCCURRENCE: a tree cultivated in the East Indies, India and Sri Lanka.

PARTS USED: the seeds contain a large amount of tannin, gallic acid, a fixed oil, lignin and a volatile oil. They also contain three alkaloids, arcoline, arecain and guracine with the second listed being the active principle.

MEDICINAL USES: aromatic, astringent, taenacide and mydriatic. The native people chew these nuts, which stain the teeth, lips and excrement red. Taken internally, the seeds expel tapeworms and cause contraction of the pupil of the eye. Areca nut is also made into a toothpaste in Britain.

ADMINISTERED AS: powdered nut, fluid extract.

Arnica *Arnica montana*. COMMON NAME: Mountain tobacco, leopard's bane.

OCCURRENCE: indigenous to central Europe but found in England and southern Scotland.

PARTS USED: the rhizome and flowers. They contain arnicin, tannin, phullin and a volatile oil.

MEDICINAL USES: stimulant, vulnerary and diuretic. It is used in external application to bruises and sprains but is rarely used internally as it irritates the stomach, and may cause severe poisoning. A tincture of arnica has been used to treat epilepsy and seasickness.

ADMINISTERED AS: tincture, poultice.

Arrach *Chenopodium olidum.* COMMON NAME: Stinking motherwort, arrach/goosefoot, dog's arrach, goat's arrach, netchweed.

OCCURRENCE: an annual herb found on waste ground or roadsides throughout Great Britain.

PARTS USED: herb. contains trimethylamine, osmazome and nitrate of potash.

MEDICINAL USES: nervine, emmenagogue, anti-spasmodic. This is used in female hysteria and was formerly said to cure barrenness.

ADMINISTERED AS: an infusion, fluid extract or injection.

Arrowroot *Maranta arundinacea.* COMMON NAME: *Maranta indica, M. ramosissima*, maranta starch or arrowroot, araruta, Bermuda arrowroot, Indian arrowroot.

OCCURRENCE: indigenous to the West Indies and central America. It is cultivated in Bengal, Java, the Philippines, mauritius and West Africa.

PARTS USED: the dried, powdered starch from the rhizome.

MEDICINAL USES: nutritive, demulcent, non-irritating. Well suited for infants and convalescents, particularly after bowel complaints. The jelly made of water or milk may be flavoured with sugar, lemon juice or fruit. The fresh rhizomes are mashed and applied to wounds from poisoned arrows, scorpion or spider bites and to stop gangrene. The freshly expressed juice of the rhizome, when mixed with water, is said to be a good antidote against vegetable poisons.

ADMINISTERED AS: fresh root, expressed juice, dietary item.

Asarabacca *Asarum europaeum.* COMMON NAME: Hazelwort, wild nard.

OCCURRENCE: Asarabacca is the only British species of the birthwort family and is very rare. It is found in woodlands.

PARTS USED: the root and herb.

MEDICINAL USES: stimulant, tonic, emetic, purgative, aromatic and sternulatory. As dried powdered leaves of the herb, it is used in the preparation of snuffs, causing sneezing and giving relief to headaches and weak eyes. It has been utilized to remove mucus from the respiratory passages and may be an antidote to the bite of venomous snakes. The herb was formerly used as an emetic or purgative but its use has been replaced by safer drugs.

ADMINISTERED AS: tincture, emulsion.

Asparagus *Asparagus officinalis.* COMMON NAME: Sparrow grass.

OCCURRENCE: a rare native in Britain, but found wild on the south-west coast of England. It is cultivated as a food crop in parts of Scotland.

PARTS USED: the root.

MEDICINAL USES: this plant has diuretic, laxative, cardiac and sedative effects. It is recommended in cases of dropsy.

ADMINISTERED AS: expressed juice, decoction or made in a syrup.

Avens *Geum urbanum.* COMMON NAME: Colewort, herb bennet, city Avens, wild rue, way bennet, goldy star, clove root.

OCCURRENCE: a common hedgerow plant in Britain and Europe.

PARTS USED: the herb and root. The herb contains a volatile oil composed of eugenol and a glucoside, while the root also contains tannin.

MEDICINAL USES: an astringent, styptic, febrifuge, sudorific, stomachic, antiseptic, tonic and aromatic. It is useful in diarrhoea, sore throat, chills, fevers and headache amongst other complaints. An infusion may be used for skin problems, as a wash.

ADMINISTERED AS: an infusion, decoction or tincture.

Balm *Melissa officinalis.* COMMON NAME: Sweet balm, lemon balm, honey plant, cure-all.

OCCURRENCE: a common garden plant in Great Britain, which was naturalized into southern England at a very early period.

PARTS USED: the herb.

MEDICINAL USES: as a carminative, diaphoretic, or febrifuge. It can be made into a cooling tea for fever patients and balm is often used in combination with other herbs to treat colds and fever.

ADMINISTERED AS: an infusion.

Baneberry *Actaea spicata.* COMMON NAME: Herb Christopher, bugbane, toadroot.

OCCURRENCE: a rare plant in Britain, found only in limestone districts of the Lake District and Yorkshire.

PARTS USED: the root.

MEDICINAL USES: antispasmodic. The plant is acrid and poisonous. The root is used as a remedy for catarrh and some nervous disorders, but the plant must be used with great caution.

ADMINISTERED AS: infusion, dried or fresh root.

Barberry *Berberis vulgaris.* COMMON NAME: Berbery, pipperidge bush, *Berberis dumetorum.*

OCCURRENCE: a common bush that grows wild in some parts of England but is unlikely to be native to Scotland and Ireland.

PARTS USED: the root, root-bark and berries. The bark contains berberine, a bitter alkaloid, along with several other compounds.

MEDICINAL USES: as a tonic, purgative and antiseptic. It is normally used to treat jaundice and liver complaints, and is an aid to regulating digestion and stopping constipation. The berries are used to produce an acid drink that helps ease diarrhoea and fevers.

ADMINISTERED AS: powdered bark, fluid extract and solid extract.

Barley *Hordeum distichon* and *Hordeum vulgare.* COMMON NAME: Pearl barley, *Perlatum*

OCCURRENCE: throughout Britain.

PARTS USED: decorticated seeds; composed of eighty per cent starch and six per cent proteins, cellulose, etc.

MEDICINAL USES: Barley is used to prepare a nutritive and demulcent drink for ill and fevered patients. Barley water is given to sick children suffering from diarrhoea or bowel inflammation etc. malt extract is also used medicinally.

ADMINISTERED AS: an infusion and beverage.

Basil *Ocimum basilicum.* COMMON NAME: Sweet basil, garden basil.

OCCURRENCE: as a garden plant throughout Britain.

PARTS USED: the herb, which contains a volatile, camphoraceous oil.

MEDICINAL USES: aromatic with carminative and cooling properties. It is used to treat mild nervous disorders and an infusion of basil is said to be good for obstructions of the internal organs and in stopping vomiting and nausea.

ADMINISTERED AS: a flavouring in food, dried leaves or an infusion.

Bayberry *Myrica corifera*. COMMON NAME: Candleberry, waxberry, tallow shrub, wax myrtle.

OCCURRENCE: widely distributed through America, Europe and Great Britain.

PARTS USED: the bark, which contains volatile oil, starch, lignin, tannic and gallic acids along with lesser compounds.

MEDICINAL USES: a powerful stimulant, astringent and tonic. The powdered bark may be used in poultices, often together with elm. A decoction is used to treat the throat and sore gums.

ADMINISTERED AS: an infusion, decoction, powder and injection.

Bearberry *Archostaphylos uva-ursi*. COMMON NAME: *Arbutus uva-ursi, uva-ursi*.

OCCURRENCE: on heaths of the Scottish Highlands, south to Yorkshire, and in high mountains of Europe, Asia and America.

PARTS USED: the leaves, which contain arbutin as the chief constituent.

MEDICINAL USES: when made into an infusion, the leaves have a soothing, astringent and diuretic effect. This is of benefit in diseases affecting the bladder, and the kidneys, e.g. urethritis, cystitis, etc.

ADMINISTERED AS: an infusion.

Beech *Fagus Sylvatica*. COMMON NAME: Buche, boke, faggio, fagos.

OCCURRENCE: found in Europe, including Britain, although only indigenous to England.

PARTS USED: the oil of beech nuts, and beech tar.

MEDICINAL USES: beech tar is stimulating and antiseptic so is used internally as a stimulating expectorant to treat chronic bronchitis. It is used externally applied to various skin diseases.

ADMINISTERED AS: beech oil or beech tar.

Beetroot *Beta vulgaris*. COMMON NAME: Spinach beet, sea beet, garden beet, whit beet, mangel-wurzel.

OCCURRENCE: *Beta vulgaris* is native to southern Europe and is derived from the sea beet, *Beta maritima* which grows wild on the coasts of Europe, England, North Africa and Asia. There are many cultivated forms and varieties of beetroot with similar properties.

PARTS USED: the leaves and root. The root contains a pure fruit sugar which is easily taken up by the body, as well as starch and gum.

MEDICINAL USES: the juice of the white beet was said to be of a 'cleansing, digestive quality' to 'open up obstructions of the liver and spleen' and ease headaches. Beetroot is used to produce refined sugar, as a vegetable and to make wine or ale.

ADMINISTERED AS: dietary item, decoction, expressed juice.

Belladonna *Atropa belladonna*. COMMON NAME: Deadly nightshade, devil's cherries, dwale, black cherry, devil's herb, great morel.

OCCURRENCE: native to central and southern Europe but commonly grows in England.

PARTS USED: the roots and leaves. The root contains several alkaloid compounds including hyoscyamine, atropine and belladonnine. The same alkaloids are present in the leaves but the amount of each compound varies according to plant type and methods of storing and drying leaves.

MEDICINAL USES: as a narcotic, diuretic, sedative, mydriatic, antispasmodic. The drug is used as an anodyne in febrile conditions, night-sweats and coughs. It is valuable in treating eye diseases and is used as a pain-relieving lotion to treat neuralgia, gout, rheumatism and sciatica. Belladonna is an extremely poisonous plant and should always be used under medical supervision. cases of accidental poisoning and death are well-known. despite this, it is a valuable drug used to treat a wide range of disease.

ADMINISTERED AS: a liquid extract which is used to produce alcoholic extracts, plasters, liniment, suppositories, tincture and ointment.

Bergamot *Monarda didyma*. COMMON NAME: Scarlet monarda, oswego tea, bee balm.

OCCURRENCE: a plant which is indigenous to North America.

PARTS USED: the oil extracted from the whole plant, and the leaves.
MEDICINAL USES: used in a similar manner to other plants containing thymol as an active chemical. Oil of bergamot has antiseptic, aromatic, carminative, tonic and antispasmodic properties. An infusion of the young leaves was a common beverage in the USA before tea became more common. The infusion is also good for coughs, sore throats, fevers and colds.
ADMINISTERED AS: essential oil, infusion, fluid extract.

Bethroot *Trillium pendulum, Trillium erectum.* COMMON NAME: Indian shamrock, birthroot, lamb's quarters, wake-robin, Indian balm, ground lily.
OCCURRENCE: a native North American plant found in the western and middle United States.
PARTS USED: the dried root and rhizome; the leaves.
MEDICINAL USES: antiseptic, astringent, tonic, expectorant, pectoral and alterative. It is useful in all cases of internal bleeding, profuse menstruation and pulmonary complaints. It is used to promote safe childbirth and delivery. The leaves may be applied to ulcers and tumours while the root makes a good antiseptic poultice to stop gangrene spreading or for skin diseases. It was used by the native Americans as a medicine.
ADMINISTERED AS: the powdered root, fresh leaves and infusion.

Betony, Wood *Stachys bentonica, Betonica officinalis.* COMMON NAME: Bishopswort.
OCCURRENCE: found wild in woodlands, or on heath or moorland but less common in Scotland.
PARTS USED: the herb.
MEDICINAL USES: aromatic, astringent and alterative. Betony was thought to be one of the best treatments for headaches and hangover. It is normally combined with other herbs to produce a tonic for nervous affections, dyspepsia and rheumatism. The dried herb was also used to make a tea substitute and was smoked as tobacco.
ADMINISTERED AS: an infusion.

Bindweed, Greater *Convolvulus sepium.* COMMON NAME: Hedge convolvulus, old man's night cap, hooded bindweed, bearbind.

OCCURRENCE: a native of Britain which is abundant in England but rarer in Scotland.

PARTS USED: the resin produced from the roots.

MEDICINAL USES: the resin is normally made into a tincture. This preparation is then applied internally and has a purgative effect. The effects are not as pronounced as in the related plant species *Convulvus jalapa* (jalap bindweed) and *Convulvus scammonia* (Syrian bindweed).

ADMINISTERED AS: tincture.

Birch, Common *Betula alba*. COMMON NAME: White birch, bouleau, berke, bereza.

OCCURRENCE: common in Europe, from Sicily to Iceland and also found in northern Asia.

PARTS USED: the bark and leaves. The bark contains tannic acid, behilin and behils camphor while the leaves contain betulorentic acid.

MEDICINAL USES: bitter and astringent. The bark yields oil of birch tar upon destructive distillation, which is very similar to oil of WINTERGREEN. The oil is used in skin disease ointments, e.g. treating eczema while it is also used as a component of insect repellent. Birch tea made of the leaves is recommended for gout, rheumatism and dropsy and is also said to be good for breaking up kidney stones. Sap from the tree is used to produce beer, wine, spirits and vinegar in various parts of Europe.

ADMINISTERED AS: oil, infusion.

Birthwort *Aristolochia longa*. COMMON NAME: Long-rooted birthwort.

OCCURRENCE: throughout Europe and Great Britain.

PARTS USED: the root, which contains aristolochine.

MEDICINAL USES: aromatic and stimulant. It is useful in treating gout and rheumatism and may be used to clear obstructions after childbirth.

ADMINISTERED AS: powdered root.

Bistort *Polygonum bisorta*. COMMON NAME: Snakeweed, adderwort, twice writhen, osterick, Easter marigiant, English sepentary.

OCCURRENCE: a native of many parts of northern Europe, common in the north of England and southern Scotland.

PARTS USED: the root-stock which contains tannin, starch, gallic acid and gum.

MEDICINAL USES: a strong astringent and is mainly used in external and internal bleeding and haemorrhages from the lungs or stomach. Can be used to treat diarrhoea, dysentery, cholera and bowel complaints. Bistort is important in alleviating diabetes and as a mouth wash or gargle to 'fasten loose teeth' and heal gum problems.

ADMINISTERED AS: a powder, fluid extract, decoction or injection.

itter root *Apocynum androsaemifolium.* COMMON NAME: milkweed, dogsbane, fly-trap, wild cotton.

OCCURRENCE: found in mountainous regions of Europe and North America.

PARTS USED: the dried rhizome and roots. The active chemicals in the plant are a bitter principle called cymarin, and to a lesser extent the glucoside apocynamarin.

MEDICINAL USES: cardiac tonic, hydragogue, alterative. Bitter root is similar to foxglove in action and is very powerful in slowing the pulse and it also has a strong action on the vaso-motor system. It may irritate the mucous membranes, causing nausea and purging of the bowels, so that it cannot be tolerated by all people. As a powerful hydrogogue it is good against fluid accumulation in the abdomen (ascites), particularly when it is linked to liver cirrhosis. It is also highly effective in treating dropsy which is related to heart failure. The plant's alterative powers are used against syphilis, scrofula and rheumatism. Because of irregular absorption of the drug through the gastro-intestinal tract, great care must be taken with the dosage administered and the patient's condition.

ADMINISTERED AS: powdered root, liquid extract.

ittersweet *Solanum dulcamara.* COMMON NAME: Woody nightshade, violet bloom, scarlet berry, felonwood, felonwort, dulcamara.

OCCURRENCE: a climbing plant found in hedgerows in Britain

PARTS USED: the twigs and root-bark. The twigs contain the alkaloid solamine and the glucoside dulcamarine which gives

bittersweet its characteristic taste. It also contains sugar, gur
starch and resin.

MEDICINAL USES: narcotic, resolvent, diuretic and alterative. Bi
tersweet promotes all secretions, particularly of the skin an
kidneys, and is generally used to clear up stubborn skin infe
tions and eruptions, scrofula and ulcers and has been recom
mended in chronic bronchial catarrh, asthma or whoopir
cough. In large doses, the drug can cause paralysis of the cer
tral nervous system and lead to death.

ADMINISTERED AS: a fluid extract, decoction.

Blackberry *Rubus fructicosus*. COMMON NAME: Bramble, bumble-kit
bramble-kite, bly, brummel, brameberry, scaldhead, bramblebern
OCCURRENCE: common throughout Britain in hedgerows an
ditches.

PARTS USED: the root and leaves, which both contain tannin.

MEDICINAL USES: as astringent and tonic. It is valuable against dy
entery and diarrhoea. A decoction of the root was used to tre
whooping cough. A cordial or vinegar drink was made and is us
ful in treating looseness of the bowels, piles or a feverish cold.

ADMINISTERED AS: decoction, fluid extract or made into cordia
wine or vinegar.

Blackcurrant *Ribes nigrum*. COMMON NAME: Quinsy berrie
squinancy berries.

OCCURRENCE: a common garden plant throughout Britain, b
is only truly native to Yorkshire and the Lake District. It is als
found in Europe.

PARTS USED: the fruit, leaves, bark and root.

MEDICINAL USES: diuretic, diaphoretic, febrifuge, refrigerar
detergent. The fruit juice is excellent in febrile diseases ar
can be made to an extract which is good for sore throats. Th
leaves when infused are cleansing while a root infusion is use
in eruptive fevers and has been used to treat cattle. A decoctic
of the bark is effective against calculus, oedema ar
haemorrhoids. The fruit was commonly used to make jelly, win
and cheese.

ADMINISTERED AS: juice, infusion or decoction.

adderwrack *Fucus vesiculosus*. COMMON NAME: Bladder fucus, seawrack, kelp ware, black-tang, cutweed, seetang, blasentang, meeriche.

OCCURRENCE: common around the coasts of the North Atlantic Ocean including Britain.

PARTS USED: the root, stem and leaves, the thallus. The seaweed contains a volatile oil, cellulose, mucilage, mannite, soda and iodine along with the bromine compounds of sodium and potassium.

MEDICINAL USES: a deobstruent, antifat. It has been used to cause weight loss and reduce obesity by stimulation of the thyroid gland. The wine made from grapes and dried fucus has been of benefit in diseases of the hip, joints and bones in children. It may also be applied externally as a poultice to treat enlarged glands.

ADMINISTERED AS: a liquid extract, decoction, infusion, fluid extract, or charcoal derived from *Fucus vesiculosus*.

uebell *Scilla nutans, Hyacinthus nonscriptus*. COMMON NAME: Calverkeys, culverkeys, auld man's bell, ring-o' bells, jacinth, wood bells, *Agraphis nutans*.

OCCURRENCE: abundant in western Europe, Great Britain and Italy.

PARTS USED: the bulb, dried and powdered.

MEDICINAL USES: diuretic, styptic. This medicine is little used today but it was considered a very powerful remedy for leucorrhoea. It may also have been used to cure snake bite. The fresh bulbs are poisonous, so the plant is always used when dried.

ADMINISTERED AS: powdered bulb.

ue flag *Iris versicolor*. COMMON NAME: Poison flag, flag lily, liver lily, snake lily, dragon flower, dagger flower, water flag.

OCCURRENCE: indigenous to North America and was introduced into Britain and Europe and is now a common garden plant.

PARTS USED: the rhizome which contains starch, gum, tannin, isophthalic acid, salicylic acid and oleoresin of which the latter compound contains the medicinal properties.

MEDICINAL USES: alterative, diuretic, cathartic, stimulant. It is

chiefly used for its alterative properties being useful as a pu
gative in disorders of the liver and the duodenum. Also, con
bined with other herbs as a blood purifier, or used alone again
syphilis, scrofula, skin afflictions and dropsy.

ADMINISTERED AS: powdered root, solid extract, fluid extract
tincture.

Bogbean *Menyanthes trifoliata*. COMMON NAME: Buckbean, mars
trefoil, water trefoil, marsh clover, boonan.

OCCURRENCE: found in spongy bogs, marshes and shallow wat
throughout Europe and is more common in northern Englar
and Scotland.

PARTS USED: the herb which consists of volatile oil and a gluc
side called menyanthin.

MEDICINAL USES: as a tonic, cathartic, deobstruent and febrifug
A liquid extract is used to treat rheumatism, scurvy and sk
complaints. It has also been recommended as an external a
plication to reduce glandular swelling. In the Highlands of Sco
land it was used to remedy stomach pains, particularly due
ulcers, and bogbean was also brewed into beer and smoked
herb tobacco. It is thought to cure ague (malaria) where
other cures have failed.

ADMINISTERED AS: the liquid extract, infusion or as tea.

Borage *Borago officinalis*. COMMON NAME: Burrage.

OCCURRENCE: naturalized in Britain and Europe and is found
gardens, rubbish heaps and near houses.

PARTS USED: the leaves and flowers consist of potassium, ca
cium, mineral acids along with nitrogen salts.

MEDICINAL USES: diuretic, demulcent, emollient, refrigerant.
is effective in treating fevers and pulmonary complaints as
activates the kidneys. It is applied externally as a poultice again
inflammation and swelling and has been developed into a crea
which treats itch and skin complaints, e.g. eczema and psori
sis. The flowers may be eaten raw, candied or made into a co
serve to strengthen people weakened by prolonged illness.

ADMINISTERED AS: an infusion, poultice or lotion.

Brooklime *Veronica beccabunga*. COMMON NAME: Water pimperne becky leaves, cow cress, horse cress, housewell grass, limewort, brooklembe, limpwort, wall-ink, water-pumpy, well-ink.

OCCURRENCE: very common in all parts of Great Britain.

PARTS USED: the herb. This plant contains tannin, a bitter principle, a volatile oil and sulphur.

MEDICINAL USES: alterative, diuretic. It is used as an infusion as an antiscorbutic and to treat impurities of the blood.

ADMINISTERED AS: infusion or poultice.

Broom *Cytisus scoparius.* COMMON NAME: Broom tops, Irish tops, basam, bizzom, browne, brum, bream, green broom.

OCCURRENCE: indigenous to England and commonly found on heathland throughout Britain, Europe and northern Asia.

PARTS USED: the young herbaceous tops which contain sparteine and scoparin as the active components.

MEDICINAL USES: diuretic and cathartic. The broom tops may be used as a decoction or infusion to aid dropsy while if the tops are pressed and treated broom juice is obtained. This fluid extract is generally used in combination with other diuretic compounds. An infusion of broom, AGRIMONY and DANDELION root is excellent in remedying bladder, kidney and liver trouble. *Cytisus* should be used carefully as the sparteine has a strong effect on the heart and, depending upon dose, can cause weakness of the heart similar to that caused by HEMLOCK (*Conium maculatum*). Death can occur in extreme cases if the respiratory organ's activity is impaired.

ADMINISTERED AS: fluid extract and infusion.

Bryony, Black *Tamus communis.* COMMON NAME: Blackeye root.

OCCURRENCE: native to Great Britain and is common in woods and hedges.

PARTS USED: the root.

MEDICINAL USES: as a rubefacient and diuretic. The drug is seldom used internally now due to its poisonous nature, but was formerly used to treat asthmatic complaints. Externally the fresh root is scraped, pulped and applied as a plaster to areas affected by gout, rheumatism or paralysis. A root pulp poultice was used on bruises and black eyes to remove discolouration from the skin. Chilblains were treated using a tincture made from the roots.

ADMINISTERED AS: a plaster, poultice, tincture, rarely as expressed juice.

Bryony, White *Bryonia dioica, Bryonia alba.* COMMON NAME: English mandrake, wild vine, wild hops, lady's seal, tetterbury, wild nep, tamus.

OCCURRENCE: a native of Europe, frequently found in England but rare in Scotland

PARTS USED: the root.

MEDICINAL USES: irritative, hydragogue, cathartic. It was previously used as a purgative drug but these and other uses have been discontinued on account of its highly irritant nature. It is still used in small doses for coughs, influenza, bronchitis and pneumonia. It is useful in cardiac disorders caused by gout or rheumatism and in malarial and contagious diseases. Care should be taken when used, due to its poisonous nature.

ADMINISTERED AS: liquid extract.

Bugle *Ajuga reptans.* COMMON NAME: Common bugle, carpenter's herb, middle confound, middle comfrey, sicklewort, herb carpenter, bugula.

OCCURRENCE: abundant throughout Great Britain in damp pastures and woods.

PARTS USED: the herb.

MEDICINAL USES: bitter, astringent and aromatic. As an infusion this herb is considered very good in arresting haemorrhages, easing irritation and coughs. It acts in a similar way to that of FOXGLOVE (*Digitalis purpurea*) in lowering the pulse rate and is said to be one of the mildest and best narcotics in existence. It is also considered good for the bad effects of excessive drinking.

ADMINISTERED AS: a decoction and infusion.

Burdock *Artium lappa.* COMMON NAME: Lappa, fox's clote, thorny burr, beggar's buttons, cockle buttons, love leaves, philanthropium, personata, happy major, clot-bur.

OCCURRENCE: freely found in ditches and hedgerows throughout England and Europe but rare in Scotland.

PARTS USED: the root, herb and seeds (fruits). They contain the chemicals inulin, mucilage, sugar and tannic acid along with a crystalline glucoside, lappin.

MEDICINAL USES: alterative, diuretic and diaphoretic. It is an excellent blood purifier and very effective in remedying all skin diseases. The root is most powerful and has anti-scorbutic properties which make it very useful for boils, scurvy and rheumatism. Also used as a wash for ulcers, a poultice for tumours, gouty swellings and bruises. An infusion of the leaves aids the stomach and eases indigestion. The tincture obtained from the seeds is relaxant, demulcent and a tonic for the skin.

ADMINISTERED AS: a fluid extract, infusion, tincture and solid extract.

Burnet, Greater *Sanguisorba officinalis*. COMMON NAME: garden burnet, common burnet, salad burnet.

OCCURRENCE: found in moist meadows and shady areas almost all over Europe and in British gardens.

PARTS USED: the herb and root.

MEDICINAL USES: astringent and tonic. Decoction of the whole herb is useful in haemorrhages. Both the herb and root are taken internally to treat abnormal discharges such as diarrhoea, dysentery and leucorrhoea. It is also used to make herb beer.

ADMINISTERED AS: a powder and infusion.

Burr Marigold *Bidens Impartica*. COMMON NAME: Water agrimony.

OCCURRENCE: commonly found in wet places in England but less frequently seen in Scotland.

PARTS USED: the whole plant.

MEDICINAL USES: astringent, diaphoretic, diuretic. This plant has been useful in dropsy, gout, haematuria and fevers. It is very good in treating diseases of the respiratory organs where bleeding occurs and also in uterine haemorrhage.

ADMINISTERED AS: an infusion.

Butcher's Broom *Ruscus aculeatus*. COMMON NAME: Kneeholm, knee holy, jew's myrtle, sweet broom, pettigree.

OCCURRENCE: a low shrubby plant found in woods and waste ground, primarily in the south of England.

PARTS USED: the herb and root.

MEDICINAL USES: diaphoretic, diuretic, deobstruent and aperient. It is used in jaundice, gravel, urinary and female obstructions and is said to be good in clearing phlegm from the chest and relieving difficult breathing.

ADMINISTERED AS: a decoction.

Butterbur *Petasites vulgaris.* COMMON NAME: Langwort, umbrella plant, bog rhubarb, plapperdock, blatterdock, capdockin, bogshorns, butterdock.

OCCURRENCE: in low wet grounds, marshy meadows and riversides in Great Britain.

PARTS USED: the rhizome or root-stock.

MEDICINAL USES: as a cardiac tonic, stimulant, and diuretic. It is good as a remedy for fevers, asthma, colds, urinary complaints gravel and plague. It is also taken as a homeopathic remedy for severe neuralgia in the back and loins. Recently, the use of butterbur has been recommended in easing the pain of migraine and painful menstruation. One of the most important developments is the treatment of cancer with *petasites* where the drug attacks tumours and abnormal cell changes very strongly and, in clinical tests, it has been shown to slow or stop the cancer spreading through the body. It has also become an effective remedy for severe asthma.

ADMINISTERED AS: a decoction and tincture.

Buttercup, Bulbous *Ranunculus bulbosus.* COMMON NAME: St Antony's turnip, crowfoot, frogsfoot, goldcup.

OCCURRENCE: found in meadows and fields throughout Britain

PARTS USED: the juice and herbs.

MEDICINAL USES: this plant has various uses including easing headaches and as a cure for shingles. The herb inflames and blisters the skin upon contact and is used to aid gout, sciatic and rheumatism. It has also been used as a poultice on the stomach.

ADMINISTERED AS: a poultice, decoction and tincture.

Cacao *Theobroma cacao.* COMMON NAME: Cocoa, chocolate tree

OCCURRENCE: found in tropical America and cultivated in most tropical countries, e.g. Sri Lanka and Java

PARTS USED: the seed which contain about two per cent of the chemical theobromine and forty to sixty per cent solid fat.

MEDICINAL USES: emollient, diuretic, stimulant and nutritive. The seeds are ground into a paste between hot rollers, with sugar and starch being added to produce cocoa. The cocoa butter (or oil of theobroma) produced forms a hard solid which is used in cosmetics, suppositories and coating pills. It has very good emollient qualities and is used to soften chapped hands and lips. The alkaloid, theobromine, which is contained in the beans is similar to caffeine in action on the central nervous system, but less powerful. It acts on the heart, kidneys and muscle and is used as a diuretic and stimulant of the kidneys. This is useful after fluid has accumulated in the body after heart failure and it is given in conjunction with digitalis (FOXGLOVE). The drug is also of benefit in high blood pressure.

ADMINISTERED AS: expressed oil, theobromine.

Calamint *Calamintha officinalis*. COMMON NAME: Mill mountain, mountain balm, basil thyme, mountain mint.

OCCURRENCE: a bushy plant found in hedgerows and lanes all over Great Britain and Europe.

PARTS USED: the herb. This contains a camphoraceous, volatile, stimulating oil similar to those found in other mint plants.

MEDICINAL USES: diaphoretic, expectorant and aromatic. It can be infused into a tea to treat weak stomachs, colic and flatulence. Can also be brewed into a syrup or decoction to heal the spleen, gall bladder and jaundice.

ADMINISTERED AS: an infusion, decoction and syrup.

Calamus *Aconus calamus*. COMMON NAME: Sweet flag, sweet sedge, sweet root, gladdon, sweet rush, sweet cane, myrtle grass, sweet myrtle, cinnamon sedge, myrtle wedge.

OCCURRENCE: grows freely in all European countries except Spain and it is common on river banks in Great Britain

PARTS USED: the rhizome, which produces a volatile oil after steam distillation, which is made up of pinene and asaryl aldehyde. It also contains alkaloidal material including choline and the glucoside acorin.

MEDICINAL USES: aromatic, carminative, stimulant, tonic and stomachic. It is used to remove the discomfort of flatulence, wind, colic, ague and dyspepsia. It can increase the appetite and aid digestion. Calamus oil is used in inhalations.

ADMINISTERED AS: a fluid extract, infusion, tincture and distilled oil.

Camphor *Cinnamonum camphora*. COMMON NAME: gum Camphor, laurel camphor, camphire, *Laurus camphora*, *Camphora officinarum*.

OCCURRENCE: found in China, Japan and parts of East Asia.

PARTS USED: the gum and distilled oil.

MEDICINAL USES: sedative, anodyne, antispasmodic, diaphoretic, anthelmintic, aromatic. It is mainly used in colds, chills, fevers, inflammatory complaints and for severe diarrhoea. It is taken internally for hysteria, nervousness, neuralgia and is used as an excitant in cases of heart failure due to infections, fever and pneumonia. Camphor is highly valued in all irritations of the sexual organs. Large doses of camphor should be avoided as they can cause vomiting, palpitations and convulsions due to the effects it has on the human brain.

ADMINISTERED AS: tincture, distilled oil, injection, capsules.

Caraway *Carum Carvi*. COMMON NAME: Caraway seed, caraway fruit, alcaravea.

OCCURRENCE: common in Europe and Asia and naturalized in Britain.

PARTS USED: the fruit, which produces a volatile oil containing hydrocarbon, carvene and an oxygenated oil, carvol.

MEDICINAL USES: aromatic, stimulant and carminative. It was widely used as a cordial to ease dyspepsia and hysteria. The oil is applied to treat flatulence and stomach disorders. Distilled caraway water is used to ease flatulent colic in infants and is an excellent children's medicine. The bruised fruits were used to remove pain from bad earache and was also used as a poultice to take away bruises. Caraway is widely as a flavouring for cheeses and seed-cakes.

ADMINISTERED AS: a liquid extract and poultice.

Cardamom *Elettaria cardamomum.* COMMON NAME: Mysore cardamon seeds, malabar cardamom, ebil, kakelah seghar, capalaga, gujalatti elachi, ilachi, ailum, *Amomum cardamomum, A. repens, Alpina cardamom, matonia Cardamomum, Cardamomum minus, Cardamomi Semina.*

OCCURRENCE: native to southern India and cultivated in Sri Lanka.

PARTS USED: the dried ripe seed containing volatile and fixed oil, starch, mucilage, potassium salts, resin and lignin.

MEDICINAL USES: carminative, stimulant, aromatic. They have a warming aromatic effect which is useful in indigestion and flatulence. If chewed, they are said to be good for colic and headaches. Cardamom is used chiefly as a flavouring for cakes, liqueurs, etc. and forms part of curry powder mixtures used in cookery.

ADMINISTERED AS: powdered seeds, tincture and fluid extract.

Caroba *jacaranda procera.* COMMON NAME: Carob tree, carobinha, caaroba, *jacaranda caroba, Bignonia caroba.*

OCCURRENCE: found in South America and Africa.

PARTS USED: the leaves contain many compounds including caroba balsam, caroborelinic acid, carobic acid, steocarobic acid, caroban and carobin.

MEDICINAL USES: alterative, diaphoretic, diuretic. The active principles have proved to be of benefit in treating syphilis and other venereal diseases. The soothing qualities of the herb have also been used to help epilepsy, as it has a sedative effect upon the nervous system. Caroba is rarely used in medicine today.

ADMINISTERED AS: dried, powdered leaves.

Carrot *Daucus carota.* COMMON NAME: Philtron, bird's nest, bee's nest.

OCCURRENCE: a native wild plant common everywhere in Great Britain. The wild and cultivated parts both exist today.

PARTS USED: the whole herb, seeds and root.

MEDICINAL USES: diuretic, stimulant, deobstruent. The herb infused in water is an active remedy in treating dropsy, chronic kidney infections and bladder disorders. Carrot tea was good for gout, while a strong decoction is good against gravel and flatulence. The roots have antiseptic properties and were formerly used as a laxative, vermifuge or a poultice. The wild carrot was particularly well thought of as a poultice for cancerous sores, while the seeds act in a similar manner to CARAWAY in treating stomach and gastric complaints. Carrot seed also has properties as an emmenagogue and in clearing obstructions of the viscera and jaundice. Carrots are made into jam, wine, spirit and can be roasted to produce a coffee substitute.

ADMINISTERED AS: an infusion, tea and poultice.

Cassia *Cinnamomum cassia.* COMMON NAME: Bastard cinnamon, Chinese cinnamon, cassia bark, canton cassia, *Cassia lignea, Cassia aromaticum.*

OCCURRENCE: indigenous to China and cultivated in Japan, Sumatra, Java, South America, Mexico and Sri Lanka.

PARTS USED: the bark. The bark of this tree is regarded as a substitute for cinnamon and it produces a volatile oil similar to oil of cinnamon. Cassia oil contains cinnamic aldehyde, cinnamylacetate, cinnamic acid, tannic acid and starch amongst other compounds.

MEDICINAL USES: stomachic, carminative, tonic, astringent and emmenagogue. The tincture is used in uterine haemorrhage, menorrhagia and to decrease the flow of breast milk. It is also used to assist and flavour other drugs and benefits diarrhoea, vomiting, nausea and flatulence. Cassia oil is a powerful germicide but is not normally used in medicine as such as it is very irritant. It may be used for gastric pain, flatulent colic and gastric debility as it is a strong local stimulant.

ADMINISTERED AS: expressed oil, powdered bark.

Castor oil plant *Ricinus communis.* COMMON NAME: palma Christi, castor oil bush.

OCCURRENCE: a native of India, but has been cultivated in many tropical, sub-tropical and temperate countries around the globe.

PARTS USED: the oil expressed from the seeds.

MEDICINAL USES: cathartic, purgative, laxative, vermifuge, galactogogue. Castor oil is regarded as one of the best laxative and purgative preparations available. It is of particular benefit for children and pregnant women due to its mild action in easing constipation, colic and diarrhoea due to slow digestion. The oil expels worms from the body, after other suitable remedies have been given. When applied externally, Castor oil eases cutaneous complaints such as ringworm, itch and leprosy, while it is used as a carrier oil for solutions of pure alkaloids, e.g. atropine or cocaine, from BELLADONNA (*Atropa belladonna*), that these drugs can be used in eye surgery. Castor oil is used for a range of industrial purposes from soap-making to varnishes.

ADMINISTERED AS: expressed oil.

Catmint *Nepeta cataria.* COMMON NAME: Catnep, nep.

OCCURRENCE: a wild English plant in hedges, field borders and waste ground. It is found on a localized basis in Scotland.

PARTS USED: the herb.

MEDICINAL USES: carminative, tonic, diaphoretic, refrigerant, mildly stimulating and slightly emmenagogue. This herb is good in treating colds, fevers, restlessness and colic. It is also used in nervousness and insanity and to calm children and soothe nightmares when taken as an infusion or conserve. Catmint can be applied to swellings and bruises as a poultice.

ADMINISTERED AS: an infusion, injection or poultice.

Cayenne *Capsicum minimum, Capsicum frutescens.* COMMON NAME: African pepper, chillies, bird pepper.

OCCURRENCE: native to Zanzibar but is now cultivated in most tropical and sub-tropical countries, e.g. Sierra Leone, Japan and Madagascar

PARTS USED: the fruit, both fresh and dried.

MEDICINAL USES: stimulant, tonic, carminative, rubefacient. It is possibly the purest and best stimulant in herbal medicine. It produces natural warmth and helps the blood circulation, and eases weakness of the stomach and intestines. Cayenne is added to tonics and is said to ward off disease and can prevent development of colds and fevers.

ADMINISTERED AS: powdered fruit, tincture, capsules, dietary item.

Cedar, Yellow *Thuja occidentalis.* COMMON NAME: Tree of life,

arbor vitae, false white cedar, *Cedrus lycea*, hackmatack, thuia
de Canada, Lebensbaum.

OCCURRENCE: the United States and Canada.

PARTS USED: the leaves and twigs. The plant contains the bitter
principle pinipicrin, volatile oil, sugar, wax, resin and a colouring
principle called thujin. The leaves and twigs yield an essential
oil similar to camphor, which contains pinene, fenchone,
thujone and carvone.

MEDICINAL USES: aromatic, astringent, diuretic, anthelmintic,
irritant, expectorant, emmenagogue. A decoction of the twigs
can help intermittent fevers, coughs, gout, amenorrhoea, dropsy
and scurvy. When made into an ointment, the leaves ease rheumatism. An infusion is good at removing warts and fungal
growths. A preparation of the twigs may induce abortion by reflex action on the uterus from severe gastro-intestinal irritation. This plant should be used with some care.

ADMINISTERED AS: infusion, decoction, injection, poultice, tincture, ointment.

Celandine *Chelidonium majus.* COMMON NAME: Garden celandine, common celandine, greater celandine.

OCCURRENCE: common all over Great Britain and Europe.

PARTS USED: the herb, which contains the alkaloids chelidanine,
chelerythrin (of which the latter is narcotic), homochelidonine
A and B. Three other major chemicals are found in the plant.

MEDICINAL USES: alterative, diuretic and purgative. It is of benefit to jaundice, eczema, scrofulous diseases and scurvy. The
fresh juice was used to cure warts, ringworm and corns but
should not otherwise be allowed to come into direct contact
with the skin. In various forms, it has previously been effective
against itching, piles, toothache and cancer.

ADMINISTERED AS: infusion, fluid extract, decoction, lotion, poultice.

Celery *Apium graveolens.* COMMON NAME: Smallage, wild celery.

OCCURRENCE: native to southern Europe and cultivated in Britain.

PARTS USED: the ripe seeds, herb and root of which the seeds
contain two oils and apiol.

MEDICINAL USES: carminative, stimulant, diuretic, tonic, nervine and aphrodisiac. It is utilised as a tonic in combination with other herbs, promoting restfulness, sleep and lack of hysteria and is excellent in relieving rheumatism.

ADMINISTERED AS: fluid extract, essential oil and powdered seeds.

Chamomile, Camomile *Anthemis nobilis.* COMMON NAME: Roman chamomile, double chamomile, manzanilla (Spanish), maythen (Saxon).

OCCURRENCE: a low growing plant found wild in the British Isles.

PARTS USED: the flowers and herb. The active principles therein are a volatile oil, anthemic acid, tannic acid and a glucoside.

MEDICINAL USES: tonic, stomachic, anodyne and anti-spasmodic. An infusion of chamomile tea is an extremely effective remedy for hysterical and nervous afflictions in women, as well as an emmenagogue. Chamomile has a powerful soothing and sedative effect which is harmless. A tincture is used to cure diarrhoea in children and it is used with purgatives to prevent griping, and as a tonic it helps dropsy. Externally, it can be applied alone or with other herbs as a poultice to relieve pain, swellings, inflammation and neuralgia. Its strong antiseptic properties make it invaluable for reducing swelling of the face due to abscess or injury. As a lotion, the flowers are good for resolving toothache and earache. The herb itself is an ingredient in herb beers. The use of chamomile can be dated back to ancient Egyptian times when they dedicated the plant to the sun because of its extensive healing properties.

ADMINISTERED AS: decoction, infusion, fluid extract and essential oil.

Cherry laurel *Prunus laurocerasus*

OCCURRENCE: native to Russia and now cultivated in many temperate European countries.

PARTS USED: the leaves. The main constituent is prulaurasin which resembles amygdalin and hydrocyanic acid.

MEDICINAL USES: sedative, narcotic. The leaves are used to produce a distilled water which is the main herbal preparation used of this herb. It is good against coughs, dyspepsia, indigestion, whooping cough and asthma.

ADMINISTERED AS: cherry laurel water.

Chestnut, Horse *Aesculus hippocastanum*. COMMON NAME: *Hippocastanum vulgare*.

OCCURRENCE: a tree native to northern and central Asia from which it was introduced into England and Scotland.

PARTS USED: the bark and fruit, from both of which a fluid extract is made.

MEDICINAL USES: tonic, narcotic, febrifuge and astringent. The bark is used in intermittent fevers as an infusion, while it is also used externally to treat ulcers. The fruits are employed in easing neuralgia, rheumatism as well as rectal complaints and haemorrhoids.

ADMINISTERED AS: an infusion and fluid extract.

Chestnut, Sweet *Castanea vesca*. COMMON NAME: *Fagus castanea*, sardia nut, Jupiter's nut, hushed nut, Spanish chestnut, *Castanea vulgaris*.

OCCURRENCE: very common in Britain, Europe and North America.

PARTS USED: the leaves.

MEDICINAL USES: tonic, astringent. It is used in a popular remedy to treat fever and ague. Its reputation is due to the great effectiveness in treating violent and convulsive coughs, particularly whooping cough and in other irritable respiratory organ conditions. The nut is commonly eaten as food or as a stuffing for meat.

ADMINISTERED AS: an infusion.

Chickweed *Stellania media*. COMMON NAME: Starweed, star chickweed, *Alsine media*, passerina.

OCCURRENCE: native to all temperate and North Arctic regions and is naturalized wherever Man has settled. A common weed.

PARTS USED: the whole herb, both fresh and dried.

MEDICINAL USES: demulcent, refrigerant. It is good as a poultice to reduce inflammation and heal indolent ulcers, but is most important as an ointment in treating eye problems and cutaneous diseases. It will also benefit scurvy and kidney disorders as an infusion.

ADMINISTERED AS: an infusion, poultice and ointment.

hicory *Cichonium intybus*. COMMON NAME: Succory, wild succ-ory, hendibeh, barbe de capucin.

OCCURRENCE: common in England and Ireland but rarer in Scotland.

PARTS USED: the root.

MEDICINAL USES: tonic, diuretic and laxative. A decoction of the root has benefit in jaundice, liver problems, gout and rheumatic complaints. The root, when dried, roasted and ground, may be added to coffee or may be drunk on its own as a beverage.

ADMINISTERED AS: a decoction, poultice, syrup or distilled water.

hives *Allium schoenoprasum*. COMMON NAME: Cives.

OCCURRENCE: native to temperate and northern Europe and Great Britain and has been cultivated over a large area of the northern hemisphere.

PARTS USED: the herb.

MEDICINAL USES: this herb stimulates the appetite and helps digestion during convalescence. It is also said to be effective against infections and prevent anaemia. They are also widely used in food dishes and add vitamins and colour to many meals.

ADMINISTERED AS: fresh herbs.

icely, Sweet *Myrrhis odorata*. COMMON NAME: Smooth cicely, British myrrh, anise, great sweet chervil, smelt chervil, sweet bracken, sweet-fern, sweet humlock, sweets, The Roman plant, shepherd's needle, cow chervil.

OCCURRENCE: native to Great Britain and also found in mountain pastures across Europe.

PARTS USED: the root and herb.

MEDICINAL USES: aromatic, carminative, stomachic, expectorant. The fresh root may be eaten or used as a tonic in brandy. It eases coughs, flatulence, indigestion and stomach upsets. The herb, as an infusion, is good for anaemia and a tonic for young girls. The antiseptic roots have been used for snake or dog bites while the distilled water is diuretic and effective in treating pleurisy. Sweet Cicely essence is said to have aphrodisiac properties.

ADMINISTERED AS: a root infusion, herb infusion, decoction, es
sence and distilled water.

Cinnamon *Cinnamomum zeylanicum.* COMMON NAME: Lauri
cinnamomum.

OCCURRENCE: native to Sri Lanka but is cultivated in other East
ern countries.

PARTS USED: the bark.

MEDICINAL USES: carminative, astringent, stimulant, antiseptic
aromatic. It is used as a local stimulant as a powder and infu
sion, generally combined with other herbs. Cinnamon stop
vomiting and nausea, relieves flatulence and diarrhoea and ca
also be employed to stop haemorrhage of the womb.

ADMINISTERED AS: powder, distilled water, tincture or an essen
tial oil.

Clematis *Clematis recta.* COMMON NAME: Upright virgin's bowe
Clammula jovis.

OCCURRENCE: a perennial plant common to Europe.

PARTS USED: the roots and stem.

MEDICINAL USES: diuretic, diaphoretic. When bruised, the leave
and flowers irritate the eyes and throat prompting tears an
coughing. If applied to the skin, it produces inflammation an
blisters appear. The herb is used both as a local external appli
cation, and internally against syphilis, cancer and other ulcer
It is used by homeopaths for eye complaints, gonorrhoea an
inflammatory conditions.

ADMINISTERED AS: dried leaves, fluid extract.

Clivers *Galium aparine.* COMMON NAME: Cleavers, goosegras
borweed, hedgesheriff, hayriffe, eriffe, grip grass, hayruf
catchweed, scratweed, mutton chops, robin-run-in-the-gras
love-man, goosebill, everlasting friendship.

OCCURRENCE: an abundant hedgerow weed in Europe, Grea
Britain and North America.

PARTS USED: the herb, which contains chlorophyll, starcl
galitannic acid, citric acid and rubichloric acid.

MEDICINAL USES: diuretic, tonic, aperient and alterative. It is su
cessfully administered to treat obstruction of the urinary organ

gravel, suppression of urine, etc. A wash of the herb helps sunburn and freckles, while an ointment provides benefit against cancerous growths and tumours. The expressed juice or infusion will help scurvy, scrofula, psoriasis and other skin complaints as well as stopping insomnia and inducing sleep.

ADMINISTERED AS: an infusion, decoction, ointment, expressed juice or lotion.

Clover, Red *Trifolium pratense*. COMMON NAME: Trefoil, purple clover.

OCCURRENCE: widely distributed in Britain and Europe.

PARTS USED: the flowers.

MEDICINAL USES: alterative, sedative, antispasmodic. The fluid extract or infusion are excellent in treating bronchial and whooping coughs. External applications of the herb in a poultice has been used on cancerous growths.

ADMINISTERED AS: fluid extract and infusion.

Cloves *Eugenia caryophyllata*. COMMON NAME: *Eugenia aromatica*, *Eugenia caryophyllus*, clavos.

OCCURRENCE: grows on the Molucca Islands in the southern Philippines.

PARTS USED: the underdeveloped flowers.

MEDICINAL USES: stimulating, carminative, aromatic. It is given as powder or an infusion for nausea, vomiting, flatulence, languid indigestion and dyspepsia. The volatile oil contains the medicinal properties and it is a strong germicide, antiseptic and a local irritant. It has been used as an expectorant to aid bronchial troubles. Clove oil is often used in association with other medicines.

ADMINISTERED AS: powdered cloves, infusion, essential oil, fluid extract.

Club moss *Lycopodium clavatum*. COMMON NAME: Lycopodium, lycopodium seed, vegetable sulphur, wolf's claw, muscus terrestris repens.

OCCURRENCE: occurs throughout Great Britain being most plentiful on heath or moorland in northern countries and is also found all over the world.

PARTS USED: the fresh plant and spores.

MEDICINAL USES: spores are diuretic, nervine and aperient. The fresh plant has been used as a stomachic and a diuretic herb in calculus and kidney complaints. The spores are currently applied externally to wounds and taken internally for diarrhoea, dysentery, gout and scurvy.

ADMINISTERED AS: dried spores, fresh moss.

Coca, Bolivian: *Erythroxylum coca*; **Peruvian**: *Erythroxylum truxillense*. COMMON NAME: Cuca, cocaine.

OCCURRENCE: native to Peru and Bolivia; cultivated in Java and Sri Lanka.

PARTS USED: the leaves. They contain the alkaloids cocaine, amamyl cocaine and truxilline or cocamine when grown in South America. Eastern-grown plants contain additional chemicals and glucosides.

MEDICINAL USES: nerve stimulant, anodyne, tonic, aphrodisiac. The leaves are used as a cerebral and muscle stimulant during convalescence relieving nausea, vomiting and stomach pain. It is utilized as a general nerve tonic and in treating asthma. In South America, the locals chew the leaves to relieve hunger and fatigue, but this does cause health damage when done over a long period of time. There is a danger of developing an addictive habit to this drug and the possible medicinal benefits are less than the potential health damage. People with a cocaine habit can appear emaciated, suffer loss of memory, sleeplessness and delusions. In Great Britain, the distribution and use of this drug is controlled by the Dangerous Drugs Act.

ADMINISTERED AS: tincture, powdered leaves, fluid extract.

Coffee *Coffea arabica*. COMMON NAME: Caffea.

OCCURRENCE: native to a province of Abyssinia and cultivated throughout the tropics.

PARTS USED: the seed and leaves. When roasted, coffee contains oil, wax, caffeine, aromatic oil, tannic acid, caffetannic acid, gum, sugar and protein.

MEDICINAL USES: stimulant, diuretic, anti-narcotic, anti-emetic. Coffee is commonly used as a beverage but it can also be applied as a medicine. It is a brain stimulant, causing sleeplessness

and hence is useful in cases of narcotic poisoning. For this reason it is very good against snake bite in that it helps stop people
falling into a coma. Caffeine can be valuable for heart disease,
fluid retention and it is used against drunkenness. As a powerful diuretic, it can help ease gout, rheumatism, gravel and
dropsy.

ADMINISTERED AS: beverage, caffeine preparation.

Cohosh, Black *Cimicifuga racemosa.* COMMON NAME: Black sna-
keroot, bugbane, rattleroot, rattleweed, squawroot, *Actaea
racemosa, Macrotys actaeoides.*

OCCURRENCE: a native of the United States and Canada and was
introduced into England around 1860.

PARTS USED: the rhizome. The main constituents are a resinous
substance known as cimicifuga (or macrotin) and racemosin
which gives the drug its bitter taste.

MEDICINAL USES: astringent, emmenagogue, diuretic, alterative,
expectorant. This root is said to be effective in many disorders
including whooping cough and rheumatism. It is supposed to
be an antidote to poison and rattlesnake bites. The drug can
help ease children's diarrhoea, and in consumption acts by slowing the pulse rate, inducing perspiration and easing the cough.
In overdoses, black Cohosh can cause vomiting and nausea.

ADMINISTERED AS: tincture, infusion, decoction, powdered root.

Cohosh, Blue *Caulophyllum thalictroides.* COMMON NAME: Pa-
poose root, squawroot, blueberry root, *Leontice thalichoides.*

OCCURRENCE: found in the United States and Canada.

PARTS USED: the rhizome. It contains gum, starch, salts, soluble
resin and a chemical similar to saponin.

MEDICINAL USES: diuretic, antispasmodic, vermifuge, emmenagogue, athelmintic, diaphoretic. This drug has been used in
rheumatism, epilepsy, uterine inflammation, hysteria and
dropsy. It is also taken to expedite childbirth and induce menstruation.

ADMINISTERED AS: decoction, infusion, tincture, solid extract.

Coltsfoot *Tussilago farfara.* COMMON NAME: Coughwort, hallfoot,
horsehoof, ass's foot, foals-wort, fieldhove, bullsfoot, donnhove.

OCCURRENCE: commonly found wild on waste ground an
riverbanks in Great Britain.

PARTS USED: the leaves, flowers and root.

MEDICINAL USES: demulcent, expectorant and tonic. Coltsfoot
one of the most popular cough remedies and is generally take
in conjunction with HOREHOUND, MARSHMALLOW or GROUND IVY.
has been called 'nature's best herb for the lungs' and it w
recommended that the leaves be smoked to relieve a coug
Today, it forms the basis of British herb tobacco along wit
BOGBEAN, EYEBRIGHT, WOOD BETONY, ROSEMARY, THYME, LAVEND
and CHAMOMILE which is said to relieve asthma, catarrh, bron
chitis and lung troubles.

ADMINISTERED AS: syrup or smoked when dried.

Columbine *Aquilegia vulgaris*. COMMON NAME: Culverwort.

OCCURRENCE: found as both a wild and garden plant in Gre
Britain.

PARTS USED: the leaves, roots and seeds.

MEDICINAL USES: astringent. It must be administered in sma
doses where it is used as a lotion for sore mouths and throat
It was also used for stone, jaundice and liver obstructions. Larg
doses can cause poisoning, so care must be taken in utilizin
this drug.

ADMINISTERED AS: fresh root and infusion.

Comfrey *Symphytum officinale*. COMMON NAME: Common com
frey, knitbone, knitback, bruisewort, slippery root, gum plan
consolida, ass ear, blackwort.

OCCURRENCE: a native of Europe and temperate Asia but is con
mon throughout England by rivers and ditches.

PARTS USED: the root and leaves. The roots contain a large quan
tity of mucilage, choline and allantoin.

MEDICINAL USES: demulcent, mildly astringent, expectorant an
vulnerary. It is frequently used in pulmonary complaints,
soothe intestinal trouble and is a gentle remedy for diarrho
and dysentery. A strong decoction or tea is administered in cas
of internal haemorrhage whether it is the lungs, stomach, bow
els or haemorrhoids. Externally, the leaves have been used as

poultice to promote healing of severe cuts, ulcers and abscesses and to reduce swelling, sprains and bruises. Allantoin is known to reduce swelling round damaged or fractured bones, thus allowing healing to occur faster and more thoroughly.

ADMINISTERED AS: a decoction, poultice and liquid extract.

Coriander *Coriandrum sativum*

OCCURRENCE: indigenous to southern Europe and found occasionally in Britain, at riversides, fields and waste ground.

PARTS USED: the fruit and leaves.

MEDICINAL USES: stimulant, aromatic and carminative. It is generally used with active purgatives as flavouring and to lessen their griping tendencies. Coriander water was formerly used for windy colic.

ADMINISTERED AS: powdered fruit, fluid extract.

Cornflower *Centaurea cyanus.* COMMON NAME: bluebottle, bluebow, hurtsickle, blue cap, bluet.

OCCURRENCE: common in cultivated fields and roadsides in Britain.

PARTS USED: the flowers.

MEDICINAL USES: tonic, stimulant and emmenagogue properties. A water distilled from cornflower petals was said to be a remedy for eye inflammation and weak eyesight.

ADMINISTERED AS: distilled water and infusion.

Costmary *Tanacetum balsamita.* COMMON NAME: Alecost, balsam herb, costmarie, mace, balsamita.

OCCURRENCE: an old English herb, naturalized from the Orient in the sixteenth century.

PARTS USED: the leaves.

MEDICINAL USES: it was formerly used as an aperient, antiseptic and astringent herb in treating dysentery. Used as an infusion to heal stomach and head problems but also as flavouring for ale and in salads.

ADMINISTERED AS: infusion and tincture.

Cotton root *Gossypium herbaceum* (and other species)

OCCURRENCE: indigenous to India and cultivated in Greece, Turkey, Sicily and Malta.

PARTS USED: the root-bark which contains a peculiar acid resin, sugar, gum, chlorophyll, fixed oil and tannin.

MEDICINAL USES: this drug is used to induce abortion or miscarriage as it causes contraction of the uterus. It is useful in treating abnormal uterine bleeding particularly when linked to fibroids, and in cases of difficult or obstructed menstruation. A preparation is given to induce labour (at full term) to aid safe delivery. It is said to be of use in sexual lassitude.

ADMINISTERED AS: fluid extract, decoction, solid extract.

Couchgrass *Agropyrum repens.* COMMON NAME: Twitchgrass, Scotch quelch, quickgrass, dog's grass, *Triticum repens.*

OCCURRENCE: abundant in fields and waste ground in Britain, Europe, northern Asia and North and South America

PARTS USED: the rhizome, which contains triticin (a carbohydrate).

MEDICINAL USES: diuretic, demulcent, aperient. Widely used in complaints of the urinary organs and bladder. Also recommended for gout and rheumatism.

ADMINISTERED AS: an infusion, decoction and liquid extract.

Cowslip *Primula veris.* COMMON NAME: Herb peter, paigle, peggle, key flower, key of heaven, fairy cups, petty mulleins, patsywort, plumrocks, mayflower, Our Lady's keys, arthritica.

OCCURRENCE: a common wild flower in all parts of Great Britain

PARTS USED: the flower.

MEDICINAL USES: sedative, antispasmodic. It is very good in relieving restlessness and insomnia. Commonly brewed into wine which was a good children's medicine in small doses.

ADMINISTERED AS: an infusion or wine.

Croton *Croton tiglian.* COMMON NAME: Tiglium, *Tiglium officinale.*

OCCURRENCE: a tree found on the Malabar coast of India and on the Indian archipelago.

PARTS USED: the oil expressed from the seeds, croton oil contains glycerides of stearic, palmitic, myristic, lauric and oleic acids; the glycerin ethers of formic, acetic, isobutyric and isovaleranic acids. The active principle is probably Crotonic acid.

MEDICINAL USES: irritant, rubefacient, cathartic, purgative. A drastic purgative drug which acts quickly, often evacuating the bowels in less than one hour. In large doses, it causes vomiting and severe griping pains which can possibly be fatal. The drug is only used in cases of obstinate constipation where other drugs have failed. It is applied externally as a counter-irritant to relieve rheumatism, gout, neuralgia and bronchitis. The use of this oil should be monitored most carefully, only administered in small doses, and never given to children or pregnant women.
ADMINISTERED AS: expressed oil.

Crowfoot, Upright meadow *Ranunculus acris.* COMMON NAME: gold cup, grenouillette.
OCCURRENCE: native in meadows, pastures and fields in all parts of northern Europe and Great Britain.
PARTS USED: the whole herb.
MEDICINAL USES: the expressed juice is used to remove warts. A poultice of the fresh herb is good at removing violent, painful headaches or in relieving gout. The fresh herb once formed part of a famous cure for cancer practised in 1794.
ADMINISTERED AS: fresh leaves, expressed juice.

Cuckoopint *Arum maculatum.* COMMON NAME: Lords and Ladies, starchwort, arum, adder's root, friar's cowl, kings and queens, parson and clerk, ramp, Quaker, wake robin.
OCCURRENCE: the sole British species of the arum, aroidae family and is also widely distributed over Europe.
PARTS USED: the root. This contains starch, albumen, sugar, lignin, saponin a an unidentified alkaloid.
MEDICINAL USES: diaphoretic, expectorant, diuretic, stimulant. The fresh root can be prepared into a tincture and given to remedy sore, feverish throats. The dried root can be stored for long periods, but is rarely employed as a medicine today. An ointment prepared of the fresh root was used to cure ringworm.
ADMINISTERED AS: tincture, expressed juice and ointment.

Cucumber *Cucumis sativa.* COMMON NAME: Cowcumber.
OCCURRENCE: a native of the East Indies, but was first cultivated in Britain around 1573.

PARTS USED: the whole fruit, peeled or unpeeled, raw and cooked
MEDICINAL USES: the seeds are diuretic and are an excellent tae
niacide and purge. The fruit is very good as a skin cosmetic a
it has cooling, healing and soothing effects on irritated skin
Cucumber juice is widely utilised in emollient ointments o
creams and is good for sunburn.

ADMINISTERED AS: expressed juice, lotion or ointment.

Cudweed *Graphalium uliginosum*. COMMON NAME: Cottonweed
marsh everlasting, cotton dawes.

OCCURRENCE: found in marshy areas in all parts of Europe.

PARTS USED: the herb.

MEDICINAL USES: astringent. It is a very good remedy for quinsy
when used as a gargle and can also be taken internally.

ADMINISTERED AS: an infusion.

Cumin *Cuminum cyminum*. COMMON NAME: Cummin, *Cumino
aigro*.

OCCURRENCE: indigenous to upper Egypt and is cultivated i
Arabia, India, China and Mediterranean countries since early
times.

PARTS USED: the fruit. The chief constituents are a volatile oil, a
fatty oil with resin, mucilage, gum, malates and albuminous
matter.

MEDICINAL USES: stimulant, carminative, antispasmodic. This
herb has similar effects to FENNEL and CARAWAY but its use ha
declined due to its disagreeable taste. It had a considerable
reputation in helping correct flatulence due to languid diges
tion and as a remedy for colic and dyspeptic headache. Applied
externally as a plaster, it eased stitches and pains in the side
and has been combined with other herbs to form a stimulating
liniment.

ADMINISTERED AS: dried, powdered fruit, whole fruit.

Cup moss *Cladonia pyxidata*. COMMON NAME: Chin cups.

OCCURRENCE: indigenous to north-west America but is also
common weed through Great Britain and Europe.

PARTS USED: the whole plant.

MEDICINAL USES: expectorant – used as a decoction to trea

children's coughs and whooping cough with great effectiveness.

ADMINISTERED AS: decoction.

Daffodil *Narcissus pseudo-narcissus.* COMMON NAME: Narcissus, porillion, daffy-down-dilly, fleur de coucou, Lent lily.

OCCURRENCE: found wild in most European countries including the British Isles.

PARTS USED: the bulb, leaves and flowers. The bulbs contain an alkaloid called lyconine.

MEDICINAL USES: the flowers, when powdered, have emetic properties and as an infusion are used in pulmonary catarrh. The bulbs are also emetic and, indeed, can cause people to collapse and die due to paralysis of the central nervous system due to the action of lyconine, which acts quickly. Accidents have resulted from daffodil bulbs being mistaken for ONIONS and eaten. Since high temperatures and cooking does not break down the poisonous alkaloid, considerable care should be taken to avoid problems. The bulbs are used externally as an astringent poultice to dissolve hard swellings and aid wound healing.

ADMINISTERED AS: powder and extract.

Daisy, Ox-eye *Chrysanthemum leuconthemum.* COMMON NAME: great ox-eye, goldens, marguerite, moon daisy, horse gowan, maudlin daisy, field daisy, dun daisy, butter daisy, horse daisy, maudlinwort, white weed, gowan.

OCCURRENCE: found in fields throughout Europe and northern Asia.

PARTS USED: the whole herb, flowers and root.

MEDICINAL USES: antispasmodic, diuretic, tonic. This herb's main use has been in whooping cough, asthma and nervous excitability. When taken as a tonic, it acts in a similar way to chamomile flowers and calms night-sweats and nightmares. An infusion of ox-eye daisy flowers is good at relieving bronchial coughs and catarrh. It is also used as a lotion for wounds, bruises and ulcers.

ADMINISTERED AS: an infusion and lotion.

Damiana *Turnera aphrodisiaca* or *Turnera diffusa* var. *aphrodisiaca.*

OCCURRENCE: indigenous to Texas and Mexico; cultivated in other areas of sub-tropical America and Africa.

PARTS USED: the leaves which contain a volatile oil, resins, tannin and the bitter principle damianin.

MEDICINAL USES: mild purgative, diuretic, tonic, stimulant, aphrodisiac. This drug acts as a tonic to the nervous system and has a direct and general beneficial effect on the reproductive organs.

ADMINISTERED AS: fluid extract, solid extract.

Dandelion *Taraxacum officinale.* COMMON NAME: priest's crown, swine's snout.

OCCURRENCE: widely found across the northern temperate zone in pastures, meadows and waste ground.

PARTS USED: the root and leaves. The main constituents of the root are taraxacin, a bitter substance, and taraxacerin, an acid resin, along with the sugar inulin.

MEDICINAL USES: diuretic, tonic and slightly aperient. It acts as a general body stimulant, but chiefly acts on the liver and kidneys. Dandelion is used as a bitter tonic in atonic dyspepsia as a mild laxative and to promote increased appetite and digestion. The herb is best used in combination with other herbs and is used in many patent medicines. Roasted dandelion root is also used as a coffee substitute and helps ease dyspepsia, gout and rheumatism.

ADMINISTERED AS: fluid and solid extract, decoction, infusion and tincture.

Dill *Peucedanum graveolus, Fructus anethi.* COMMON NAME: Dill seed, dill fruit, *Anethum graveolus, Fructus anethi.*

OCCURRENCE: indigenous to Mediterranean districts and South Russia and is cultivated in England and Europe.

PARTS USED: the dried ripe fruit. An oil obtained from the fruit is almost identical to oil of CARAWAY, both containing limonene and carvone.

MEDICINAL USES: stimulant, aromatic, carminative and stomachic. It is usually given as dillwater which is very good for children's flatulence or disordered digestion. Oil of dill is used in medicine in largely the same way, but is also used in perfuming soaps.

ADMINISTERED AS: distilled water, essential oil.

Dock, Yellow *Rumex crispus.* COMMON NAME: Curled dock.

OCCURRENCE: normally found on roadside ditches and waste ground, all over Great Britain.

PARTS USED: the root and whole herb.

MEDICINAL USES: the root has laxative, alterative and a mildly tonic action and is used in rheumatism, bilious complaints and haemorrhoids. It is very useful in treating jaundice, diseases of the blood, scurvy, chronic skin diseases and as a tonic on the digestive system. Yellow dock is said to have a positive effect on slowing the development of cancer, due to its alterative and tonic properties. It has similar effects to that of RHUBARB and has been used in treating diphtheria.

ADMINISTERED AS: dried extract, syrup, infusion, tincture, ointment, fluid extract and solid extract.

Dodder *Cuscuta europea.* COMMON NAME: Lesser dodder, dodder of thyme, beggarweed, hellweed, strangle tare, scaldweed, devil's guts.

OCCURRENCE: a parasitic plant found in most areas of the world.

PARTS USED: the herb.

MEDICINAL USES: hepatic, laxative, purgative. A decoction made with dodder, GINGER and ALLSPICE has been used against urinary complaints, kidney, spleen and liver disorders. The herb is good in treating sciatica, scorbutic problems, scrofulous tumours and it acts as a purge due to its very bitter taste.

ADMINISTERED AS: decoction, infusion.

Dog-rose *Rosa canina.* COMMON NAME: Wild briar, hip tree, cynosbatos.

OCCURRENCE: indigenous to Great Britain.

PARTS USED: the ripe fruit which contain invert fruit sugars, a range of mineral salts and a large proportion of vitamin C or ascorbic acid.

MEDICINAL USES: astringent, refrigerant and pectoral. The fruit is used in strengthening the stomach and digestion, as well as easing coughs. It is made into an uncooked preserve, a syrup which is excellent for infants and children and rose-hip tea has very beneficial effects. An infusion of dog-rose leaves has been used as a tea substitute and has a pleasant aroma.

ADMINISTERED AS: an infusion, syrup or dietary item.

Dropwort, Hemlock water *Œnanthe crocata*. COMMON NAME: Horsebane, deadtongue, five-fingered root, water lovage, yellow water dropwort.

OCCURRENCE: common in ditches and watering places in England, particularly the southern counties.

PARTS USED: the roots.

MEDICINAL USES: the beneficial uses are few because this plant is virulently poisonous. A tincture is used to treat eruptive diseases of the skin, but with very small dosages and great caution. Poultices have been used to heal whitlows or ulcers. This wild plant is the most poisonous of our indigenous plants and many deaths have resulted from adults and children eating the leaves or roots mistakenly.

ADMINISTERED AS: tincture, poultice.

Dropwort, Water *Œnanthe phellandrium*. COMMON NAME: fine-leaved water dropwort, water fennel, fine-leaved oenanthe, *Phellandrium aquaticum*.

OCCURRENCE: a common plant in ditches and water courses across Europe and Great Britain.

PARTS USED: the fruit, which yields an ethereal oil called water fennel oil. The main chemical in the oil is the terpene phellandrene.

MEDICINAL USES: expectorant, alterative, diuretic. The fruits are used to ease chronic pectoral conditions like bronchitis, consumption and asthma and also works well against dyspepsia, intermittent fevers and ulcers. Applied externally, the root has been utilized as a remedy for haemorrhoids. When taken in too large amounts, causing an overdose, the fruit prompts vertigo, intoxication and other narcotic effects. If the root is eaten by mistake, it can prove fatal in the same manner as with HEMLOCK WATER DROPWORT (*Oenanthe crocata*) where stomach irritation, circulation failure, giddiness, convulsions and coma can occur.

ADMINISTERED AS: powdered fruit, tincture, essence.

Dwarf elder *Sanbucus ebulus.* COMMON NAME: Danewort, wallwort, ground elder, walewort, blood hilder.

OCCURRENCE: found in ruins and waste ground throughout Europe and the British Isles.

PARTS USED: the leaves, roots and berries.

MEDICINAL USES: expectorant, diuretic, diaphoretic, purgative. The leaves are used internally to ease inflammation of the kidney and liver, and have a healing effect when used as a poultice on swellings and contusions. Dwarf elder tea was prepared from the dried root, when ground, and is one of the finest remedies for dropsy. The fresh root, when used as a decoction, is a drastic purgative. Overall, the dwarf elder is much more drastic in action than the common ELDER (*Sambucus nigra*).

ADMINISTERED AS: fresh root, decoction, poultice, infusion.

Echinacea *Echinacea angustifolia.* COMMON NAME: Black sampson, coneflower, rudbeckia, *Brauneria pallida*.

OCCURRENCE: a native plant of the prairie regions of the United states, west of Ohio. Also cultivated in Britain.

PARTS USED: the dried root and the rhizome. The wood and the bark contain oil, resin and large quantities of inulin, inuloid, sucrose, betaine, two phytosterols and oleic, cerotic, linolic and palmatic fatty acids.

MEDICINAL USES: alterative, antiseptic. This herb is considered sacred by many North American Indian tribes including the Sioux Indians. The herb boosts the immune system and increases bodily resistance to infection. It is used for boils, septicaemia, cancer, syphilis and gangrene. Echinacea is of particular value in treating diphtheria, typhoid and other infectious fevers. The herb can be used to improve appetite and digestion and can ease haemorrhoids when administered via injection.

ADMINISTERED AS: poultice, infusion, injection, fresh herb.

Elder *Sambucus nigra.* COMMON NAME: Black elder, common elder, european elder, pipe tree, bore tree, bour tree.

OCCURRENCE: frequently seen in Europe and Great Britain.

PARTS USED: the bark, leaves, flowers and berries.

MEDICINAL USES: the bark is a strong purgative and in large doses is emetic. It has been used successfully in epilepsy, and a tincture of the young bark relieves asthmatic symptoms and croup in children. A tea made from elder roots was highly effective against dropsy. The leaves are used both fresh and dried and contain the alkaloid sambucine, a glucoside called sambunigrin, as well as hydrogenic acid, cane sugar and potassium nitrate amongst other compounds. The leaves are used in preparation of green elder ointment which is used domestically for bruises, haemorrhoids, sprains, chilblains and applied to wounds. Elder leaves have the same purgative effects as the bark (but produce more nausea) and have expectorant, diaphoretic and diuretic actions.

The elder flowers are either distilled into elderflower water or dried. The water is used in eye and skin lotions as it is mildly astringent and a gentle stimulant. When infused, the dried flowers make elderflower tea which is gently laxative, aperient and diaphoretic. It is an old-fashioned remedy for colds and influenza when taken hot, before bed. The tea is also recommended to be drunk before breakfast as a blood purifier. Elder flowers would also be made into a lotion or poultice for use on inflamed areas and into an ointment which was good on wounds, scalds and burns. The ointment was used on the battlefields in World War I and at home for chapped hands and chilblains.

ADMINISTERED AS: an infusion, tincture, ointment, syrup, lotion, distilled water, poultice and dried powder.

Elecampane *Inula helenium.* COMMON NAME: Scabwort, elf dock, wild sunflower, horseheal, velvet dock.

OCCURRENCE: a true native of southern England, temperate Europe and Asia, but cultivated for medicinal purposes in northern England and Scotland.

PARTS USED: the root. This plant is a rich source of the drug inulin.

MEDICINAL USES: diuretic, tonic, diaphoretic, expectorant, antiseptic, astringent, and gently stimulant. It is used principally in coughs, consumption and pulmonary complaints, e.g. bronchitis. It is also used in acute catarrhal afflictions, dyspepsia ans asthma. Internally, it is normally combined with other herbs, as a decoction. Applied externally, it is rubefacient, and used in treating sciatica and facial neuralgia. The active bitter principle in the herb, helenin, is a very powerful antiseptic and bacterial chemical. This has meant elecampane has been used against the Tubercle bacteria and in surgical dressings.

ADMINISTERED AS: powdered root, fluid extract, tincture, poultice, infusion.

lm, Common *Ulmus campestris.* COMMON NAME: Field elm, ulmi cortex, broad-leaved elm.

OCCURRENCE: common in Britain, Europe, Asia and North Africa.

PARTS USED: the dried inner bark.

MEDICINAL USES: tonic, demulcent, astringent and diuretic. It was formerly employed as an antiscorbutic decoction recommended in skin diseases such as ringworm. Also used as a poultice to relieve pain from gout or rheumatism.

ADMINISTERED AS: tincture, fluid extract or tea.

phedra *Ephedra vulgaris.* COMMON NAME: Ephedrine, epitonin, mattuang.

OCCURRENCE: grows in west central China, southern Siberia and Japan.

PARTS USED: the stems, of which ephedrine is the active alkaloidal chemical.

MEDICINAL USES: nerve stimulant, antispasmodic. The herb resembles adrenaline in effect and it relieves swellings of the mucous membranes quickly. It has been used to treat asthma, hay fever and rheumatism as well as being a prophylactic drug to help low blood pressure in influenza or pneumonia.

ADMINISTERED AS: tablets, injection.

rgot *Claviceps purpurea.* COMMON NAME: Ergot of rye, smut of rye, spurred rye, *Serale cornutum.*

OCCURRENCE: this herbal remedy is the fungal mycelium which grows parasitically on rye, wheat and other grasses.

PARTS USED: ergot contains two alkaloids – ergotoxine and ergotamine as the active chemicals.

MEDICINAL USES: emmenagogue, haemostatic, uterine, stimulant,

and sedative It is normally used as a muscle stimulant in men
strual disorders such as leucorrhoea and painful or lacking men
struation and can be used to stop internal haemorrhage with bes
results against uterine haemorrhage. It is used as a sedative in
cases of delirium, asthma or hysteria and also acts as a galactogogue
ADMINISTERED AS: extract, infusion, tincture, liquid extract.

Eryngo *Eryngicum campestre*. COMMON NAME: Sea holly, eringo
sea hulver, sea holme.

OCCURRENCE: found on sandy soils and seashores around En
gland and the rest of Europe's coastline, but rare in Scotland
PARTS USED: the root.

MEDICINAL USES: diaphoretic, diuretic, aromatic, stimulant, ex
pectorant. It is good in dealing with coughs, consumption, pa
ralysis and chronic nervous diseases. It has effective result
against all diseases of the bladder, scorbutic complaints, jaun
dice and liver problems.

ADMINISTERED AS: decoction.

Eucalyptus *Eucalyptus globulus*. COMMON NAME: Blue gum tree
stringy bark tree.

OCCURRENCE: native to Australia and Tasmania; now introduce
into North and South Africa, India and southern Europe.

PARTS USED: the oil distilled from the leaves. The oil contain
eucalyptol, which is the important medically-active chemical.

MEDICINAL USES: antiseptic, antispasmodic, stimulant, aromatic
The oil is used as an antiseptic and stimulant gargle; it increase
the action of the heart and is said to have some antimalaria
properties. It is taken internally in pulmonary tuberculosis, scar
let, typhoid and intermittent fevers. The oil is used as an inhal
ant to clear catarrh and used externally to ease croup and throa
troubles. However, in large doses it can irritate the kidneys
depress the nervous system and possibly stop respiration an
breathing. Despite its harmless appearance, care should be use
when administering the drug internally.

ADMINISTERED AS: distilled oil, emulsion.

Euphorbia *Euphorbia hirta*. COMMON NAME: Asthma-wee
catshair, *Euphorbia pilulifera*.

OCCURRENCE:grows in India and other tropical countries.

PARTS USED: the herb.

MEDICINAL USES: anti-asthmatic, pectoral. It is highly effective in treating paroxysmal asthma, coughs and bronchial and pulmonary disorders. In India it is used against syphilis.

ADMINISTERED AS: tincture, liquid extract.

vening primrose *Oenothera biennis.* COMMON NAME: Tree primrose, sun drop.

OCCURRENCE: native to North America but has been naturalized to British and European gardens.

PARTS USED: the bark and leaves.

MEDICINAL USES: astringent, sedative. The drug from this herb is not extensively used but has been of benefit in treating gastro-intestinal disorders, dyspepsia, liver torpor and in female problems in association with pelvic illness. It has also been successfully used in whooping cough and spasmodic asthma.

ADMINISTERED AS: liquid extract.

yebright *Euphrasia officinalis.* COMMON NAME: Euphrasia.

OCCURRENCE: a wild plant growing in meadows and grasslands in England and Europe.

PARTS USED: the herb. This plant contains various chemicals including euphrasia-tannin, mannite and glucose.

MEDICINAL USES: slightly tonic and astringent. As its name suggests, eyebright is recommended in treating diseases of the sight, weak eyes, etc. It is generally used as an infusion in water or milk and is combined in a lotion with GOLDEN SEAL, the pairing said to be highly effective.

ADMINISTERED AS: infusion, ointment or expressed juice.

ennel *Foeniculum vulgare.* COMMON NAME: Hinojo, fenkel, sweet fennel, wild fennel.

OCCURRENCE: found wild in most areas of temperate Europe and generally considered indigenous to the shores of the Mediterranean. It is cultivated for medicinal benefit in France, Russia, India and Persia.

PARTS USED: the seeds, leaves and roots. The roots are rarely used in herbal medicine today. The essential oil is separated by

distillation with water. Fennel oil varies widely in quality an
composition dependent upon where and under what condition
the fennel was grown.

MEDICINAL USES: aromatic, stimulant, carminative and stomachi
The herb is principally used with purgatives to allay their ten
dency to griping, and the seeds form an ingredient of the com
pound liquorice powder. Fennel water also acts in a simila
manner to DILL water in correcting infant flatulence.

ADMINISTERED AS: fluid extract, distilled water, essential oil.

Fenugreek *Trigonella foenum-graecum.* COMMON NAME: Bird
foot, Greek hay-seed.

OCCURRENCE: indigenous to eastern Mediterranean countrie
but is cultivated in India, Africa and England.

PARTS USED: the seeds. These contain mucilage, two alkaloid
trigonelline and choline – phosphates, lecithin an
nucleoalbumin.

MEDICINAL USES: a preparation where seeds are soaked in wate
until they swell and form a thick paste is used to prevent fever
is comforting to the stomach and has been utilized for diabete
Alcoholic tinctures are used to prepare emollient cream, oin
ments and plasters while the mucilage is used externally as
poultice for skin infections such as abscesses, boils and ca
buncles. It is also good at relieving rickets, anaemia and scroful
while, combined with the normal dosage of conventional med
cine e.g insulin, it is helpful in gout, diabetes and neurastheni
It is widely used as a flavouring for both human and cattle fee

ADMINISTERED AS: poultice, ointment, infusion or tincture.

Feverfew *Chrysanthemum parthenium.* COMMON NAM
Featherfew, featherfoil, flirtwort, bachelor's buttons, pyrethru
parthenium.

OCCURRENCE: a wild hedgerow plant found in many areas
Europe and Great Britain.

PARTS USED: the herb.

MEDICINAL USES: aperient, carminative, bitter, stimulant, emme
nagogue. It is employed in hysterical complaints, nervousnes
and low spirits as a general tonic. A decoction is made and

useful in easing coughs, wheezing and difficult breathing. Ear-ache was relieved by a cold infusion while a tincture of feverfew eased the pain and swelling caused after insect or vermin bites. The herb was planted around dwellings to purify the atmosphere and ward off disease. Today, it is used to prevent or ease migraines or headaches.

ADMINISTERED AS: warm or cold infusion, poultice, tincture, decoction.

Fig *Ficus carica.* COMMON NAME: Common fig.

OCCURRENCE: indigenous to Persia, Asia minor and Syria, but cultivated in most of the Mediterranean countries and England.

PARTS USED: the fleshy inflorescence (so-called fruit)

MEDICINAL USES: nutritive, emollient, demulcent, laxative. It is normally utilized in laxative confections and syrups with SENNA and carminatives. Demulcent decoctions are prepared from figs and are used in treating catarrhal afflictions of the nose and throat. Roasted figs, when split open, are used as a poultice to gumboils, dental abscesses, boils and carbuncles. The fruit is used both fresh and dried.

ADMINISTERED AS: poultice, syrup, decoction.

Figwort *Scrophularia nodosa.* COMMON NAME: Rose noble, throatwort, carpenter's square, kernelwort, scrofula plant.

OCCURRENCE: a wild plant of Great Britain and Europe.

PARTS USED: the herb

MEDICINAL USES: diuretic, anodyne, depurative. Due to this herb's beneficial action on skin abscesses, eruptions and wounds, it has been termed the scrofula plant. The fresh leaves are used as a poultice on sprains, swellings, inflammation, wounds, gangrene and scrofulous sores to great effect.

ADMINISTERED AS: decoction, fresh leaves, dried herb, ointment and fluid extract.

Flax *Linum usitatissimum.* COMMON NAME: Linseed.

OCCURRENCE: grows in most temperate and tropical countries.

parts used: the seeds and oil expressed from the seeds, a cake remains which can be ground up to form linseed meal.

MEDICINAL USES: emollient, demulcent, pectoral. A poultice of linseed meal, either alone or with mustard, is effective in relieving pain and irritation from boils, ulcers, inflamed areas and abscesses. Flax is normally utilized as an addition to cough medicines, while linseed oil is sometimes given as a laxative or to remove gravel and stones. When mixed with lime water the oil is excellent on burns and scalds.

administered as: essential oil, ground seed coats (meal), infusion, syrup and poultice.

Foxglove *Digitalis purpurea.* COMMON NAME: Witch's gloves, dead men's bells, fairy's glove, gloves of Our Lady, bloody fingers, virgin's glove, fairy caps, folk's glove, fairy thimbles, fair women's plant.

OCCURRENCE: indigenous and widely distributed throughout Great Britain and Europe.

PARTS USED: the leaves, which contain four important glucoside – digitoxin, digitalin, digitalein and digitonin – of which the first three listed are cardiac stimulants.

MEDICINAL USES: cardiac tonic, sedative, diuretic. Administering digitalis increases the activity of all forms of muscle tissue, particularly the heart and arterioles. It causes a very high rise in blood pressure and the pulse is slowed and becomes regular. Digitalis causes the heart to contract in size, allowing increased blood flow and nutrient delivery to the organ. It also acts on the kidneys and is a good remedy for dropsy, particularly when it is connected with cardiac problems. The drug has benefits in treating internal haemorrhage, epilepsy, inflammatory diseases and delirium tremens. Digitalis has a cumulative action whereby it is liable to accumulate in the body and then have poisonous effects. It should only be used under medical advice. Digitalis is an excellent antidote in aconite poisoning when given as a hypodermic injection.

ADMINISTERED AS: tincture, infusion, powdered leaves, solid extract, injection.

Fumitory *Fumaria officinalis.* COMMON NAME: Earth smoke, beggary, fumus, vapor, nidor, fumus terrae, fumiterry, scheitereg, taubenkropp, kaphnos, wax dolls.

OCCURRENCE: a common weed plant in Great Britain and Europe.

which has been naturalized into North America; originally from Asia and Greece.

PARTS USED: the herb and the expressed juice and fluid extract derived from it.

MEDICINAL USES: weak tonic, diaphoretic, diuretic, aperient. This herb is valuable in all internal obstructions, particularly those of the liver and stomach and is also of benefit in scorbutic afflictions and skin eruptions including leprosy. It is the preferred herb to purify the blood in France and Germany, and in some areas it is smoked as tobacco. It was said to aid removal of skin blemishes and freckles and was also used to ease dyspepsia and headaches.

ADMINISTERED AS: expressed juice, essence, syrup, distilled water, decoction, dried herb, several different tinctures, powdered seed.

Gale, Sweet *Myrica gale*. COMMON NAME: bayberry, English bog myrtle, dutch myrtle, gale palustris.

OCCURRENCE: a bushy shrub found in higher latitudes of the northern hemisphere; abundant in Scottish moors and bogs.

PARTS USED: the shrub.

MEDICINAL USES: aromatic, astringent. The leaves have been used as an emmenagogue and an abortifacient (induces abortion or miscarriage).

ADMINISTERED AS: dried leaves and infusion.

Garlic *Allium sativum*. COMMON NAME: Poor man's treacle.

OCCURRENCE: cultivated throughout Europe since antiquity.

PARTS USED: the bulb.

MEDICINAL USES: antiseptic, diaphoretic, diuretic, expectorant, stimulant. It may be externally applied as ointment, lotion, antiseptic or as a poultice. Syrup of garlic is very good for asthma, coughs, difficulty in breathing and chronic bronchitis, while fresh juice has been used to ease tubercular consumption. The essential oil is commonly taken as a supplement in the form of gelatine capsules. Several species of wild garlic are utilized for both medicinal and dietary purposes.

ADMINISTERED AS: expressed juice, syrup, tincture, essential oil, poultice, lotion and ointment.

Gentian, Yellow *Gentiana lutea.*

OCCURRENCE: native to alpine regions of central and southern Europe

PARTS USED: the root. The dried root contains gentian, gentiamarin, bitter glucosides, gentianic acid and various sugars. The fresh root also contains gentiopicrin, another bitter glucoside.

MEDICINAL USES: bitter tonic, stomachic, febrifuge, emmenagogue, anthelmintic and antiseptic. This drug is probably the most effective bitter tonic of use in exhaustion from chronic disease, general debility, weakness of the digestive organs and lack of appetite. It acts to strengthen the whole body and is a very good tonic to combine with purgative drugs in order to temper their debilitating effects. Yellow gentian is useful in many dyspeptic complaints, hysteria, female weakness, intermittent fevers and jaundice. The roots have also been used to make an alcoholic beverage in Germany and Switzerland.

ADMINISTERED AS: infusion, tincture, solid extract, fluid extract

Germander, Wall *Teucrium chamaedys.* COMMON NAME: Petit chêne, chasse fièvre.

OCCURRENCE: a native of many parts of Europe, the Greek Islands and Syria but is an escape from garden cultivation in England.

PARTS USED: the whole herb, dried.

MEDICINAL USES: stimulant, tonic, diaphoretic, diuretic, aperient. Germander has a reputation as a specific cure for gout dating back to the sixteenth century. It has been used as a tonic in treating intermittent fevers and uterine obstructions and a decoction of the fresh herb is good against asthmatic afflictions and coughs. The expressed juice is taken for obstructions of the viscera, while the herb has also been used for jaundice, as a vermifuge, ulcers, continual headache and cramps.

ADMINISTERED AS: expressed juice, poultice, decoction, powdered seeds.

Ginger *Zingiber officinale.*

OCCURRENCE: a native of Asia, it is now cultivated in the West Indies, Jamaica and Africa.

PARTS USED: the root, which contains volatile oil, two resins, gum, starch, lignin, acetic acid and asmazone as well as several unidentified compounds.

MEDICINAL USES: stimulant, carminative, expectorant. A valuable herb in dyspepsia, flatulent colic, alcoholic gastritis and diarrhoea. Ginger tea is taken to relieve the effects of cold temperatures including triggering normal menstruation patterns in women. Ginger is also used to flavour bitter infusions, cough mixtures or syrups.

ADMINISTERED AS: infusion, fluid extract, tincture and syrup.

inseng *Panax quinquefolium.* COMMON NAME: *Aralia quinquefolia,* five fingers, tartar root, red berry, man's health, panax, pannag.

OCCURRENCE: native to certain areas of China, eastern Asia and North America. It is largely cultivated in China, Korea and Japan.

PARTS USED: the root which contains a large quantity of gum, resin, volatile oil and the peculiar sweetish compound, panaquilon.

MEDICINAL USES: mild stomachic, tonic, stimulant. The generic name, *panax*, is derived from the Greek for panacea meaning 'all-healing.' The name ginseng is said to mean 'the wonder of the world' and the Chinese consider this herb a sovereign remedy in all diseases. It is good in dyspepsia, vomiting and nervous disorders, consumption and exhaustion. In the West, it is used to treat loss of appetite, stomach and digestive problems, possibly arising from nervous and mental exhaustion. Ginseng is considered to work well against fatigue, old age and its infirmities and to help convalescents recover their health. In healthy people, the drug is said to increase vitality, cure pulmonary complaints and tumours and increase life expectancy. It was also used by the native American Indians for similar problems.

ADMINISTERED AS: tincture, decoction, capsules.

ladwyn *Iris foetidissina.* COMMON NAME: Stinking gladwyn, gladwin, gladwine, stinking gladdon, spurgewort, spurge plant, roast beef plant.

OCCURRENCE: found in woods and shady parts in southern En
gland.

PARTS USED: the root.

MEDICINAL USES: antispasmodic, cathartic, anodyne. A decoctio
acts as a strong purge; has been used as an emmenagogue an
for removing eruptions. The dried powdered root can be o
benefit in hysterical disorders, fainting, nervous problems an
to relieve cramps and pain. Taken both internally and as an ex
ternal poultice, this is an excellent herb to remedy scrofula
The use of this herbal remedy can be dated back to the fourt
century before Christ.

ADMINISTERED AS: decoction, dried root, infusion.

Golden rod *Solidago virgaurea.* COMMON NAME: Verge d'or, so
idago, goldruthe, woundwort, Aaron's rod.

OCCURRENCE: normally found wild in woods in Britain, Europ
central Asia and North America but it is also a common garde
plant.

PARTS USED: the leaves contain tannin, with some bitter and as
tringent chemicals which are unknown.

MEDICINAL USES: aromatic, stimulant, carminative. This herb is as
tringent and diuretic and is highly effective in curing gravel an
urinary stones. It aids weak digestion, stops sickness and is ver
good against diphtheria. As a warm infusion it is a good diaphoreti
drug and is used as such to help painful menstruation and amer
orrhoea (absence or stopping of menstrual periods).

ADMINISTERED AS: fluid extract, infusion, spray.

Golden seal *Hydrastis canadensis.* COMMON NAME: Orange roo
yellow root, yellow puccoon, ground raspberry, wild curcuma
tumeric root, Indian root, eyebalm, Indian paint, jaundice roo
warnera, eye root.

OCCURRENCE: a native plant of Canada and the eastern Unite
States.

PARTS USED: the rhizome which contains the alkaloids berberin
hydastine and canadine, as well as resin, albumin, starch, fatt
matter, sugar, lignin and volatile oil.

MEDICINAL USES: tonic, stomachic, laxative, alterative, detergen

Native American Indians use this plant as a source of yellow dye for clothing and weapons and also as a remedy for sore eyes, general ulceration and disordered digestion. The herb has a special action on the mucous membranes of the body, making it an excellent remedy for catarrh, dyspepsia, gastric catarrh, loss of appetite and liver problems. Given as a tonic, the root is highly effective in easing constipation and is very good at stopping sickness and vomiting. chronic inflammation of the colon and rectum can be treated by an injection of golden seal, as can haemorrhoids. When taken as an infusion, it may cure night-sweats and passive bleeding from the pelvic tissues. In large doses, *Hydrastis* is very poisonous.

ADMINISTERED AS: injection, infusion, tincture, lotion, fluid extract, dried powdered root, solid extract.

Gooseberry *Ribes grossularia.* COMMON NAME: Fea, feverberry, feabes, carberry, groseille, groset, groser, krusbaar, dewberries, goosegogs, honeyblobs, feaberry.

OCCURRENCE: a well-known shrub native to central and northern Europe, especially Great Britain.

PARTS USED: the fruit and leaves, which contain citric acid, sugar, various minerals and pectose.

MEDICINAL USES: the expressed juice is said to be a cure for all inflammations. The acid red fruit is made into a light jelly which is good for sedentary and bilious complaints as well as in cases of excess body fluid. An infusion of dried leaves is effective in treating gravel and is a useful tonic for menstruating young girls. In the Highlands of Scotland, the prickles were used as charms to remove warts and styes.

ADMINISTERED AS: an infusion, expressed juice, dietary item.

Goutwort *Aegopodium podagraria.* COMMON NAME: Goutweed, goutherb, ashweed, Jack-jump-about, herb gerard, English masterwort, pigweed, eltroot, ground elder, bishops elder, white ash, ground ash, weyl ash, bishopsweed.

OCCURRENCE: a weed plant of Europe, Great Britain and Russian Asia.

PARTS USED: the herb

MEDICINAL USES: diuretic and sedative. Taken internally fo aching joints, gouty and sciatic pain and as an external poul tice for inflamed areas. It was thought that carrying some o the herb in a pocket would prevent an attack of gout devel oping.

ADMINISTERED AS: poultice, liquid extract.

Groundsel *Senecio vulgaris*. COMMON NAME: Common ground sel, grundy, swallow, ground glutton, simson, sention, grounse
OCCURRENCE: very common weed throughout Europe and Rus sian Asia.
PARTS USED: the whole herb and fresh plant. The plant contain senecin and seniocine.
MEDICINAL USES: diaphoretic, anti scorbutic, purgative, diureti anthelmintic. It is good for sickness of the stomach, used as purgative in a weak infusion and as an emetic when in a stron infusion. This infusion removes bilious trouble and lowers bod temperature. A poultice of groundsel is used warm on boil but nursing mothers have cold poultices as a coolant on swo len, inflamed or hardened breasts. If boiling water is poured o to the fresh plant, the resulting liquid is a pleasant swab for th skin and helps soften chapped hands
ADMINISTERED AS: infusion, poultice lotion.

Hair-cap moss *Polytrichium juniperum*. COMMON NAME: Bear bed, robin's eye, ground moss, golden maidenhair, female fer herb, robinsrye, rockbrake herb.
OCCURRENCE: found in woods and hedges across Europe an Britain.
PARTS USED: the whole plant.
MEDICINAL USES: powerful diuretic. It is a very important rem edy in dropsy, urinary obstructions, gravel and suppression o urine. The herb does not cause nausea and is frequently com bined with BROOM or CARROT for best effects.
ADMINISTERED AS: infusion.

Hawthorn *Crataegus oxyacantha*. COMMON NAME: Ma mayblossom, quick, thorn, whitethorn, haw, hazels, gazel halves, hagthorn, ladies meat, bread and cheese tree, maybus

OCCURRENCE: a familiar tree in Great Britain, Europe, North Africa and Western Asia.

PARTS USED: the dried fruits which contain the chemical amyddalin.

MEDICINAL USES: cardiac, diuretic, astringent, tonic. Mainly used as a cardiac tonic in organic and functional heart problems, e.g. hypertrophy, dyspnoea, heart oppression. A decoction of the flowers and berries is good at curing sore throats, and is utilized as a diuretic in dropsy and kidney disorders.

ADMINISTERED AS: liquid extract, decoction.

Heartease *Viola tricolor.* COMMON NAME: Wild pansy, love-lies-bleeding, loving idol, call-me-to-you, three-faces-under-a-hood, godfathers and godmothers, pink-eyed-John, flower o'luce, Jack-jump-up-and-kiss-me.

OCCURRENCE: abundant all over Great Britain, in cornfields, gardens, waste ground and hedge banks. It is also distributed through Arctic Europe, North Africa, Siberia and North India.

PARTS USED: the whole herb, fresh and dried. The active chemicals within the plant include violine, mucilage, resin, salicylic acid and sugar.

MEDICINAL USES: diaphoretic and diuretic. It was formerly held in high regard as a remedy for epilepsy, asthma and catarrhal infections. It has been utilized in blood disorders and heart diseases, while a decoction of the flowers was recommended for skin diseases. In America, they use heartease as an ointment or poultice in eczema, and it is taken internally for bronchitis. People on the continent have used *Viola tricolor* for its mucilaginous, demulcent and expectorant qualities.

ADMINISTERED AS: decoction, ointment, poultice and tincture.

Hedge-hyssop *Gratiola officinalis*

OCCURRENCE: a perennial plant, native to southern Europe and found wild in damp areas in Great Britain.

PARTS USED: the root and herb. the plant contains the glucosides gratiolin and gratiosolin.

MEDICINAL USES: diuretic, cathartic, emetic. Recommended in scrofula, chronic liver complaints and enlargement of the spleen. It is also utilized in relieving dropsy and as a vermifuge.

ADMINISTERED AS: an infusion of powdered root.

Hellebore, Black *Helleborus niger*. COMMON NAME: Christe herbe, Christmas rose, melampodium.

OCCURRENCE: a native of the mountains in central and southern Europe, Greece and Asia minor, but found in Britain as a garden plant.

PARTS USED: the rhizome and root. The plant has two glucosides within it, helleborin and helleborcin, both of which are powerful poisons.

MEDICINAL USES: the drug has drastic purgative, emmenagogue and anthelmintic properties, but is a violent narcotic. It is of value in treating nervous disorders, hysteria and melancholia and was previously used in dropsy and amenorrhoea. Given externally, the fresh root is violently irritant. The drug must be administered with great care.

ADMINISTERED AS: fluid extract, tincture, solid extract, powdered root or decoction.

Hemlock *Conium maculatum*. COMMON NAME: Herb bennet, spotted conebane, musquash root, beaver poison, poison hemlock, poison parsley, spotted hemlock, vex, vecksies.

OCCURRENCE: common in hedges, meadows, waste ground and stream banks throughout Europe and is also found in temperate Asia and North Africa.

PARTS USED: the leaves, fruits and seeds. The most important constituent of hemlock leaves is the alkaloid coniine, which is poisonous, with a disagreeable odour. Other alkaloids in the plant include methyl-coniine, conhydrine, pseudoconhydrine, ethyl piperidine.

MEDICINAL USES: sedative, antispasmodic, anodyne. The drug acts on the centres of motion and causes paralysis and so it is used to remedy undue nervous motor excitability, e.g. teething, cramp and muscle spasms of the larynx and gullet. When inhaled, hemlock is said to be good in relieving coughs, bronchitis, whooping cough and asthma. The method of action of *Conium* means it is directly antagonistic to the effects of strychnine, from NUX

VOMICA (*Strychnos nux-vomica*), and hence it is used as an antidote to strychnine poisoning and similar poisons. Hemlock has to be administered with care as narcotic poisoning may result from internal application and overdoses induce paralysis, with loss of speech and depression of respiratory function leading to death. Antidotes to hemlock poisoning are tannic acid, stimulants, e.g. COFFEE, MUSTARD and CASTOR OIL.

ADMINISTERED AS: powdered leaves, fluid extract, tincture, expressed juice of the leaves and solid extract.

Henbane *Hyoscyamus niger.* COMMON NAME: Hyoscyamus, hog's bean, Jupiter's-bean, symphonica, cassilata, cassilago, deus caballinus.

OCCURRENCE: native to central and southern Europe and western Asia and was introduced to Great Britain, North America and Brazil where it is found on waste ground, ditches and near old buildings.

PARTS USED: the fresh leaves and flowering tops. The chief constituents of henbane leaves are the alkaloids hyoscyamine, atropine and hyoscine. The leaves also contain a bitter principle called hyoscytricin, choline, mucilage, calcium oxalate, potassium nitrate and fixed oil.

MEDICINAL USES: antispasmodic, hypnotic, mild diuretic, mydriatic, anodyne, sedative. The herb has a milder narcotic effect than BELLADONNA or STRAMONIUM and is utilized to lessen muscle spasms, reduce pain and can stop nervous irritation. It is used in cystitis, irritable bladder, hysteria, irritable cough, asthma, gastric ulcers and chronic gastric catarrh. When taken in small doses repeated over time, Henbane tranquillizes people affected by severe nervous irritability, enabling them to sleep without adversely affecting the digestive organs or causing headaches, which opium has the tendency to do. Thus, henbane is given to people with insomnia and to children, to which opium cannot be given. The fresh leaves of henbane can be used as a poultice to relieve local pain from gout, neuralgia, cancerous ulcers, sores and swellings. The solid extract of the drug is used to produce suppositories which are used to relieve the pain of haemorrhoids. Henbane is poisonous and should never be used except under medical advice.

ADMINISTERED AS: powdered leaves, tincture, fluid extract, expressed juice, solid extract, suppositories.

Holly *Ilex aquifolium.* COMMON NAME: Holm, hulver bush, hulm, holme chase, holy tree, Christ's thorn.

OCCURRENCE: native to central and southern Europe and grows freely in Great Britain

PARTS USED: the leaves, berries and bark

MEDICINAL USES: diaphoretic, febrifuge, cathartic, tonic. Infused holly leaves are used in catarrh, pleurisy and formerly against smallpox. Also in intermittent fevers and rheumatism where the alkaloid ilicin works to good effect. Juice expressed from fresh holly leaves is effective against jaundice. The berries have different properties and are violently emetic and purgative, but they have been utilized in dropsy and as a powder to check bleeding. Holly leaves have been utilized as a tea substitute.

ADMINISTERED AS: infusion of leaves, juice, whole or powdered berries.

Honeysuckle *Lonicera caprifolium.* COMMON NAME: Dutch honeysuckle, goat's leaf, perfoliate honeysuckle.

OCCURRENCE: grows freely in Europe, Great Britain and through the northern temperate zone.

PARTS USED: the dried flowers and leaves

MEDICINAL USES: expectorant, laxative. A syrup made of the flowers is used for respiratory diseases and asthma. A decoction of the leaves is laxative and is also good against diseases of the liver and spleen, and in gargles.

ADMINISTERED AS: syrup, decoction.

Hops *Humulus lupulus.*

OCCURRENCE: a native British plant, found wild in hedges and woods from Yorkshire southward. It is considered an introduced species to Scotland but is also found in most countries of the northern temperate zone.

PARTS USED: the flowers, which contain a volatile oil, two bitter principles – lupamaric acid, lupalinic acid- and tannin.

MEDICINAL USES: tonic, nervine, diuretic, anodyne, aromatic. The volatile oil has sedative and soporific effects while the bitter principles are stomachic and tonic. Hops are used to promote the appetite and enhance sleep. An infusion is very effective in heart disease, fits, neuralgia, indigestion, jaundice, nervous disorders and stomach or liver problems. Hop juice is a blood cleanser and is very effective in remedying calculus problems. As an external application, hops are used with CHAMOMILE heads as an infusion to reduce painful swellings or inflammation and bruises. This combination may also be used as a poultice.

ADMINISTERED AS: an infusion, tincture, poultice, expressed juice or tea.

orehound *Marrubium vulgare.* COMMON NAME: Hoarhound, white horehound.

OCCURRENCE: indigenous to Britain and found all over Europe.

PARTS USED: the herb, which contains the bitter principle marrubium, volatile oil, tannin sugar and resin.

MEDICINAL USES: tonic, expectorant, pectoral, diuretic. It is probably the most popular pectoral herbal remedy. Very valuable in coughs, asthma, consumption and pulmonary complaints. For children, it is given as a syrup to ease croup, stomach upsets and as a tonic. Taken in large doses, Horehound is a gentle purgative and the powdered leaves have been used as a vermifuge. A tea of the herb is excellent for colds. A sweetmeat candy and an ale is also made from horehound.

ADMINISTERED AS: syrup, infusion, tea, powdered leaves, ointment, expressed juice.

orsemint, American *Monarda punctata*

OCCURRENCE: native to North America and was introduced into England in 1714.

PARTS USED: the herb produces a volatile oil which is composed of thymol and higher oxygenated compounds.

MEDICINAL USES: rubefacient, stimulant, carminative, diuretic. It is used as an infusion for flatulent colic, sickness and urinary disorders and has diaphoretic and emmenagogue actions also.

It is principally used externally wherever a rubefacient is required, e.g. chronic rheumatism.

ADMINISTERED AS: a volatile oil.

Horseradish *Cochlearia armoracia*. COMMON NAME: Mountai
radish, great raifort, red cole, *Armoracia rusticara*.

OCCURRENCE: cultivated in the British Isles for centuries. Th
place of origin is unknown.

PARTS USED: the root which contains the glucoside sinigri
vitamin C, aspargin and resin.

MEDICINAL USES: stimulant, aperient, rubefacient, diuretic, an
tiseptic, diaphoretic. Horseradish is a powerful stimulant o
the digestive organs, and it acts on lung and urinary infection
clearing them away. The herb is a very strong diuretic and a
such is used to ease dropsy, gravel and calculus, as well as be
ing taken internally for gout and rheumatism. A poultice ca
be made from the fresh root and applied to rheumatic joint
chilblains and to ease facial neuralgia. Horseradish juice, whe
diluted with vinegar and glycerine, was used in children
whooping cough and to relieve hoarseness of the throat. A
infusion of the root in urine was stimulating to the entire ne
vous system and promoted perspiration, while it was also use
to expel worms in children. Care should be taken when usin
this herb because over-use of horseradish can blister the ski
and is not suitable for people with thyroid troubles.

ADMINISTERED AS: infusion, syrup, expressed juice, fluid extrac

Horsetail *Equisetum arvense*. COMMON NAME: Mare's tail, shave
grass, bottlebrush, paddock-pipes, Dutch rushes, pewterwor
OCCURRENCE: native to Great Britain and distributed throug
the temperate northern regions.

PARTS USED: the herb which is composed of silica, saponin, fla
vonoids, tannin and traces of alkaloids – nicotine, palustri
and palustrinine.

MEDICINAL USES: diuretic, astringent. Due to the herb's rich store
minerals, horsetail is given for anaemia and general debility and ca
also work to encourage the absorption and efficient use of calciu
by the body, helping prevent fatty deposits forming in the arteri

(arteriosclerosis). It helps stop bleeding and hence is good for stomach ulcers and haemorrhage as well as easing dropsy, gravel, cystitis and inflamed prostate glands due to its astringent qualities. The herb can be of benefit in the treatment of bed-wetting in children.

ADMINISTERED AS: infusion, dried herb, syrup.

Hound's tongue *Cynoglossum officinale*. COMMON NAME: dog's tongue, *Lindefolia spectabilis*.

OCCURRENCE: a common plant in Switzerland and Germany; occasionally found in Great Britain.

PARTS USED: the herb.

MEDICINAL USES: anodyne, demulcent, astringent. Used as pills or as a decoction for colds, coughs, catarrh, diarrhoea and dysentery. Administered both internally and externally to soothe the digestive organs and haemorrhoids.

ADMINISTERED AS: decoction, pills, ointment.

Houseleek *Sempervivum tectorum*. COMMON NAME: Jupiter's eye, Thor's beard, bullock's eye, sengreen, ayron, ayegreen.

OCCURRENCE: native to the mountains of central and southern Europe and the Greek islands but introduced to Britain many centuries ago.

PARTS USED: the fresh leaves.

MEDICINAL USES: refrigerant, astringent, diuretic. The bruised fresh leaves or its expressed juice are often applied as a poultice to burns, scalds, bumps, scrofulous ulcers and general skin inflammation. The juice is a cure for warts and corns. In large doses, houseleek juice is emetic and purgative. The plant was supposed to guard where it grew against fire, lightning and sorcery, hence it was grown on house roofs.

Hydrangea *Hydrangea aborescens*. COMMON NAME: Wild hydrangea, seven barks, common hydrangea, *Hydrangea vulgaris*.

OCCURRENCE: native to the United States and is cultivated across the world as a garden plant.

PARTS USED: the root which contains two resins, gum, sugar, starch, sulphuric and phosphoric acids and a glucoside called hydrangin.

MEDICINAL USES: diuretic, cathartic, tonic, nephritic. This herb is very good at preventing and removing stones in the urinary system, and relieving the pain due to urinary gravel. The fluid extract is also used to correct alkaline urine, chronic vaginal discharges and irritation of the bladder in older people. The drug was used by native American Indians and its benefits were passed on to European settlers.

ADMINISTERED AS: fluid extract, decoction, syrup.

Ipecacuanha *Cephaelis ipecacuanha*. COMMON NAME: *Psychotria ipecacuanha.*

OCCURRENCE:native to Brazil, Bolivia and parts of South America and was introduced into Europe in the seventeenth century.

PARTS USED: the chief constituents of the root are the alkaloid emetrine, cephalin and psychotrine, as well as two glucosides choline, resin, calcium oxalate and a volatile oil among other compounds.

MEDICINAL USES: diaphoretic, emetic, expectorant, stimulant. The effects of the drug on the body are entirely dependent on the dose given. In very small doses, ipecacuanha stimulate the stomach, liver and intestine aiding digestion and increasing appetite while in slightly larger doses it has diaphoretic and expectorant properties which is good for colds, coughs and dysentery. Large doses of the drug are emetic. There is a lot of historical use of this drug against amoebic (or tropical) dysentery where rapid cures can occur. Care should be taken in utilizing this drug as emetine can have a toxic effect on the heart, blood vessels, lungs and intestines and cause severe illness.

ADMINISTERED AS: powdered root, fluid extract, tincture, syrup.

Irish moss *Chondrus crispus*. COMMON NAME: Carrageen, chondrus, carrahan, carragheen.

OCCURRENCE: common at low tide on all shores of the North Atlantic.

PARTS USED: the dried plant which contains mucilage and sulphur compounds.

MEDICINAL USES: demulcent, pectoral, emollient; nutritive. A popular remedy which is made into a jelly for pulmonary complaints, kidney and bladder diseases. It is widely used as a culinary article.

ADMINISTERED AS: dietary item.

Ivy *Hedera helix*. COMMON NAME: Common ivy.

OCCURRENCE: native to many parts of Europe and northern and central Asia.

PARTS USED: the leaves and berries.

MEDICINAL USES: stimulating, diaphoretic, cathartic. The leaves have been used as poultices on enlarged glands, ulcers and abscesses and the berries ease fevers and were used extensively during the Great Plague of London.

ADMINISTERED AS: poultice, infusion.

Ivy, Ground *Glechoma Hederacea*. COMMON NAME: alehoof, gill-go-over-the-ground, haymaids, tun-hoof, hedgemaids, colts-foot, robin-run-in-the-hedge.

OCCURRENCE: very common on hedges and waste ground all over Britain.

PARTS USED: the whole herb

MEDICINAL USES: diuretic, astringent, tonic and gently stimulant. It is good in relieving kidney diseases and indigestion. Ground ivy tea is useful in pectoral complaints and in weakness of the digestive organs. The expressed juice, when sniffed up the nose, is said to successfully cure a headache and can be administered externally to ease bruises and black eyes. It also has anti-scorbutic qualities.

ADMINISTERED AS: fluid extract, expressed juice and infusion.

Ivy, Poison *Rhus toxicodendron*. COMMON NAME: Poison oak, poison vine.

OCCURRENCE: native to the United States of America.

PARTS USED: the fresh leaves which contain a resin called toxicodendron as the active principle.

MEDICINAL USES: irritant, rubefacient, stimulant, narcotic. This herb is successful in treating obstinate skin eruptions, palsy, paralysis, acute rheumatism and joint stiffness. It has also been good in treating ringworm, allergic rashes and urinary incontinence. In small doses, poison ivy is a very good sedative for the nervous system, but care must be taken in its use as it can trigger gastric and intestinal irritation, drowsiness, stupor and delirium.

ADMINISTERED AS: tincture, fluid extract, infusion.

Jaborandi *Pilocarpus microphyllus.* COMMON NAME: Arruda do mato, arruda brava, jamguarandi, juarandi.

OCCURRENCE: a native Brazilian plant.

PARTS USED: the dried leaves. The main constituents of the leaves are a volatile oil and three alkaloids – pilocarpine, isopilocarpine, pilocarpidine.

MEDICINAL USES: stimulant, diaphoretic, expectorant. This herb is used as the crude drug and as the purified alkaloid, pilocarpine. Jaborandi is used for psoriasis, deafness, baldness, chronic catarrh, tonsillitis, dropsy and catarrhal jaundice. It can also benefit fat removal from the heart in heart disease, pleurisy, chronic renal diseases and reducing thirst in fevered patients. The extracted alkaloid, Pilocarpine, has an antagonistic effect to atropine, from BELLADONNA, *Atropa belladonna* and other related plants, and causes contraction of the pupil of the eye. It is used as a fast and highly effective diaphoretic drug, increasing gland secretions and the flow of breast milk. Both the jaborandi and pilocarpine can irritate the stomach, causing vomiting even when given as an injection, so care should be advised upon using this drug.

ADMINISTERED AS: powdered leaves, tincture, injection, fluid extract.

Jacob's ladder *Polemonicum coeruleum.* COMMON NAME: Greek valerian, charity.

OCCURRENCE: found wild in ditches and streams across England and southern Scotland.

PARTS USED: the herb.

MEDICINAL USES: diaphoretic, astringent, alterative, expectorant. A useful drug in fevers and inflammatory diseases, pleurisy, etc. It induces copious perspiration and eases coughs, colds, bronchial and lung complaints.

ADMINISTERED AS: an infusion.

Jewelweed *Impatiens aurea, Impatiens biflora.* COMMON NAME:
Wild balsam, balsamweed, pale-touch-me-not, slipperweed,
silverweed, wild lady's slipper, speckled jewels, wild celandine,
quick in the hand, *Impatiens pallida, I. fulva.*

OCCURRENCE: members of the genus *Impatiens* are found distributed across the northern temperate zone and South Africa; mostly
natives of mountainous regions in tropical Asia and Africa.

PARTS USED: the herb.

MEDICINAL USES: aperient, diuretic, emetic, cathartic. The diuretic
qualities of the herb make it useful against dropsy and jaundice
while the fresh juice is reputed to remove warts, corns and cure
ringworm. The fresh herb was made into an ointment with lard
and used for piles. Due to its acrid taste and strong action, jewelweed is rarely used in herbal medicine today.

ADMINISTERED AS: expressed juice, ointment.

Juniper *Juniperus communis*

OCCURRENCE: a common shrub native to Great Britain and widely
distributed through many parts of the world.

PARTS USED: the berry and leaves.

MEDICINAL USES: the oil of juniper obtained from the ripe berries is stomachic, diuretic and carminative and is used to treat
indigestion, flatulence as well as kidney and bladder diseases.
The main use of juniper is in dropsy, and aiding other diuretic
herbs to ease the disease.

ADMINISTERED AS: essential oil from berries, essential oil from
wood, fluid extract, liquid extract, solid extract.

Kava-kava *Piper methysticum.* COMMON NAME: Ava, ava pepper,
kava, intoxicating pepper.

OCCURRENCE: indigenous to Polynesia, Sandwich Islands, South
Sea Islands and Australian colonies.

PARTS USED: the peeled, dried rhizome. The plant contains two
resins, one called kavine, a volatile oil, starch and an alkaloid
termed kavaine methysticcum yangonin.

MEDICINAL USES: tonic, stimulant, diuretic. There is a long history of use against gonorrhoea, vaginitis, leucorrhoea, nocturnal incontinence and other problems of the urinary-genital tract.

As a strong diuretic, kava is good for gout, rheumatism, bron
chial problems and heart trouble. kava acts on the nerve cen
tres in a stimulating, then depressing manner, and has been
used as a local anaesthetic as it causes paralysis of the respira
tory centre. It relieves pain and has an aphrodisiac effect.

ADMINISTERED AS: powdered root, fluid extract, solid extract.

Knapweed, Greater *Centaurea scabiosa*. COMMON NAME: Hard
head, ironhead, hard irons, churls head, logger head, horse
knops, mat fellon, bottleweed, bullweed, cowede, bottsede.

OCCURRENCE: a perennial plant frequently seen in field borders
and waste ground in England, but rare in Scotland.

PARTS USED: the root and seeds.

MEDICINAL USES: diuretic, diaphoretic and tonic. Formerly greatly
appreciated as a vulnerary herb and used to cure loss of appe
tite. When taken as a decoction, it is good for catarrh; as an
ointment for wounds, bruises and sores, etc.

ADMINISTERED AS: decoction and ointment.

Knotgrass *Polyganum ariculare*. COMMON NAME: Centuriode
ninety-knot, nine-joints, allseed, bird's tongue, sparrow tongue
red robin, armstrong, cowgrass, hogweed, pigrush, swynel grass
swine's grass.

OCCURRENCE: native around the globe; abundant on arable land
waste ground and roadside verges.

PARTS USED: the whole herb.

MEDICINAL USES: astringent, diuretic, anthelmintic, vulnerary and
styptic. An infusion of the herb was used in diarrhoea, bleed
ing haemorrhoids and all haemorrhages. As a diuretic, it was
said to expel stones and also parasitic worms. The fresh juice
stops nosebleeds, if squirted up the nose and applied to the
temples. As an ointment, it heals sores very well.

ADMINISTERED AS: expressed juice, infusion, decoction and oint
ment.

Kola nuts *Kola vera*. COMMON NAME: Guru nut, cola, kola seeds
gurru nuts, bissy nuts, cola seeds, *Cola acuminata*, *Sterculi
acuminata*.

OCCURRENCE: native to Sierra Leone and North Ashanti an

cultivated in tropical western Africa, West Indies, Brazil and Java.

PARTS USED: the seeds.

MEDICINAL USES: nerve stimulant, diuretic, cardiac tonic. This drug is a good overall tonic, largely due to the caffeine it contains. It has been used as a remedy for diarrhoea and for those with an alcoholic habit.

ADMINISTERED AS: powdered seeds, tincture, fluid and solid extract.

Laburnum *Cytisus laburnam*. COMMON NAME: Yellow laburnum.

OCCURRENCE: indigenous to high mountain regions of Europe and widely cultivated across the globe as a garden plant.

PARTS USED: the alkaloid, obtained from the plant, called cytisine.

MEDICINAL USES: all parts of the laburnum are thought to be poisonous, particularly the seeds. The alkaloid has been recommended in whooping cough and asthma, and also as an insecticide, but it has not been used due to the very poisonous nature of the compound. Laburnum poisoning symptoms include intense sleepiness, vomiting, convulsive movements, coma and unequally dilated pupils. Laburnum is also poisonous to cattle and horses and deaths of both livestock and humans have resulted from ingestion of this plant.

Lady's mantle *Alchemilla vulgaris*. COMMON NAME: Lion's foot, bear's foot, nine hooks, stellaria.

OCCURRENCE: native to mountainous districts of Britain and widely distributed over northern or Arctic Europe, Asia and greenland.

PARTS USED: the herb.

MEDICINAL USES: astringent, styptic, vulnerary. Herbalists used to say that lady's mantle was one of the best herbs for wounds. In modern times, it is used as a cure for excessive menstruation as an infusion or injection. The root is very good for stopping all bleeding and may also act as a violent purge. The herb is also said to promote quiet sleep.

ADMINISTERED AS: decoction, infusion, injection, tincture, fluid extract, dried root.

Larch *Pinus larix.* COMMON NAME: *Larix europaea, Abies larix, Larix decidua, Laricus cortex,* European larch, Venice turpentine.

OCCURRENCE: indigenous to hilly regions of central Europe, but was introduced into Britain in 1639.

PARTS USED: the inner bark which contains tannic acid, larixinic acid and turpentine.

MEDICINAL USES: stimulant, diuretic, astringent, balsamic and expectorant. It is very useful as an external application for eczema and psoriasis. However, it is mainly used as a stimulant expectorant in chronic bronchitis, internal haemorrhage and cystitis. Larch turpentine has also been suggested as an antidote in cyanide or opium poisoning and has been used as a hospital disinfectant.

ADMINISTERED AS: fluid extract or syrup.

Larkspur *Delphinicum consolida.* COMMON NAME: Field larkspur, lark's chaw, lark's heel, knight's spur.

OCCURRENCE: found wild in fields through Europe and Great Britain.

PARTS USED: the seeds. The active principle in the plant is delphinine, an irritant poison also found in STAVESACRE.

MEDICINAL USES: parasiticide, insecticide. The tincture of the seeds is used to destroy lice and nits in the hair and given internally in spasmodic asthma and dropsy. The expressed juice from the leaves was applied to bleeding piles and an infusion of the whole plant was said to benefit colic.

ADMINISTERED AS: infusion, tincture, expressed juice.

Laurel *Laurus nobilis.* COMMON NAME: bay, sweet bay, true laurel, laurier d'apollon, roman laurel, noble laurel, lorbeer, laurier sauce, daphne.

OCCURRENCE: native to the shores of the Mediterranean and cultivated in Britain.

PARTS USED: the leaves, fruit and essential oil. The volatile oil contains pinene, geraniol, eugenol, cineol, bitter principles and tannin.

MEDICINAL USES: stomachic, narcotic, diaphoretic, emetic. In ancient times, laurel was highly valued as a medicine but now laurel is only selectively utilized. The leaves were formerly used in hysteria, flatulent colic and in treating the absence of menstrual periods, but now are only used to stimulate the digestion. The oil of bays is also used for earache, sprains and bruises and rheumatism.

ADMINISTERED AS: essential oil, infusion.

Lavender, English *Lavandula vera*

OCCURRENCE: indigenous to mountainous regions in the western Mediterranean and is cultivated extensively in France, Italy, England and Norway.

PARTS USED: the flowers and the essential oil which contains linalool, linalyl acetate, cineol, pinene, limonene and tannin

MEDICINAL USES: aromatic, carminative, stimulant, nervine. It is mainly used as a flavouring agent for disagreeable odours in ointments or syrups. The essential oil when taken internally is restorative and a tonic against faintness, heart palpitations, giddiness and colic. It raises the spirits, promotes the appetite and dispels flatulence. When applied externally, the oil relieves toothache, neuralgia, sprains and rheumatism. The oil is utilized widely in aromatherapy, often to very beneficial effects.

ADMINISTERED AS: fluid extract, tincture, essential oil, spirit, infusion, tea, poultice, distilled water.

Lemon *Citrus limonica*. COMMON NAME: Limon, *Citrus medica*, *Citrus Limonum*, citronnier, neemoo, leemoo, limoun, limone.

OCCURRENCE: indigenous to northern India and widely cultivated in Mediterranean countries.

PARTS USED: the fruit, rind, juice and oil. Lemon peel contains an essential oil and a bitter principle, while lemon juice is rich in citric acid, sugar and gum. Oil of lemon contains the aldehyde, citral and the oils pinene and citronella.

MEDICINAL USES: antiscorbutic, tonic, refrigerant, cooling. Lemon juice is the best preventative drug for scurvy and is also very valuable in fevers and allaying thirst. It is recommended in acute rheumatism and may be given to counteract narcotic poisons such as opium. It is used as an astringent gargle in sore throats, for uterine haemorrhage after childbirth, as a lotion in sunburn and as a cure for severe hiccoughs. The juice is also good for jaundice and heart palpitations. A decoction of lemon is a good antiperiodic drug and can be used to replace quinine in malarial injections, or to reduce the temperature in typhoid fever. Lemon oil is a strong external rubefacient and also has stomachic and carminative qualities.

ADMINISTERED AS: syrup, decoction, fresh juice, tincture, essential oil, dietary item.

Lettuce, Wild *Lactuca virosa*. COMMON NAME: Lachicarium, strong-scented lettuce, green endive, lettuce opium, acrid lettuce, laitue vireuse.

OCCURRENCE: found in western and southern Europe, including Great Britain.

PARTS USED: the leaves, dried milk juice – lactuarium. Lactuarium is obtained by cutting the stem in sections and collecting the latex juice. It turns reddish-brown in colour when dried.

MEDICINAL USES: anodyne, sedative, narcotic, mild diaphoretic, diuretic. The drug resembles a weak opium, without opium's tendency to upset the digestive system. It is used to allay irritable coughs and as a sedative and narcotic, but only infrequently. It is also used for dropsy, inducing sleep and easing colic.

ADMINISTERED AS: powder, tincture, fluid extract, syrup, alcoholic extract.

Lilac *Syringa vulgaris*. COMMON NAME: Common lilac.

OCCURRENCE: a shrub native to Persia and the mountains of eastern Europe.

PARTS USED: the leaves and fruit.

MEDICINAL USES: as a vermifuge, tonic, antiperiodic and febrifuge. It may be used as a substitute for ALOES (*Aloe vera*/*Aloe perryi*) and in the treatment of malaria.

ADMINISTERED AS: an infusion.

Lily of the valley *Convallaria magalis*. COMMON NAME: May lily, convarraria, Our Lady's tears, conval-lily, lily constancy, ladder to heaven, Jacob's ladder.

OCCURRENCE: native to Europe and distributed over North America and northern Asia. It is a very localized plant in England and Scotland.

PARTS USED: the flowers, leaves and whole herb. The chief constituents are two glucosides – convallamarin (the active principle) and convallarin, as well as tannin and mineral salts.

MEDICINAL USES: cardiac tonic, diuretic. A similar drug to digitalis, from the FOXGLOVE, although it is less powerful. Strongly recommended in valvular heart disease, cardiac debility, dropsy and it slows the action of a weak, irritated heart. Lily of the valley does not have accumulatory effects and can be taken in full and frequent doses without harm. A decoction of the flowers is good at removing obstructions in the urinary canal.

ADMINISTERED AS: fluid extracts, decoction tincture, powdered flowers.

Lily, Madonna *Lilium candidum.* COMMON NAME: White lily, meadow lily.

OCCURRENCE: a southern European native which has been cultivated in Great Britain and America for centuries.

PARTS USED: the bulb.

MEDICINAL USES: demulcent, astringent, mucilaginous. The bulb is mainly used as an emollient poultice for ulcers, tumours and external inflammation. When made into an ointment, Madonna lily removes corns and eliminates pain and inflammation from burns and scalds, reducing scarring. When used in combination with life root (*Senecio aureus*), Madonnna lily is of great value in treating leucorrhoea, prolapse of the womb and other female complaints. The bulb is very often eaten as food in Japan.

ADMINISTERED AS: poultice, ointment, decoction.

Lime fruit *Citrus medica* var. *acida.* COMMON NAME: *Citrus acris, Citrus acida,* limettae fructus.

OCCURRENCE: a native Asian tree which is cultivated in many warm countries including the West Indies and Italy.

PARTS USED: the fruit and juice.

MEDICINAL USES: refrigerant, antiscorbutic. The juice of the lime contains citric acid and is a popular beverage, sweetened as syrup. It is used to treat dyspepsia.

ADMINISTERED AS: fresh juice, syrup

Lime tree *Tilia europoea.* COMMON NAME: Linden flowers, linn flowers, common lime, tilleul, flores tiliae, *Tilia vulgaris, T intermedia, T. cordata, T. platyphylla.*

OCCURRENCE: native to the British Isles and the northern temperate zone.

PARTS USED: the lime flowers, bark, powdered charcoal. The flowers contain volatile oil, flavonid glucosides, saponins, condensed tannins and mucilage.

MEDICINAL USES: nervine, stimulant, tonic. An infusion of the flowers is good for indigestion, hysteria, nervous vomiting colds, 'flu and catarrh. They can also help calm overactive children and relax the nervous system. Lime flower tea eases headaches and insomnia. The flowers are said to lower blood pressure (possibly due to the bioflavonoids they contain) and are said to remedy arteriosclerosis. The inner bark of the lime has a diuretic effect and is utilized for gout and kidney stones as well as treating coronary artery disease by dilating the coronary arteries. The powdered charcoal was used in gastric and dyspeptic disorders and applied to burnt or sore areas.

ADMINISTERED AS: infusion, powdered charcoal, dried inner bark tea.

Liquorice *Glycyrrhiza glabra.* COMMON NAME: Licorice, lycorys *Liquiriha officinalis.*

OCCURRENCE: a shrub native to south-east Europe and south west Asia and cultivated in the British Isles

PARTS USED: the root. The chief compound in the root is glycyr rhizin along with sugar, starch, gum, asparagus, tannin and resin.

MEDICINAL USES: demulcent, pectoral, emollient. A very popular and well-known remedy for coughs, consumption and chest complaints. Liquorice extract is included in cough lozenge and pastilles, with sedatives and expectorants. An infusion of bruised root and FLAX (linseed) is good for irritable coughs sore throats and laryngitis. Liquorice is used to a greater extent as a medicine in China and other eastern countries. The herb is used by brewers to give colour to porter and stout and is employed in the manufacture of chewing or smoking tobacco.

ADMINISTERED AS: powdered root, fluid extract, infusion, solid extract.

liverwort, English *Peltigera canina*. COMMON NAME: Lichen caninus, lichen cinereus terrestris, ash-coloured ground liverwort, liverleaf, *Hepatica triloba*.

OCCURRENCE: grows in moist, shady places in Britain and Europe.

PARTS USED: the whole lichen.

MEDICINAL USES: deobstruent, slightly purgative, *Peltigera canina* is held in esteem as a cure for liver complaints and was formerly regarded as a remedy for hydrophobia.

ADMINISTERED AS: infusion and fluid extract.

Lobelia *Lobelia inflata*. COMMON NAME: Indian tobacco, asthma weed, pukeweed, jagroot, vomitwort, bladderpod, *Rapuntium inflatum*.

OCCURRENCE: native to North America and grown in British gardens for many years.

PARTS USED: the herb, which contains the alkaloids, lobeline, isolobeline, lobelanidine and lobinaline along with fixed oil, gum, resin and lignin.

MEDICINAL USES: expectorant, emetic, diaphoretic, anti-asthmatic, stimulant. The use of this plant was passed to Europeans from native American Indians and it has been used as a major relaxant remedy used to treat pain caused by muscle spasms. Thus it is highly effective against asthma, bronchial complaints and lung problems. Lobelia may be given to ease convulsive and inflammatory disorders such as epilepsy, tonsillitis, diphtheria and tetanus. Externally, the herb is used for eye complaints, insect bites, POISON IVY irritation, ringworm, sprains, bruises and muscle spasms. The use of lobelia as an emetic is debatable as to whether it would benefit the patient, and its use is encouraged or discouraged by different herbals. Lobelia is a very important herbal remedy in modern usage.

ADMINISTERED AS: tincture, infusion, powdered bark, syrup and fluid extract.

Loosestrife *Lysimachia vulgaris*. COMMON NAME: Yellow loosestrife, yellow willow herb, herb willow, willow-wort, wood pimpernel.

OCCURRENCE: grows in shady banks and riversides in England.

PARTS USED: the herb.

MEDICINAL USES: astringent, expectorant. This herb is good at stopping bleeding of any kind, particularly of the mouth, nose and wounds. It is also used to restrain profuse menstrual bleeding and calm severe diarrhoea. Distilled water made with loosestrife was utilized to clean ulcers and reduce inflammation and to clear spots, marks and scabs from the skin. An infusion was used as a gargle in relaxed throat and quinsy.

ADMINISTERED AS: distilled water, dried herb, infusion and ointment.

Lovage *Levisticum officinale*. COMMON NAME: *Ligusticum levisticum*, old English lovage, Italian lovage, Cornish lovage, Chinese tang kui, man-mu.

OCCURRENCE: one of the old English herbs which was very generally cultivated; it was not indigenous to Great Britain but native to the Mediterranean region.

PARTS USED: the root, leaves, young stems and seeds. The plant contains a volatile oil, angelic acid, a bitter extract and resin.

MEDICINAL USES: the young stems are used in a similar manner to ANGELICA for flavouring and confectionery. The roots and fruit are aromatic, stimulant, diuretic and carminative in action. They are generally used in stomach disorders, and feverish attacks including those with colic and flatulence. The fresh leaves are eaten as a salad and when dried are infused into a pleasant tea with emmenagogue properties. An infusion of the root was recommended by old herbalists for gravel, jaundice and urinary problems and the sudorific nature of the roots and seeds meant they were highly favoured in treating 'pestilential disorders'.

ADMINISTERED AS: infusion of leaves and root infusion.

Lucerne *Medicago sativa*. COMMON NAME: Purple medick, cultivated lucern, alfalfa, purple medicle.

OCCURRENCE: an ancient herb, of unknown origin. It has been cultivated in Europe, Great Britain, Peru and Persia for hundreds of years.

PARTS USED: the herb.

MEDICINAL USES: this herb is used, as an infusion, to encourage weight gain and flesh development. It has also been used to feed cattle and horses.

ADMINISTERED AS: infusion.

upin, White *Lupinus albus*. COMMON NAME: Lupine, wolfsbohne.

OCCURRENCE: native to southern Europe and parts of Asia and is now extensively cultivated in Italy.

PARTS USED: the seeds, herb. The main compounds within the plant are the glucoside, lupinin; the alkaloids lupinidine and luparine.

MEDICINAL USES: anthelmintic, diuretic, emmenagogue. The bruised seeds, when soaked in water, are applied to ulcers and sores and when taken internally the seeds kill parasitic worms and excite the menstrual discharge. It was used by the Romans as food and can also be used for fibres to make cloth, paper and adhesive.

ADMINISTERED AS: poultice, infusion.

lace *Myristica fragrans*. COMMON NAME: Macis, muscadier, *Arillus myristicae*, *Myristica officinalis*, *Myristica moschata*.

OCCURRENCE: native to the Molucca Islands, New Guinea, bondy Islands and introduced into Sri Lanka and the West Indies.

PARTS USED: the growth outside the shell of the nutmeg seed – called the arillus. The main constituents of mace are a volatile oil, protein, gum, resins, sugars and two fixed oils. The volatile oil contains a lot of pinene and some myristicin.

MEDICINAL USES: stimulant, tonic, carminative, flavouring agent. This herb is used to help digestion and stomach weakness and increase the blood circulation and body temperature. Mace has been used against putrid and pestilential fevers and, combined with other herbs, intermittent fevers.

ADMINISTERED AS: powdered herb.

agnolia Magnolia Virginiana. COMMON NAME: Cucumber tree, blue magnolia, swamp sassfras, *Magnolia glauca*, *M. acuminata*, *M. tripetata*.

OCCURRENCE: native to the USA but is cultivated in Great Brit ain.

PARTS USED: the bark of stem and root.

MEDICINAL USES: mild, diaphoretic, tonic, aromatic, stimulant The bark is used against rheumatism and malaria, and the cone of the tree are steeped in spirit to make a tonic tincture. A warm infusion of bark is laxative and sudorific while a cold infusio is antiperiodic and tonic in effect.

ADMINISTERED AS: tincture, infusion, fluid extract.

Maidenhair *Adiantum capillus-veneris.* COMMON NAME: Tru maidenhair, hair of venus, rock fern, capillaire common o capillaire de montpellier.

OCCURRENCE: this grows wild in southern Europe and souther and central Britain.

PARTS USED: the herb, which contains tannin and mucilage bu has not yet been fully investigated.

MEDICINAL USES: pectoral, expectorant, mucilaginous. The fer has been used as a remedy in chest complaints, coughs an throat problems. It is an ingredient of cough mixtures, its flavou masked by sugar and orange-flower water. Maidenhair is goo at easing pulmonary catarrh and is used in Europe as an em menagogue.

ADMINISTERED AS: infusion, syrup.

Mandrake *Atropa mandragora.* COMMON NAME: Mandragor satan's Apple.

OCCURRENCE: a plant native to southern Europe but it can b cultivated in Great Britain.

PARTS USED: the herb and root.

MEDICINAL USES: emetic, purgative, cooling, anodyne, hypnotic The fresh root is a very powerful emetic and purgative dru and the dried bark of the root also shares the purgative quali ties. Ancient herbalists used mandrake to kill pain and to giv rest and sleep to patients, as well as using it for melanchol convulsions, rheumatic pain and scrofulous tumours. The administered the drug as the bark of the root, expressed juic or as an infusion of the root. In large doses, mandrake was sai to cause delirium and madness. The herb was used as an anaesthetic in ancient Greek medicine.

ADMINISTERED AS: infusion, fresh root, powdered bark, expressed juice.

Maple, Red *Acer rubrum.* COMMON NAME: Swamp maple, curled maple.

OCCURRENCE: a native American tree, introduced into Britain in 1656 as an ornamental tree.

PARTS USED: the bark.

MEDICINAL USES: astringent. The native American Indians used an infusion of the bark as an application for sore eyes.

ADMINISTERED AS: an infusion.

Mare's Tail *Hippuris vulgaris.* COMMON NAME: Female horsetail, marsh barren horsetail.

OCCURRENCE: a native British aquatic flowering plant found in shallow ponds, rivers, ditches and lake margins.

PARTS USED: the herb.

MEDICINAL USES: vulnerary. Old herbalists viewed mare's tail as good for stopping bleeding, be it internal or external. It was said to be used to heal ulcers, green wounds in children, ruptures and urinary stones. The herb was also used to strengthen the intestinal system, for head colds and as a warm poultice on skin eruptions and inflammations.

ADMINISTERED AS: poultice, decoction.

Marigold *Calendula officinalis.* COMMON NAME: *Caltha officinalis*, golds, ruddes, marg gowles, oculus Christi, marygold, garden marigold, solis sponsa.

OCCURRENCE: a native of southern Europe and a common garden plant in Great Britain.

PARTS USED: the petals and herb. Only the deep orange-flowered variety is of medicinal use.

MEDICINAL USES: stimulant, diaphoretic. Mainly used as a local remedy. Taken internally, an infusion of the herb prevents pus formation and externally is good in cleaning chronic ulcers and varicose veins. Formerly considered to be of benefit as an aperient and detergent to clear visceral obstructions and jaundice.

A marigold flower, when rubbed onto a bee or wasp sting, was
known to relieve pain and reduce swelling, while a lotion from
the flowers was good for inflamed and sore eyes. The expressed
juice of the plant was used to clear headaches and remove warts.
ADMINISTERED AS: infusion, distilled water and lotion.

Marjoram *Origanum vulgare*

OCCURRENCE: generally distributed over Asia, Europe and North
Africa and also found freely in England.

PARTS USED: the herb and volatile oil.

MEDICINAL USES: the oil has stimulant, carminative, diaphoretic,
mildly tonic and emmenagogue qualities. As a warm infusion
it is used to produce perspiration and bring out the spots of
measles as well as giving relief from spasms, colic and dyspeptic pain. The oil has been used externally as a rubefacient and
liniment, and on cotton wool placed next to an aching tooth it
relieves the pain. The dried herb may be utilized as a hot poultice for swellings, rheumatism and colic, while an infusion of
the fresh plant will ease a nervous headache.

ADMINISTERED AS: essential oil, poultice and infusion.

Marjoram, Sweet *Origanum marjorana*. COMMON NAME: knotted
marjoram, *Majorana hortensis*.

OCCURRENCE: native to Portugal and grown as an annual plant
through the rest of Europe and Great Britain.

PARTS USED: the herb and leaves. The plant contains tannic acid,
mucilage, bitter substances and an essential oil.

MEDICINAL USES: tonic, stimulant, emmenagogue. The essential
oil, oleum majoranae when extracted from the leaves, makes a
good external application for sprains and bruises, and acts as
an emmenagogue when taken internally. Sweet marjoram is
widely used in cookery and aids digestion of food.

ADMINISTERED AS: essential oil, dried or fresh leaves.

Marshmallow *Althaea officinalis*. COMMON NAME: Mallards, mauls,
schloss tea, cheeses, mortification, root, guimauve.

OCCURRENCE: a native of Europe, found in salt marshes, meadows, ditches and riverbanks. It is locally distributed in England
and has been introduced to Scotland.

PARTS USED: the leaves, root and flowers. Marshmallow contains starch, mucilage, pectin, oil, sugar, asparagin, glutinous matter and cellulose.

MEDICINAL USES: demulcent, emollient. Very useful in inflammation and irritation of the alimentary canal and the urinary and respiratory organs. A decoction of the root is effective against sprains, bruises of any muscle aches. When boiled in milk or wine marshmallow relieves diseases of the chest, e.g. coughs, bronchitis or whooping cough and it eases the bowels after dysentery without any astringent effects. It is frequently given as a syrup to infants and children.

ADMINISTERED AS: infusion, decoction, syrup, fluid extract.

Masterwort *Imperatoria ostruthium*

OCCURRENCE: native to central Europe and alpine regions; cultivated in Great Britain for many years.

PARTS USED: the rhizome.

MEDICINAL USES: stimulant, antispasmodic, carminative. Masterwort has been used in asthma, stroke, dyspepsia and menstrual problems. A decoction of the herb in urine was considered beneficial against dropsy, cramp, epilepsy, flatulence, gout and kidney and uterine problems.

ADMINISTERED AS: distilled water, decoction, fluid extract.

Mayweed *Anthemis cotula*. COMMON NAME: Maroute, cotula, dog chamomile, wild chamomile, foetid or stinking chamomile (or mayweed), dog's fennel, maithes, mathor, *Maruta cotula*, *Maruta foetida*, *Manzilla loca*, *Camomille puante*.

OCCURRENCE: frequently grows in fields and wild places in Great Britain and Europe.

PARTS USED: the flowers and leaves. The flowers contain volatile oil, oxalic, valeric and tannic acids, a bitter extractive and salts of iron, potassium, calcium and magnesium.

MEDICINAL USES: tonic, antispasmodic, emmenagogue and emetic. The smell of the flowers is still repulsive, but it is less offensive than that of the rest of the plant, so the flowers are mainly used in medicine. It is used in hysteria, as a poultice for haemorrhoids and as an infusion in the bath. The flowers have also been used in sick headaches, menstrual problems, scrofula, gastric troubles and dysentery; to induce sleep in asthma and in convalescence after fevers.

ADMINISTERED AS: fluid extract, poultice, infusion, decoction.

Meadowsweet *Spiraea ulmaria*. COMMON NAME: Meadsweet, dolloff, queen of the meadow, bridewort, lady of the meadow.

OCCURRENCE: common in the British Isles in meadows or woods.

PARTS USED: the herb

MEDICINAL USES: aromatic, astringent, diuretic, alterative. This herb is good against diarrhoea, stomach complaints and blood disorders. It is highly recommended for children's diarrhoea and dropsy and was used as a decoction in wine to reduce fevers. Meadowsweet makes a pleasant everyday drink when infused and sweetened with honey. It is also included in many herb beers.

ADMINISTERED AS: infusion, decoction.

Melilot *Melilotus officinalis*, *Melilotus alba*, *Melilotus arvensis*. COMMON NAME: King's clover, king's chafer, yellow melilot, white melilot, corn melilot, sweet clover, plaster clover, sweet lucerne, wild laburnham hart's tree

OCCURRENCE: naturalized in all parts of the British Isles.

PARTS USED: the dried herb containing coumarin, hydrocoumaric acid, orthocoumaric acid and melilotic anhydride.

MEDICINAL USES: aromatic, emollient, carminative. When applied as a plaster, ointment or poultice, the herb is good at relieving abdominal or rheumatic pain. It is taken internally to relieve flatulence. The herb was formerly used for clearing the eyesight, headaches, wounds, ulcers and inflammation.

ADMINISTERED AS: poultice, expressed juice, infusion.

Mercury, Dog's *Mercurialis perennis*.

OCCURRENCE: a common plant in woods and shady places in Europe and Russian Asia.

PARTS USED: the herb.

MEDICINAL USES: purgative. Recommended for use externally to treat sore, watery eyes, deafness, pains in the ear, ague, jaundice and women's diseases. The fresh juice of the plant is used to remove warts and to cleanse inflammatory and discharging sores and swellings. A lotion is made for antiseptic external dressings while the juice is used as a nasal douche for catarrh.

ADMINISTERED AS: expressed juice, lotion, fresh herb.

Mistletoe *Viscum album*. COMMON NAME: European mistletoe, bird lime mistletoe, herbe de la croix, mystyldene, lignum crucis.

OCCURRENCE: an evergreen, true parasitic plant found on several tree species including fruit and oak trees. It is found throughout Europe and Britain except in Scotland, where it is very rare.

PARTS USED: the leaves and young twigs. They contain mucilage, sugar, fixed oil, tannin and viscin, the active part of the plant.

MEDICINAL USES: nervine, antispasmodic, tonic and narcotic. It is highly recommended for epilepsy and other convulsive disorders, along with stopping internal haemorrhage. It has also been used in delirium, hysteria, neuralgia, nervous debility, urinary disorders and many other complaints arising from a weakened state of the nervous system. The berries are taken to cure severe stitches in the side, and the plant produces a sticky substance called bird-lime which is applied to ulcers and sores. Mistletoe is excellent for reducing blood pressure and has been indicated to be a successful cure for chronic arthritis and in treating malignant tumours in the body.

ADMINISTERED AS: tincture, powdered leaves, infusion, fluid extract.

Mountain flax *Linum catharticum*. COMMON NAME: Purging flax, dwarf flax, fairy flax, mill mountain.

OCCURRENCE: a common plant in meadows and pastures across Europe and Great Britain.

PARTS USED: the herb which contains a bitter resin and a crystalline principle called linin.

MEDICINAL USES: purgative, laxative, cathartic. It is a gentle cathartic drug with a laxative action preferred to SENNA. As an infusion, the dried herb has been used internally to treat muscular rheumatism and catarrhal infections. It can also be beneficial in liver complaints and jaundice.

ADMINISTERED AS: infusion, dried herb.

Mugwort *Artemisia vulgaris*. COMMON NAME: Felon herb, St. John's plant, moxa, cirigulum Sancti Johannis.

OCCURRENCE: this grows wild in Great Britain on roadsides and hedgerows.

PARTS USED: the leaves, which contain volatile oil, flavonoids, tannin and a bitter principle called absinthin; the roots.

MEDICINAL USES: emmenagogue, stimulant, tonic, nervine, diuretic, diaphoretic. As a nervine, this herb is good in palsy, fits, epilepsy and for people with a feeble constitution. An infusion of the herb is used for intermittent fevers and the ague and given as a tonic. Mugwort's main use is as an emmenagogue to provoke delayed or absent periods and therefore it should not be used during pregnancy, except under the guidance of a qualified herbal practitioner. However, it does help during and after childbirth in speeding up the birth process and to expel the afterbirth. Mugwort acts on the digestive process and stimulates the liver and is used to treat gout and rheumatism. in China, the dried herb is burnt on or near the skin to stop rheumatic pain caused by damp and cold conditions. In China mugwort is taken during pregnancy to prevent miscarriage, differing from the Western viewpoint.

ADMINISTERED AS: dried herb, fluid extract.

Mulberry *Monus nigra*. COMMON NAME: Common mulberry, black mulberry, purple mulberry.

OCCURRENCE: a native of Turkey, Armenia, Persia and is cultivated throughout Europe and Britain.

PARTS USED: the fruit which contains glucose, protein, pectin, tartaric and malic acids and ash.

MEDICINAL USES: laxative, refrigerant, nutritive. The fruit juice is a beneficial drink for convalescent people, as it checks the thirst and cools the blood after fevers. The fruits are made into wine, jam and conserve. The bark of the tree has a purgative and vermifuge effect on the body.

ADMINISTERED AS: syrup, expressed juice, infusion of bark.

Mullein *Verbascum thapsus*. COMMON NAME: Blanket herb, beggar' blanket, Aaron's rod, lady's foxglove, donkey's ears, torches candlewick plant, wild ice leaf, Jupiter's staff, clown's lungwort, velvet plant, clot.

OCCURRENCE: widely distributed through Europe, temperate Asia, North America, Ireland and Great Britain.

PARTS USED: the leaves and flowers. The plant contains saponins, mucilage, gum volatile oil, flavonoids and glucosides.

MEDICINAL USES: demulcent, emollient, astringent, sedative, narcotic. This herb is very useful in pectoral complaints, hoarseness, bronchitis, asthma, whooping-cough, wasting diseases and bleeding of the lungs and bowels. It can also be good for diarrhoea, mild catarrh, colic, inflammation of the urinary system, and as a poultice for boils and sores. The dried leaves may be smoked to remove irritation of the mucous membranes, the cough associated with consumption and spasmodic coughs in general. After placing bruised mullein leaves in olive oil and leaving it for a period, the oil can be used for relieving pain from bruises, frostbite and earache. Water distilled from the flowers was recommended for gout, burns and the condition called erysipelas, where the skin and tissue is infected with the bacterium *Streptococcus pyogenes* and the affected areas are red and swollen.

ADMINISTERED AS: fluid extract, distilled water, poultice, tincture, decoction.

Musk seed *Hibiscus abelmoschus.* COMMON NAME: Ambretta, Egyptian alcée, bisornkorner, target-leaved hibiscus, galu gastrin, *Abelmoschus moschatus.*

OCCURRENCE: native to India and grown in Egypt and the East and West Indies.

PARTS USED: the seeds. They contain fixed oil, a resin and a volatile body.

MEDICINAL USES: antispasmodic, aromatic, stomachic, nervine, aphrodisiac, insecticide. An emulsion of the seeds is regarded as anti-spasmodic and the seeds were chewed to benefit the nerves and stomach. The seeds are dusted over woollens to protect the fibre from moths.

ADMINISTERED AS: whole seeds, emulsion.

Mustard, Black *Brassica nigra, Siriapis nigra.* COMMON NAME
Brassica sinapioides.

OCCURRENCE: it grows wild throughout Europe, South Siberia
Turkey and North Africa and is cultivated in England, Italy
Germany and the Netherlands as a condiment.

PARTS USED: the seeds which contain an acrid, volatile oil, a
active principle, the glucoside sinigrin and the enzyme myrosin
When the seeds are crushed with water, these latter two chemi
cals come into contact and form oil of mustard.

MEDICINAL USES: irritant, stimulant, diuretic and emetic. Mainly
used as a poultice to relieve acute local pain, e.g. pneumonia
bronchitis and other respiratory organ diseases. The herb draw
blood to the skin surface, easing congestion of the organs, head
aches, neuralgia and spasms. The oil of mustard is a powerfu
irritant and rubefacient when undiluted, but is very useful whe
dissolved in spirit for chilblains, rheumatism and colic. A ho
infusion of the seed is a stimulating footbath and aids remov
of colds or headaches. Mustard flour, when taken internall
can act as an emetic, aperient and alterative herb and may als
cure hiccups. It is also a very good antiseptic and sterilizin
agent and deodorizer.

ADMINISTERED AS: poultice, infusion, essential oil, seed flou
leaves.

Myrrh *Commiphora molmol.* COMMON NAME: *Balsamodendro*
myrrha, Commiphora myrrha var. *molmol,* mira, morr.

OCCURRENCE: obtained from bushes in North-East Africa an
in Arabia.

PARTS USED: the oleo-gum-resin which contains volatile oil, res
ins and gum.

MEDICINAL USES: stimulant, tonic, healing, antiseptic, astringen
expectorant, emmenagogue. Myrrh has a long history of us
incountering poisons and putrid tissues throughout the bod
It is used in leucorrhoea, chronic catarrh, thrush, athlete's foo
absence of menstrual periods, ulcers and as a vermifuge. Th
resin acts as a tonic in dyspepsia, stimulates the circulatio
appetite and the production of gastric juices. It makes a ver

good gargle or mouthwash for an inflamed sore throat, spongy gums and mouth ulcers.

ADMINISTERED AS: fluid extract, tincture, pills.

Nettle *Urtica dioica, Urtica urens.* COMMON NAME: Common nettle, stinging nettle.

OCCURRENCE: widely distributed throughout temperate Europe and Asia, Japan, South Africa and Australia.

PARTS USED: the whole herb, which contains formic acid, mucilage, mineral salts, ammonia and carbonic acid.

MEDICINAL USES: astringent, stimulating, diuretic, tonic. The herb is anti-asthmatic and the juice of the nettle will relieve bronchial and asthmatic troubles, as will the dried leaves when burnt and inhaled. The seeds are taken as an infusion or in wine to ease consumption or ague. Nettles are used widely as a food source and can be made into puddings, tea, beer, juice and used as a vegetable. A hair tonic or lotion can also be made from the nettle. In the Highlands of Scotland, they were chopped, added to egg white and applied to the temples as a cure for insomnia.

ADMINISTERED AS: expressed juice, infusion, decoction, seeds, dried herb, dietary item.

Nightshade, Black *Solarum nignum.* COMMON NAME: garden nightshade, petty morel.

OCCURRENCE: a common plant in south England, seen less frequently in northern England and Scotland.

PARTS USED: the whole plant, fresh leaves. Both contain the active principle, solanine which is found in variable quantities within the plant, throughout the year.

MEDICINAL USES: the bruised fresh leaves are used external to the body to ease pain and reduce inflammation. Juice of the leaves has been used for ringworm, gout and earache and is supposed to make a good gargle or mouthwash when mixed with vinegar. This species of plant is reputed to be very poisonous, narcotic and sudorific, so is only utilized in very small doses, under careful supervision.

ADMINISTERED AS: infusion, expressed juice and fresh leaves.

Nutmeg *Myristica fragrans.* COMMON NAME: Nux moschata, *Myristica officinalis, M. aromata,* myristica

OCCURRENCE: native to the Banda Islands, Malayan Archipelago and the Molucca Islands. It is cultivated in Java, West Indies, Sumatra and French Guiana.

PARTS USED: the dried kernel of the seed which contains a volatile and a fixed oil, starch, gum, various acids and terpenes.

MEDICINAL USES: carminative, stomachic, stimulant. The grated or powdered kernel is used to relieve flatulence, vomiting and nausea. It is mainly used as an ingredient of various medicines and as a culinary spice. Nutmeg has similar properties to MACE but mace has a stronger flavour. Large doses of nutmeg can be toxic, producing disorientation, double vision and convulsions.

ADMINISTERED AS: expressed oil, powdered kernel.

Nux vomica *Strychnos Nux-vomica.* COMMON NAME: Poison nut, semen strychnox, Quaker buttons.

OCCURRENCE: a tree indigenous to India and now grown in Burma, China, Australia and the Malay Archipelago.

PARTS USED: the dried ripe seeds. They contain the alkaloids strychnine, brucine and strychnicine, fatty matter, caffeotannic acid and the glucoside, loganin.

MEDICINAL USES: tonic, bitter, stimulant. Nux vomica is utilized as a general tonic, mainly when combined with other herbal remedies, to treat neuralgia, dyspepsia, impotence, chronic constipation and general debility. This drug can also be of benefit in cardiac failure, surgical shock or poisoning by chloroform where it raises blood pressure and increases pulse rate but it can also cause violent convulsions. *Nux vomica* should only be used in limited circumstances and under strict control as strychnine is very poisonous.

ADMINISTERED AS: fluid extract, tincture.

Oak *Quercus robur.* COMMON NAME: Common oak, tanner's bark

OCCURRENCE: a tree widely dispersed over Europe.

PARTS USED: the bark.

MEDICINAL USES: slightly tonic, strongly astringent, antiseptic. It is very good in chronic diarrhoea, dysentery as a decoction and used as a gargle for sore throats. May also be used as an injection for leucorrhoea and applied locally for piles and bleeding gums. Water distilled from the oak buds was said to be good on any kind of inflammation.

ADMINISTERED AS: fluid extract, infusion, tincture, injection.

Oats *Avena sativa.* COMMON NAME: Groats, oatmeal.

OCCURRENCE: distributed across Europe, Britain and the USA.

PARTS USED: the seeds which are made up of starch, gluten, albumen and other proteins, sugar, gum oil and salts.

MEDICINAL USES: nervine, stimulant, antispasmodic, *Avena* forms a nutritious and easily digested food for convalescent patients and exhaustion after fevers. It can be made into a demulcent enema, or a good emollient poultice. Oat extract or tincture is useful as a nerve and uterine tonic.

ADMINISTERED AS: fluid extract, tincture, enema, dietary item.

Olive *Olea Europea.* COMMON NAME: *Olea oleaster, Olea larcifolia, Olea gallica,* oliver.

OCCURRENCE: native to the Mediterranean countries, Syria and Turkey. Now cultivated in Chile, Peru and Australia.

PARTS USED: the oil expressed from the ripe fruit, the leaves.

MEDICINAL USES: the oil is emollient, demulcent, laxative and aperient. It is a good substitute for CASTOR OIL when given to children, but its value in clearing parasitic worms or gallstones is unsure. The oil is a good ingredient in liniments or ointment and is used for bruises, sprains, cutaneous injuries and rheumatic problems. It is also utilized externally in joint, kidney and chest complaints or for chills, typhoid and scarlet fevers, plague and dropsy. When combined with alcohol, the oil is good as a hair tonic. Olive leaves have astringent and antiseptic properties, and an infusion of these leaves has proved beneficial in obstinate fevers.

ADMINISTERED AS: expressed oil, infusion, ointment.

Onion *Allium cepa.*

OCCURRENCE: originally native to south-west Asia and now cultivated around the globe.

PARTS USED: the bulb.

MEDICINAL USES: diuretic, expectorant, antiseptic. Although onions are extensively used in cookery, they also have medicinal uses. A roasted onion is applied to tumours or earache to remove the pain and onions steeped in gin produce a fluid extract which is given for gravel and dropsy. A homeopathic remedy is made from red onions and is useful in neuralgic pain, colds, hay fever, toothache and in the early stages of laryngitis with hoarseness.

ADMINISTERED AS: poultice, tincture.

Orange, Bitter *Citrus aurantium* subsp. *amara*. **Orange, Sweet** *Citrus vulgaris*. COMMON NAME: (bitter orange) *Citrus bigaradia*, *Citrus vulgaris*, *Bi garadier*, bigarade orange, Seville orange, naranja. (sweet orange) Portugal orange, China orange, *Citrus dulcis*.

OCCURRENCE: the bitter orange originated from northern India but is now grown in Mediterranean countries. The sweet orange is grown in Sicily, Africa and the West Indies.

PARTS USED: the fruit, peel and flowers. Oil is extracted from the peel of both types of orange – bitter orange produces oil of bigarde and the sweet orange oil is oil of Portugal. Distillation of the bitter orange flowers with water produces orange flower water and an essential oil called neroli.

MEDICINAL USES: tonic, stomachic, carminative, aromatic. Both sweet and bitter orange oils are used as flavouring agents for medicinal compounds but may be used in a similar manner to oil of TURPENTINE in treating chronic bronchitis. An infusion of dried flowers can be taken as a mild nervous stimulant and a tonic may be given of bitter orange peel, either on its own or as an infusion. In China, the dried peel of the sweet orange is used as a diuretic and to aid digestion. Oil of neroli is used in aromatherapy for treating anxiety and nervous depression.

ADMINISTERED AS: infusion, dried peel, essential oil, distilled water.

Orris *Iris florentina* (and other species). COMMON NAME: Florentine orris, orris root.

OCCURRENCE: grown in Italy and Morocco and to a smaller extent in England.

PARTS USED: the root, which contains oil of orris, fat, resin, starch, mucilage, a glucoside called iridin and a bitter extractive substance.

MEDICINAL USES: Orris root is rarely used in medicine today. The fresh root has emetic, diuretic and cathartic properties and was formerly used against congested headache, dropsy, bronchitis and chronic diarrhoea. It is more generally used in perfumery, as it strengthens the odour of other fragrant herbs and acts as a fixative in perfumes and pot pourri. It is also part of dusting powders, toilet powders and tooth powders.

Parsley *Carum petroselinum*. COMMON NAME: *Apium petroselinum*, *Petroselinum lativum*, petersylinge, persely, persele.

OCCURRENCE: this was first cultivated in Britain in 1548, now completely naturalized through England and Scotland.

PARTS USED: the root, seeds and leaves. The root is slightly aromatic and contains starch mucilage, sugar, volatile oil and apiin. Parsley seeds contain more volatile oil, which consists of terpenes and apiol, an allyl compound.

MEDICINAL USES: carminative, tonic, aperient, diuretic. A strong decoction of the root is used in gravel, stone, kidney congestion, jaundice and dropsy. Bruised parsley seeds used to be given against plague and intermittent fevers, while the external application of the leaves may help to dispel tumours. A poultice of the leaves is effective against bites and stings of poisonous insects.

ADMINISTERED AS: fluid extract, essential oil, infusion, ointment and poultice.

Parsley piert *Alchemilla arvensis*. COMMON NAME: Parsley breakstone, parsley piercestone, field lady's mantle.

OCCURRENCE: common across Great Britain, Europe and North Africa and was introduced into North America.

PARTS USED: the herb.

MEDICINAL USES: diuretic, demulcent, refrigerant. This herb is mainly employed in gravel, stone, dropsy and in bladder and kidney problems. It can effect results even in seemingly incurable cases. It can also help jaundice and clearing obstructions of the liver. To limit its irritancy, it is sometimes combined with demulcent or diuretic herbs for best effect, e.g. BROOM, JUNIPER, CARROT, COMFREY or MARSHMALLOW.

ADMINISTERED AS: fresh herb or infusion.

Parsnip *Pastinaca sativa*. COMMON NAME: Le panais, die pastinake.

OCCURRENCE: native European, cultivated commercially as food.

PARTS USED: the root.

MEDICINAL USES: nutritive. The parsnip exceeds almost all other vegetables in terms of food value (except potatoes) and is very nourishing for humans and animals alike. They are preferred to carrots for fattening pigs and given to cattle. Some old herbalists saw parsnips as a cure for asthma, cancer and consumption and used bruised parsnip roots as an application on bruises. In many areas, parsnips were made into a preserve, a beer or wine. They are also used extensively in salads, soups, as a vegetable and in cakes.

Passionflower *Passiflora incarnata*. COMMON NAME: passion vine, granadilla, maracoc, maypops.

OCCURRENCE: a native of Virginia in the United States.

PARTS USED: the flower and the dried vine. The plant contains flavonoids, sugars, sterols and gum as well as the alkaloids harmone, harmol, harmaline, harmine and harmalol.

MEDICINAL USES: antispasmodic, sedative, narcotic. This drug relaxes the nervous system and the sedative effects are good as well. It is non-addictive. It is a very good remedy for anxiety, tension, insomnia, diarrhoea, dysentery, neuralgia and painful menstruation. The alkaloids have tranquillizing effects and it is used to reduce high blood pressure.

ADMINISTERED AS: fluid extract.

Peach *Prunus persica*. COMMON NAME: *Persica vulgaris, Amygdalus persica*.

OCCURRENCE: cultivated in Asia for centuries and introduced into Europe from Persia.

PARTS USED: the bark, leaves and the oil expressed from the weeds.

MEDICINAL USES: demulcent, sedative, diuretic, expectorant. The leaves or bark, when used as an infusion, are almost a specific for irritation and congestion of the gastric surfaces. The infusion is also good for chronic bronchitis, whooping cough and ordinary coughs. A syrup or infusion made of the peach flowers was thought to be a mild acting purgative for children, as well as good for jaundice and giving health to a poorly child. The kernel oil was thought to induce sleep and rest if rubbed on to the temples. The oil is also used as a substitute for the more expensive ALMOND oil.

ADMINISTERED AS: infusion, fresh leaves, powdered leaves, oil.

ellitory-of-the-wall *Parietaria officinalis*. COMMON NAME: Parietaria diffusa, lichwort, paritary.

OCCURRENCE: a common wild plant in Europe and Great Britain.

PARTS USED: the herb, which contains a bitter glucoside, tannin, sulphur, mucilage and flavones among its chemical constituents.

MEDICINAL USES: diuretic, laxative, refrigerant, demulcent. It is given as an infusion or decoction to treat urine retention, cystitis, nephritis, dropsy, prostate inflammation, urinary stones and gravel. In the form of an ointment, this herb was used for haemorrhoids, gout and fistulas. The fresh herb is more effective than the dried herb.

ADMINISTERED AS: infusion, syrup, poultice, decoction.

ennyroyal *Mentha pulegium*. COMMON NAME: Pulegium, run-by-the-ground, pudding grass, lurk-in-the-ditch, piliolerial.

OCCURRENCE: a native plant of most of Europe and parts of Asia and commonly grown in gardens.

PARTS USED: the herb and the oil distilled from the herb called oil of pulegiam.

MEDICINAL USES: carminative, diaphoretic, stimulant, emmenagogue. The herb is mainly used to bring on menstruation which has been obstructed by cold or chills. It is also beneficial in spasms, flatulence, hysteria, sickness, colds, headaches and is a blood purifying herb. Pennyroyal is supposed to encourage sleep and was hung in bedrooms for that purpose. The oil has

been used to prevent mosquito and gnat bites for many years
If taken internally, the oil can be highly toxic and death ca
result. This herb should not be taken by pregnant women as
promotes menstruation and may cause haemorrhage and death
ADMINISTERED AS: dried herb, infusion, distilled oil.

Peony *Paeonia officinalis*. COMMON NAME: Paeony, paeonia, com
mon peony, piney, *Paeonia lactiflora*, *Paeonia corrallina*.

OCCURRENCE: introduced into Great Britain some centuries ag
PARTS USED: the root, which contains benzoic acid, asparagin
an alkaloid and an essential oil.

MEDICINAL USES: antispasmodic, tonic. In the past, peony ha
been used successfully in spasmodic nervous problems suc
as epilepsy and spasms as well as lunacy. An infusion of th
powdered root is recommended for liver obstructions, and help
kidney and gall bladder diseases. Since this plant is poisonou
it is rarely utilized in modern herbal medicine.

ADMINISTERED AS: infusion.

Pepper *Piper nigrum*. COMMON NAME: Black pepper, piper.

OCCURRENCE: grows wild in South India and Cechin-China; no
cultivated in the East and West Indies, Malay Archipelago, th
Philippines, Java, Sumatra and Borneo.

PARTS USED: the dried unripe fruits. White pepper comes fro
the same plant, except that the pericarp of the fruit has bee
removed prior to drying. The active chemicals in black or whi
pepper are piperine, volatile oil, starch, cellulose and a res
called chavicin.

MEDICINAL USES: aromatic, stimulant, carminative, febrifuge. Th
herb is useful in treating constipation, gonorrhoea, prolapse
rectum, paralysis of the tongue and acts on the urinary organ
The stimulant properties of pepper work on the gastro-intest
nal system to aid digestion, ease dyspepsia, torbid stomach con
ditions, and relieve flatulence and nausea. Pepper has also bee
recommended in diarrhoea, cholera, scarlatina, vertigo an
paralytic and arthritic disorders. Peppercorns, as the dried fru
is known, are used both whole and ground in many culina
dishes and are used as a condiment. In the Siege of Rome

408 AD, pepper was so highly priced that it was used as a form of currency.

ADMINISTERED AS: powdered dried fruits, gargle.

eppermint *Mentha piperita*. COMMON NAME: Brandy mint, curled mint, balm mint.

OCCURRENCE: found across Europe, was introduced into Britain and grows widely in damp places and waste ground.

PARTS USED: the herb and distilled oil. The plant contains peppermint oil, which is composed of menthol, menthyl acetate and isovalerate, menthone, cineol, pinene and limonene. The medicinal qualities are found in the alcoholic chemicals.

MEDICINAL USES: stimulant, antispasmodic, carminative, stomachic, oil of peppermint is extensively used in both medicine and commerce. It is good in dyspepsia, flatulence, colic and abdominal cramps. The oil allays sickness and nausea, is used for chorea and diarrhoea but is normally used with other medicines to disguise unpalatable tastes and effects. Peppermint water is in most general use and is used to raise body temperature and induce perspiration. Peppermint tea can help ward off colds and influenza at an early stage, can calm heart palpitations and is used to reduce the appetite.

ADMINISTERED AS: infusion, distilled water, spirit, essential oil and fluid extract.

impernel, Scarlet *Anagallis arvensis*. COMMON NAME: Shepherd's barometer, poor man's weatherglass, adder's eyes, bipinella.

OCCURRENCE: a very widely distributed plant found in all the temperate regions, in both hemispheres.

PARTS USED: the whole herb, of which little is known of the active chemicals within it. It does contain the compound, saponin.

MEDICINAL USES: diuretic, diaphoretic, expectorant. This plant has an ancient reputation for healing, particularly dealing with diseases of the brain and mental illness. It is considered beneficial in dropsy, liver obstruction, disorders of the spleen, gravel, rheumatic complaints and gout, but caution should be taken as

in experiments extracts from this plant have been found to be
poisonous to animals and its full effects on humans are not yet
known.

ADMINISTERED AS: infusion, dried herb, tincture, fluid extract.

Pine oils there are several kinds: **Siberian pine oil**, from *Abies
Sibirica*; **Pumilio pine oil**, from *Pinus muge*; **Sylvestris pine
oil**, from *Pinus sylvestris*.

PARTS USED: the oil produced from when pine wood is distilled
using steam under pressure.

MEDICINAL USES: rubefacient, aromatic. These oils are mainly used
as inhalants for bronchitis or laryngitis or as liniment plasters.

ADMINISTERED AS: distilled oil.

Pine, White *Pinus strobus.* COMMON NAME: Weymouth pine, pin
du lord, *Pinus alba*, deal pine.

OCCURRENCE: widely distributed in the northern hemisphere,
especially in North America.

PARTS USED: the bark.

MEDICINAL USES: expectorant, diuretic, demulcent. Used for the
relief of coughs, colds and chest diseases. It has a beneficial
effect on the bladder and kidney systems. A compound syrup is
the most commonly administered form of the drug, but it contains morphine so care must be taken that morphine dependence does not develop.

ADMINISTERED AS: compound syrup and fluid extract.

Plantain, Common *Plantago major.* COMMON NAME: broad-leaved
plantain, ripple grass, waybread, snakeweed, cuckoo's bread,
Englishman's foot, white man's foot, waybroad.

OCCURRENCE: a familiar weed all over Europe, Great Britain and
other parts of the world.

parts used: the root, leaves and flowers.

medicinal uses: refrigerant, diuretic, deobstruent, astringent,
cooling, alterative. The plant has been used in inflammation of
the skin, malignant ulcers, intermittent fever, applied to sores
and as a vulnerary. The fresh leaves can stop bleeding of minor
wounds, relieve the pain of insect stings, nettles, burns and
scalds.

ADMINISTERED AS: expressed juice, poultice, infusion, fresh leaves, fluid extract, decoction, ointment.

Polypody root *Polypodium vulgare*. COMMON NAME: Rock polypody, polypody of the oak, wall fern, brake root, rock brake, oak fern, rock of polypody.

OCCURRENCE: a common fern growing in sheltered places, hedgebanks, old walls and tree stumps in Great Britain and Europe.

PARTS USED: the root.

MEDICINAL USES: alterative, tonic, expectorant, pectoral. This herb is used as a laxative; as a tonic in dyspepsia and loss of appetite. It is also good for skin diseases, coughs and catarrh, consumption, hepatic complaints and some types of parasitic worm. The action of this drug is such that it may cause the formation of a rash, but these spots should disappear after a short period of time with no after effects. This fern is still used as a cure for whooping cough in many rural areas.

ADMINISTERED AS: fresh root, decoction, powdered root, fluid extract.

Poplar *Populus tremuloides*. COMMON NAME: White poplar, American aspen, quaking aspen.

OCCURRENCE: native to North America and commonly grown in Great Britain.

parts used: the bark, which is thought to contain salicin and populin.

medicinal uses: febrifuge, diuretic, stimulant, tonic. This drug is very useful against fevers, particularly those of an intermittent nature. It is often used as a substitute for Peruvian bark or quinine, as it lacks dangerous long-term side effects. Poplar bark is helpful in treating chronic diarrhoea, debility, hysteria, indigestion and faintness as well as acting as a diuretic in gleet, gonorrhoea and urinary complaints. This drug could be considered a 'universal tonic'.

ADMINISTERED AS: infusion, fluid extract.

Poppy, Red *Papaver rhoeas*. COMMON NAME: Headache, corn poppy, corn rose, flores rhoeados.

OCCURRENCE: a common flowering plant in fields and waste ground across Europe and Great Britain.

PARTS USED: flowers and petals. the fresh petals contain rhoeadi
and papaveric acids, which give the flowers their colour, an
the alkaloid rhoeadine. The amount and quantity of active ingredients in the plant is uncertain so its action is open to de-
bate.

MEDICINAL USES: very slightly narcotic, anodyne, expectorant. The
petals can be made into a syrup which is used to ease pain. I
may be used for chest complaints, e.g. pleurisy.

ADMINISTERED AS: syrup, infusion, distilled water.

Poppy, White *Papaver somniferum*. COMMON NAME: Opium poppy
mawseed.

OCCURRENCE: indigenous to Turkey and Asia, cultivated in Europe, Great Britain, Persia, India and China for opium production.

PARTS USED: the capsules and flowers. The white poppy contains twenty one different alkaloids of which morphine, narco-
tine, codeine, codamine and thebaine are the most important

MEDICINAL USES: hypnotic, sedative, astringent, expectorant, dia
phoretic, antispasmodic, anodyne. The use of this drug date
back to Greek and Roman times. It is the best possible hyp
notic and sedative drug, frequently used to relieve pain and caln
excitement. It has also been used in diarrhoea, dysentery an
some forms of cough. The tincture of opium is commonly calle
laudanum, and when applied externally with soap liniment i
provides quick pain relief.

ADMINISTERED AS: syrup, tincture, decoction and poultice.

Primrose *Primula vulgaris*.

OCCURRENCE: a common wild flower found in woods, hedgerow
and pastures throughout Great Britain.

PARTS USED: the root and whole herb. Both parts of the plan
contain a fragrant oil called primulin and the active principl
saponin.

MEDICINAL USES: astringent, antispasmodic, vermifuge, emetic
It was formerly considered to be an important remedy in mus
cular rheumatism, paralysis and gout. A tincture of the whol
plant has sedative effects and is used successfully in extrem

sensitivity, restlessness and insomnia. Nervous headaches can be eased by treatment with an infusion of the root, while the powdered dry root serves as an emetic. An infusion of primrose flowers is excellent in nervous headaches and an ointment can be made out of the leaves to heal and salve wounds and cuts.

ADMINISTERED AS: infusion, tincture, powdered root and ointment.

Puffball *Lycoperdon bovista.* COMMON NAME: *Lycoperdon giganteum.*

OCCURRENCE: grows wild throughout Great Britain and Europe.
PARTS USED: the lower section of the fungi.
MEDICINAL USES: haemostatic. This fungi grows completely enclosing its spores in fungal tissue (peridium), and then matures so that the colour changes from yellow-white to brown and then the peridium ruptures and the spores are released. When young, the spongy fungal tissue makes an excellent food and is consumed with relish by people in many European areas, including the Gaelic community in the Highlands of Scotland. Once matured, it is not edible but it can then be used to stop bleeding from wounds. It is a highly effective cure. Puffballs were also used as tinder many years ago and are burnt, producing smoke which stupefies bees so that honey can be collected safely.

ADMINISTERED AS: dried or fresh fungal tissue and spores.

Pumpkin *Cucurbita maxima.* COMMON NAME: Pumpkin seed, melon pumpkin, pompion.

OCCURRENCE: a plant grown for food and animal fodder in the United States and common in gardens in Great Britain.
PARTS USED: the seeds. They contain a fixed oil, a volatile oil, sugar, starch and an acrid resin which may be the active component.
MEDICINAL USES: taeniacide, diuretic, demulcent. This fruit has long been used as a vermifuge, removing parasitic worms including tapeworm. A mixture of the seeds, sugar, milk or water is mixed up and taken over six hours after which CASTOR OIL is

given, a few hours after the final dose of pumpkin. The vermifuge effects are thought to come from the mechanical effects of the seeds. A basic infusion of the seeds in water is used in urinary complaints.

ADMINISTERED AS: infusion.

Purslane, Golden *Portulaca sativa*. COMMON NAME: Garden purslane, pigweed.

OCCURRENCE: an herbaceous annual plant which is distributed all over the world. It is not indigenous to Great Britain.

PARTS USED: the herb, expressed juice and seeds.

MEDICINAL USES: Purslane is a herb with a great history of use for medical complaints. The expressed juice of the herb was good for strangury, dry coughs, shortness of breath, hot agues, headaches, stopping haemorrhages and as an external application to sores and inflammation. When combined with oil of ROSES, the juice was used for sore mouths, swollen gums and to fasten loose teeth. The bruised seeds were made into a decoction with wine and used to expel worms from children. The bruised herb was used as a poultice to remove heat from the head and temples and to reduce eye inflammation. It was also used on cramps or gouty areas.

ADMINISTERED AS: poultice, decoction, expressed juice.

Quince *Cydonia oblongata*. COMMON NAME: Quince seed, *Cydonica vulgaris*.

OCCURRENCE: grown in England for its fruit but is native to Persia.

PARTS USED: the fruit and seeds.

MEDICINAL USES: astringent, mucilaginous, demulcent. The fruit is used to prepare a syrup which is added to drinks when ill, as it restrains looseness of the bowels and helps relieve dysentery and diarrhoea. The soaked seeds form a mucilaginous mass similar to that produced by FLAX. A decoction of the seeds is used against gonorrhoea, thrush and in irritable conditions of the mucous membranes. The liquid is also used as a skin lotion or cream and administered in eye diseases as a soothing lotion.

ADMINISTERED AS: syrup, decoction or lotion.

Radish *Raphanus satinus*

OCCURRENCE: a native plant of China, Japan and cochin-China and widely cultivated in Europe, Great Britain and temperate Asia.

PARTS USED: the root which has been found to contain a volatile oil, an amylclytic enzyme and a chemical called phenyl-ethyl isothiocyanite.

MEDICINAL USES: antiscorbutic, diuretic. This plant is a very good food remedy for scurvy, gravel and stone. The juice has been beneficial in preventing the formation of gallstones.

ADMINISTERED AS: expressed juice, fresh root, dietary item.

Ragwort *Senecio jacobaea*. COMMON NAME: St. James's wort, stinking nanny, staggerwort, ragweed, dog standard, cankerwort, stammerwort, fireweed.

OCCURRENCE: an abundant wild plant, widely distributed over Great Britain, Europe, Siberia and north-west India.

PARTS USED: the herb.

MEDICINAL USES: diaphoretic, detergent, emollient, cooling, astringent. The leaves were used as emollient poultices, while the expressed juice of the herb was utilized as a wash in burns, eye inflammation, sores and cancerous ulcers. It has been successful in relieving rheumatism, sciatica, gout and in reducing inflammation and swelling of joints when applied as a poultice. Ragwort makes a good gargle for ulcerated throats and mouths and a decoction of its root is said to help internal bruising and wounds. The herb was previously thought to be able to prevent infection. This plant is poisonous to cattle and should be removed from their pastures. The alkaloids in the ragwort have cumulative effects in the cattle and low doses of the chemical eaten over a period of time can built up to a critical level, where the cattle show obvious symptoms and death then results. It is uncertain if sheep are also susceptible to this chemical.

ADMINISTERED AS: poultice, infusion and decoction.

Raspberry *Rubus idaeus*. COMMON NAME: American raspberry, raspbis, hindberry, bramble of Mount Ida, *Rubus strigosus*.

OCCURRENCE: found wild in Great Britain and cultivated in many parts of Europe.

PARTS USED: the leaves and fruit. The fruit contains fruit sugar, a volatile oil, pectin, mineral salts and citric and malic acids.

MEDICINAL USES: astringent and stimulant. Tea made of raspberry leaves is employed as a gargle for sore mouths, canker of the throat and as a wash for wounds and ulcers. It was also reckoned to give strength to pregnant women and encourage fast and safe delivery of the child. The leaves make a good poultice for cleaning wounds and promoting healing. Raspberry vinegar made with fruit juice, sugar and white wine vinegar makes a very good cooling drink when added to water, and is beneficial in fevers and as a gargle for sore throats. The infusion of raspberry leaves is also good in extreme laxity of the bowels and in stomach complaints of children.

ADMINISTERED AS: infusion, poultice, tea and liquid extract.

Rest-harrow *Ononis arvensis.* COMMON NAME: Wild liquorice, cammock, stinking tommy, ground furze, land whin, *Ononis spinosa.*

OCCURRENCE: a weed found on arable and waste land in Britain.

PARTS USED: the root.

MEDICINAL USES: diuretic. This herb was taken internally for dropsy, jaundice, gout, rheumatism and bladder stones. When made into a decoction, it was used as a wash for ulcers, fluid accumulation in tissues and enlarged glands. It was also proposed to subdue delirium. The young shoots were used as a vegetable or pickled, when they were said to refresh the breath and remove the smell of alcohol from the breath.

ADMINISTERED AS: decoction, dietary item.

Rhubarb, English *Rheum rhaponticum.* COMMON NAME: Garden rhubarb, bastard rhubarb, sweet round-leaved dock, *Rheum officinale.*

OCCURRENCE: its cultivation started in England around 1777 and spread throughout Great Britain. It is found growing wild or near dwellings.

PARTS USED: the rhizome and root. The stem and leaves of the plant contain potassium oxalate in quantity and some people are more sensitive to these salts and should avoid eating the plant. People with gout or those subject to urinary irritation should avoid the plant as well.

MEDICINAL USES: stomachic, aperient, astringent, purgative. This plant has a milder action than its relative, Turkey rhubarb (*Rheum palmatum*). It has a milder purgative effect and is particularly useful for stomach troubles in infants and looseness of the bowels. In large doses, rhubarb has a laxative effect. A decoction of the seed is proposed to ease stomach pain and increase the appetite. Rhubarb leaves were formerly used as a vegetable in the nineyeenth century, and several fatal cases of poisoning were recorded.

ADMINISTERED AS: decoction and powdered root.

Rice *Oryza sativa.* COMMON NAME: Nivona, dhan, bras, paddy, *Oryza montana, O. setegera, O. latifolia.*

OCCURRENCE: native to China and India; now cultivated in most sub-tropical countries.

PARTS USED: the seeds.

MEDICINAL USES: nutritive, demulcent, refrigerant. Boiled rice is good in treating upset digestion, bowel problems and diarrhoea. Rice-water, made from a decoction of the seeds, is an excellent demulcent and refrigerant drink in febrile and inflammatory diseases of the intestines, painful urination and other related conditions. It may be given as an enema for best results. Finely powdered rice flour can be used for burns, scalds and erysipelas or rice starch can be utilized in the same manner as wheat starch.

ADMINISTERED AS: poultice, decoction, dietary item, enema.

Rose, Pale *Rosa centifolia.* COMMON NAME: cabbage rose, hundred-leaved rose.

OCCURRENCE: cultivated in southern Europe and grown as a garden plant in many countries.

PARTS USED: the petals, which contain an acid red colouring matter, the glucoside quercitrin, gallic acid, tannic acid, sugar, gum and fat. Also the leaves.

MEDICINAL USES: aperient, laxative, astringent. The petals of this pink rose are rarely taken internally in modern herbal medicine, although they do have aperient properties. These flowers are mainly used for the preparation of rose-water, which is used as an eye lotion and as a carrier medium for other medicines. Cold cream is also made from rose-water and it is used on the skin of the hand and face to soothe abrasions and lesions. Rose leaves are laxative and astringent and were used to heal wounds.
ADMINISTERED AS: distilled water, ointment.

Rose, red *Rosa gallica*. COMMON NAME: Rose flowers, Provence rose, provins rose.

OCCURRENCE: a native plant of southern Europe and grown in gardens all over the world.

PARTS USED: the petals. Their composition is the same as that of the PALE ROSE, except they do not contain tannic acid.

MEDICINAL USES: tonic, astringent. Today, the petals are not normally taken internally. The petals are prepared in three manners which are then used. A confection is made of petals and sugar and this is utilized in making pills. The fluid extract is prepared using powdered rose petals, glycerine and dilute alcohol while an acid infusion is made with dried rose petals, sulphuric acid, sugar and boiling water. The infusion may be used as a flavouring for other medicines, as a lotion for eye complaints and for the treatment of night sweats relating to depression. Syrup of roses, honey of rose and rose vinegar are also preparations used medicinally in various countries around Europe. The petals are also used as flavour enhancers in two alcoholic liqueurs. *Rosa gallica* petals are used in aromatherapy.
ADMINISTERED AS: pills, lotion, infusion, poultice, syrup, fluid extract.

Rosemary *Rosmarinus officinalis*. COMMON NAME: Polar plant, compass-weed, compass plant, romero, *Rosmarinus coronarium*.

OCCURRENCE: native to the dry hills of the Mediterranean, from Spain westward to Turkey. A common garden plant in Britain, having been cultivated prior to the Norman Conquest.

PARTS USED: the herb and root. Oil of rosemary is distilled from the plant tops and used medicinally. Rosemary contains tannic acid, a bitter principle, resin and a volatile oil.

MEDICINAL USES: tonic, astringent, diaphoretic, stimulant. The essential oil is also stomachic, nervine and carminative and cures many types of headache. It is mainly applied externally as a hair lotion which is said to prevent baldness and the formation of dandruff. The oil is used externally as a rubefacient and is added to liniments for fragrance and stimulant properties. Rosemary tea can remove headache, colic, colds and nervous diseases and may also lift nervous depression.

ADMINISTERED AS: infusion, essential oil and lotion.

Rowan tree *Pyrus aucuparia.* COMMON NAME: Mountain ash, *Sorbus aucuparia, Mespilus aucuparia.*

OCCURRENCE: generally distributed over Great Britain and Europe, especially at high altitudes.

PARTS USED: the bark and fruit. The fruit may contain tartaric, citric or malic acids dependent upon its stage of ripeness. It also contains sorbitol, sorbin, sorbit, parascorbic acid and bitter, acrid colouring matters. The bark contains amygdalin.

MEDICINAL USES: astringent, antiscorbutic. A decoction of Rowan bark is given for diarrhoea and as a vaginal injection for leucorrhoea. The berries are made into an acid gargle to ease sore throats and inflamed tonsils. An infusion of the fruit is administered to ease haemorrhoids. The berries may also be made into jelly, flour, cider, ale or an alcoholic spirit. The rowan tree planted next to a house was said to protect the house against witchcraft.

ADMINISTERED AS: decoction, injection, infusion and dietary item.

Rue *Ruta graveolens.* COMMON NAME: Herb of grace, garden rue, herbygrass, ave-grace.

OCCURRENCE: indigenous to southern Europe and was introduced into Great Britain by the Romans.

PARTS USED: the herb. The herb is covered by glands which contain a volatile oil. The oil is composed of methylnonylketone, limonene, cineole, a crystalline substance called rutin and several acids. The plant also contains several alkaloids including fagarine and arborinine as well as coumarins.

MEDICINAL USES: stimulant, antispasmodic, emmenagogue, irritant, rubefacient. This is a very powerful herb and the dose administered should be kept low. It is useful in treating coughs, croup, colic, flatulence, hysteria and it is particularly good against strained eyes and headaches caused by eyestrain. An infusion of the herb is good for nervous indigestion, heart palpitations, nervous headaches and to expel worms. The chemical, rutin, strengthens weak blood vessels and aids varicose veins. In Chinese medicine, rue is a specific for insect and snake bites. When made into an ointment, rue is effective in gouty and rheumatic pains, sprained and bruised tendons and chilblains. The bruised leaves irritate and blister the skin and so can ease sciatica. This herb should not be used in pregnancy as the volatile oil, alkaloids and coumarins in the plant all stimulate the uterus and strongly promote menstrual bleeding. When a fresh leaf is chewed, it flavours the mouth and relieves headache, giddiness or any hysterical spasms quickly.

ADMINISTERED AS: fresh leaf, volatile oil, ointment, infusion, decoction, tea, expressed juice.

Rupturewort *Herniara glabra.* COMMON NAME: Herniary, breastwort.

OCCURRENCE: found in temperate and southern Europe and Russian Asia. It is a British native plant, particularly in southern and central England.

PARTS USED: the herb, which contains the alkaloid paronychine, and a crystalline principle called herniarne.

MEDICINAL USES: astringent, diuretic. This is a very active drug which has been successful in treating catarrhal infections of the bladder and oedema of cardiac or kidney origins.

ADMINISTERED AS: infusion.

Saffron *Crocus sativus.* COMMON NAME: Croccus, karcom, Alicante saffron, valencia saffron, krokos, gatinais, saffron, hay saffron, saffron crocus.

OCCURRENCE: grown from Persia and Kurdistan in the east to most European countries including Great Britain.

PARTS USED: the dried flower pistils. These parts contain an essential oil composed of terpenes, terepene alcohols and esters, a coloured glycoside called crocin and a bitter glucoside, called picrocrocin.

MEDICINAL USES: carminative, diaphoretic, emmenagogue. This herb is used as a diaphoretic drug for children and can also benefit female hysteria, absent or painful menstruation and stop chronic haemorrhage of the uterus in adults.

ADMINISTERED AS: tincture, powdered saffron.

Saffron, Meadow *Colchicum autumnale.* COMMON NAME: Colchicum, naked ladies.

OCCURRENCE: grows wild in North Africa and Europe and is found in meadows and limestone areas in the British Isles.

PARTS USED: the root and seeds.

MEDICINAL USES: cathartic, emetic, anti-rheumatic. This herb is very useful for acute rheumatic and gouty ailments, and it is normally taken along with an alkaline diuretic for best results. The active chemical in the plant is colchinine, an alkaline substance which is very poisonous. It has sedative effects and particularly acts on the bowels and kidneys. It acts as an irritant poison in large doses, and can cause undue depression. As such, care should be used when utilizing this herb.

ADMINISTERED AS: fluid extract, powdered root, tincture, solid extract.

Sage, Common *Salvia officinalis.* COMMON NAME: garden sage, red sage, saurge, broad-leaved white sage, *Salvia salvatrix.*

OCCURRENCE: native to the northern Mediterranean and cultivated through Britain, France and Germany.

PARTS USED: the leaves, whole herb. The herb contains a volatile oil, tannin and resin and is distilled to produce sage oil. This is made up of salvene, pinene, cineol, vorneol, thujone and some esters.

MEDICINAL USES: stimulant, astringent, tonic, carminative, aromatic. Sage makes an excellent gargle for relaxed throat and tonsils, bleeding gums, laryngitis and ulcerated throat. Sage tea is valuable against delirium of fevers, nervous excitement and accompanying brain and nervous diseases; as a stimulant tonic in stomach and nervous system complaints and in weak digestion. It also works as an emmenagogue, in treating typhoid fever, bilious and liver problems, kidney troubles and lung or stomach haemorrhages. The infusion is used in head colds, quinsy, measles, painful joints, lethargy, palsy and nervous head-aches. Fresh leaves are rubbed on the teeth to cleanse them and strengthen gums – even today sage is included in toothpowders. The oil of sage was used to remove mucus collections from the respiratory organs and is included in embrocations for rheumatism. The herb is also applied warm as a poultice.

ADMINISTERED AS: infusion, essential oil, tea and poultice.

Salep: early purple orchid, *Orchis mascula*; **spotted orchid**, *Orchis maculata*; **marsh orchid**, *Orchis latifolia*. COMMON NAME: Saloop, schlep, satrion, Levant salep.

OCCURRENCE: *Orchis mascula* is found in woods throughout England. *O. maculata* grows wild on heaths and commons; *O. latifolia* is found growing in marshes and damp pastures across Great Britain.

PARTS USED: the tuberous root, which contains mucilage, sugar, starch and volatile oil.

MEDICINAL USES: very nutritive, demulcent. This herb is used as a food item for convalescent people and children, made with milk or water and flavoured. It is prepared in a similar way to arrowroot. A decoction with sugar, spice or wine was given to invalids to build them up. The root is used to stop irritation of the gastro-intestinal canal and for invalids suffering from bilious fevers or chronic diarrhoea. In the old sailing ships, salep was carried and used as an emergency food source. It was sold on street corners in London as a hot drink, before COFFEE replaced its use as a beverage.

ADMINISTERED AS: decoction, dietary item.

Samphire *Crithmum maritimum*. COMMON NAME: Sea fennel, crest marine, sampier, rock fennel, rock samphire.

OCCURRENCE: found on rocks or salt marshes around the west or south of England but rare in the North and Scotland.

PARTS USED: the herb.

MEDICINAL USES: an infusion of samphire has a diuretic effect and acts on the kidneys. It is reputed to be an excellent treatment for obesity. It is eaten as a condiment, as a salad ingredient or pickled.

ADMINISTERED AS: infusion.

andalwood *Santalum album.* COMMON NAME: Santalwood, sanders-wood.

OCCURRENCE: a tree native to India and the Malay Archipelago.

PARTS USED: the wood oil.

MEDICINAL USES: aromatic, antiseptic, diuretic. The oil is given internally for chronic mucous conditions, e.g. bronchitis, inflammation of the bladder. It is also used in chronic cystitis, gleet and gonorrhoea. The oil is used in aromatherapy to lessen tension and anxiety and it was also considered a sexual stimulant in folk traditions. The fluid extract of sandalwood may be better tolerated by some people than the oil.

ADMINISTERED AS: wood oil, fluid extract.

arsaparilla, Jamaica, *Smilax ornata.* COMMON NAME: red-bearded sarsaparilla, *Smilax medica*, *Smilax officinalis*.

OCCURRENCE: a perennial climbing plant which grows in central America, primarily Costa Rica. It is termed Jamaican sarsaparilla as the plant was exported to Europe through Jamaica.

PARTS USED: the root, which is composed of starch, sarsapic acid, the glucoside sarsaponin and palmitic, stearic, behenic, oleic and linoleic fatty acids. The active principle is a crystalline compound called porillin or smilacin.

MEDICINAL USES: alterative, tonic, diaphoretic, diuretic. This root was introduced into Europe in 1563 as a remedy for syphilis. It is used in other chronic diseases, particularly rheumatism or skin diseases. It is still considered an excellent blood purifier, often given in conjunction with SASSAFRAS or BURDOCK. When smoked, Jamaican sarsaparilla was recommended for asthma.

ADMINISTERED AS: powdered root, fluid extract, solid extract.

axifrage, Burnet *Pimpinella saxifraga.* COMMON NAME: Lesser burnet, saxifrage.

OCCURRENCE: found on dry, chalky pastures throughout the British Isles.

PARTS USED: the root and the herb.

MEDICINAL USES: resolvent, diaphoretic, diuretic, stomachic, aromatic, carminative. This herb is prescribed for flatulent indigestion, toothache, paralysis of the tongue, asthma and dropsy. A decoction is used as a gargle in throat infections and hoarseness. The herb was added to casks of beer or wine to impart its aromatic flavour to the drink.

ADMINISTERED AS: fresh root, decoction dried root.

Scurvy grass *Cochlearia officinalis*. COMMON NAME: Spoonwort

OCCURRENCE: native to the coastline of Scotland, Ireland and England; also found in the sea coasts of northern and western Europe, the Arctic Circle and at altitude on the mountain chain of Europe.

PARTS USED: the herb.

MEDICINAL USES: stimulant, aperient, diuretic, antiscorbutic. It was formerly used on sea voyages to prevent scurvy. The essential oil from the herb is beneficial in cases of rheumatism or paralysis. When made into scurvy grass ale it was drunk as a tonic.

ADMINISTERED AS: infusion, essential oil.

Self-heal *Prunella vulgaris*. COMMON NAME: Prunella, all-heal, hook-heal, slough-heal, brunella, heart of the Earth, blue curls, siclewort.

OCCURRENCE: a very abundant wild plant in woods and fields all over Europe and Great Britain.

PARTS USED: the whole herb, containing a volatile oil, a bitter principle, tannin, sugar and cellulose.

MEDICINAL USES: astringent, styptic and tonic. An infusion of the herb is taken internally for sore throats, internal bleeding, leucorrhoea and as a general strengthener.

ADMINISTERED AS: infusion, injection and decoction.

Sheep's sorrel *Rumex acetosella*. COMMON NAME: Field sorrel.

OCCURRENCE: this grows in pastures and dry places around the globe, except in the tropics and is abundant in the British Isles.

PARTS USED: the herb.

MEDICINAL USES: diaphoretic, diuretic, refrigerant. The fresh juice of the herb is used for kidney and urinary diseases. Less active than SORREL (*Rumex acetosa*).

ADMINISTERED AS: expressed juice.

Shepherd's purse *Capsella bursa-pastoris*. COMMON NAME: Shepherd's bag, shepherd's scrip, lady's purse, witches' pouches, case-weed, pick-pocket, blindweed, pepper and salt, sanguinary, mother's heart, poor man's parmacettie, clappedepouch.

OCCURRENCE: native to Europe and found all over the world outside tropical zones.

PARTS USED: the whole plant which contains various chemicals which have not yet been entirely analyzed but they include an organic acid, a volatile oil, a fixed oil, a tannate, an alkaloid and a resin.

MEDICINAL USES: haemostatic, antiscorbutic, diuretic, stimulant. As an infusion of the dried plant, shepherd's purse is one of the best specifics for arresting bleeding of all kinds, particularly from the kidneys, uterus, stomach or lungs. It is said to be as effective as ergot or golden seal. It has been used for diarrhoea, haemorrhoids, dysentery, dropsy and kidney complaints. Shepherd's purse is an important remedy in catarrhal infections of the bladder and ureter and in ulcerated and abscess of the bladder where it increases the flow of urine and provides relief. Externally, the bruised herb is used as a poultice on bruised and strained areas, rheumatic joints and some skin problems. Since the herb tastes slightly unpleasant it is normally taken internally with other herbs to disguise the flavour, e.g. couch grass, juniper, pellitory-of-the-wall.

ADMINISTERED AS: fluid extract, poultice, decoction, infusion.

Silverweed *Potentilla anserina*. COMMON NAME: Trailing tansy, wild tansy, goosewort, silvery cinquefoil, goose grey, goose tansy, wild agrimony, moor grass, prince's feathers.

OCCURRENCE: very abundant in Great Britain and across temperate regions from Lapland to the Azores. It also grows in New Zealand, Chile, Armenia and China.

PARTS USED: the herb, which contains tannin.

MEDICINAL USES: astringent, tonic. an infusion is used as a lotion for bleeding haemorrhoids, as a gargle for sore throats and for cramps in the abdomen, stomach or heart. The infusion may also be used as a compress. A tea of Silverweed has been good for tetanus infections, for malarial infections, in gravel and as a specific in jaundice. A decoction of silverweed is useful for mouth ulcers, spongy gums, fixing loose teeth, toothache and preserving gums from scurvy. A distilled water made from the herb was used as a cosmetic to remove freckles, spots and pimples and to reduce the skin damage after sunburn.

ADMINISTERED AS: decoction, infusion, poultice, distilled water.

Snapdragon *Antirrhinum magus.* COMMON NAME: Calves, snout, lyons snap.

OCCURRENCE: naturalized in Great Britain and is a garden plant.

PARTS USED: the leaves.

MEDICINAL USES: bitter, stimulant. The fresh leaves have been applied as a poultice to tumours an ulcers. In old herbals, it is mentioned that the herb protects against witchcraft and that it makes the wearer 'look gracious in the sight of people.'

ADMINISTERED AS: poultice.

Soapwort *Saponaria officinalis.* COMMON NAME: Latherwort, soaproot, bruisewort, fuller's herb, crow soap, sweet betty, wild sweet william, bouncing bet.

OCCURRENCE: a common garden plant in Great Britain and also grows wild in central and southern Europe.

PARTS USED: the dried root and leaves. The root contains gum, resin, woody fibre, mucilage and saponin.

MEDICINAL USES: alterative, detergent, tonic, sternutatory. This herb has been used for scrofula and other skin complaints and in jaundice and other visceral obstructions. It is also good for venereal diseases and in rheumatism or skin eruptions due to infection with syphilis. This drug should be very carefully administered due to the very poisonous nature of saponin. In large doses, soapwort is strongly purgative so should only be given by a qualified herbalist. Soapwort is also used to clean clothes, skin and hair and is an ingredient of most herbal shampoo.

ADMINISTERED AS: decoction, expressed juice from fresh root, fluid extract.

Solomon's seal *Polygonatum multiflorum*. COMMON NAME: Lady's seals, St. Mary's seal, sigillum sanctae Mariae.

OCCURRENCE: a native plant of northern Europe and Siberia. It is found wild in some localities in England but naturalized in Scotland and Ireland.

PARTS USED: the rhizome which contains asparagin, gum, sugar, starch, pectin and convallarin, one of the active chemicals in LILY OF THE VALLEY.

MEDICINAL USES: astringent, demulcent, tonic. When combined with other herbs, it is good for bleeding of the lungs and pulmonary complaints. It is used on its own in female complaints and as a poultice for tumours, inflammations, bruises and haemorrhoids. As it is mucilaginous, it makes a very good healing and restorative tonic for inflammation of the bowels and stomach, haemorrhoids and chronic dysentery. A decoction was used to cure erysipelas and was taken by people with broken bones, as Solomon's Seal was supposed to 'encourage the bones to knit'. A distilled water prepared from the root was used as a cosmetic to remove spots, freckles and marks from the skin.

ADMINISTERED AS: decoction, infusion, poultice, distilled water.

Sorrel *Rumex acetosa*. COMMON NAME: Garden sorrel, green sauce, sour grabs, sour suds, cuckoo sorrow, cuckoo's meate, gowke-meat.

OCCURRENCE: indigenous to Britain and found in moist meadows throughout Europe.

PARTS USED: the leaves, dried and fresh.

MEDICINAL USES: refrigerant, diuretic, antiscorbutic. Sorrel is given as a cooling drink in all febrile conditions and can help correct scrofulous deposits. Its astringent qualities meant it was formerly used to stop haemorrhages and was applied as a poultice on cutaneous tumours. Sorrel juice and vinegar are said to cure ringworm, while a decoction was made to cure jaundice, ulcerated bowel, and gravel and stone in the kidneys.

ADMINISTERED AS: expressed juice, decoction, poultice and dried leaves.

Spearmint *Mentha viridis*. COMMON NAME: Mackerel mint, Our

Lady's mint, green mint, spire mint, sage of Bethlehem, fish mint, lamb mint, menthe de Notre Dame, erba Santa Maria, *Mentha spicata*, *Mentha crispa*, yerba buena.

OCCURRENCE: originally a Mediterranean native and was introduced into the British Isles by the Romans.

PARTS USED: the herb and essential oil. The main component of the essential oil is carvone along with phellandrine, limonene and dihydrocarveol acetate. The oil also has the esters of acetic, butyric and caproic acids within it.

MEDICINAL USES: antispasmodic, aromatic, carminative, stimulant. This herb is very similar to peppermint, but it seems to be less powerful. It is more suited to children's remedies. A distilled water from spearmint is used to relieve hiccoughs, flatulence and indigestion while the infusion is good for fevers, inflammatory diseases and all infantile troubles. Spearmint is considered a specific in stopping nausea and vomiting and in easing the pain due to colic. As a homeopathic remedy, spearmint has been used for strangury, gravel and as a local application for painful haemorrhoids.

ADMINISTERED AS: distilled water, infusion, tincture, fluid extract.

Spearwort, Lesser *Ranunculus flammula*.

OCCURRENCE: a very common plant throughout Britain, growing in wet and boggy heaths and commons.

PARTS USED: the whole plant.

MEDICINAL USES: rubefacient, emetic. The bruised leaves have a long history of use on the Isle of Skye and in the Highlands of Scotland in raising blisters. A distilled water from the plant is used as a painless emetic drug while a tincture is good at curing ulcers.

ADMINISTERED AS: distilled water, tincture, poultice.

Speedwell, Common *Veronica officinalis*. COMMON NAME: bird's-eye, cat's-eye.

OCCURRENCE: a common wild plant in Europe and Great Britain.

PARTS USED: the herb.

MEDICINAL USES: diaphoretic, alterative, expectorant, astringent diuretic, tonic. Lesser spearwort was formerly used in pectoral and nephritic complaints, haemorrhages, skin diseases and in treating wounds. An infusion of the dried herb is good for catarrh, coughs and most skin problems. May promote menstruation.

ADMINISTERED AS: infusion and dried herb.

Sphagnum moss *Sphagnum cymbifolium.* COMMON NAME: Bog moss.

OCCURRENCE: found in wet and boggy land, normally on peat soils on mountains and moors in Scotland, England, Ireland and parts of western Europe.

PARTS USED: the moss, which is made up of plant cells which are penetrated with a system of tubes and air spaces. This capillary tube system makes the moss resemble a very fine sponge and allows the plant to absorb huge quantities of water.

MEDICINAL USES: wound dressing. The use of sphagnum as a dressing for wounds can be dated back to the Battle of Flodden. There is a long history of use in Lapland where the dried moss is used as a mattress and blankets for infants. The moss has many advantages over other surgical dressings, e.g. cotton wool. Prepared moss can retain twice as much moisture as cotton; a 2oz dressing can absorb up to 2lb of liquid. This means that dressings need to be changed less frequently with less disturbance to the patient. In many times of war sphagnum was prepared in gauze bags, often in association with GARLIC for its antiseptic qualities. Sphagnum moss also has an antibiotic action due to micro-organisms associated with the plant which aids healing. The moss has also been used as bedding in stables and for hanging baskets and other gardening applications.

Spinach *Spinacio oleracea.*

OCCURRENCE: originally native to Persia and Asia and was introduced into Europe in the fifteenth century.

PARTS USED: the leaves, which contain iron, nitrogenous substances, hydrocarbons, chlorophyll and vitamins A and D.

MEDICINAL USES: nutritive, antiscorbutic. Spinach is primarily used as a food source as it is a good source of iron and vitamins.

Experiments have shown the benefit of eating spinach on people weakened by illness.

ADMINISTERED AS: expressed juice, dietary item.

St. John's wort *Hypericum perforatum.*

OCCURRENCE: found in woods, hedges, roadsides and meadows across Britain, Europe and Asia.

PARTS USED: the herb and flowers.

MEDICINAL USES: aromatic, astringent, resolvent, expectorant, diuretic and nervine. It is generally utilized in all pulmonary complaints, bladder trouble, suppression of urine, dysentery, diarrhoea and jaundice. It is good against hysteria, nervous depression, haemorrhages, coughing up blood and dispelling worms from the body. If children have a problem with night incontinence, an infusion of St. John's wort taken before bed will stop the problem. The herb is used externally to break up hard tissues, e.g. tumours, bruising. and swollen, hard breasts when feeding infants.

ADMINISTERED AS: an infusion and poultice.

Stockholm tar *Pinus sylvestris* (and other species). COMMON NAME: Tar, *Pix liquida.*

OCCURRENCE: obtained from various *Pinus* species grown across the northern hemisphere in Sweden, Russia, North America and Switzerland.

PARTS USED: the tar is an impure turpentine obtained from the stems and roots of *Pinus* species by destructive distillation.

MEDICINAL USES: antiseptic, diuretic, diaphoretic, expectorant, stimulant. It may be used for chronic coughs and consumption but is mainly used externally as a cutaneous stimulant and as an ointment for eczema. It is mainly used in veterinary practices.

ADMINISTERED AS: ointment, fluid extract.

Stramonium *Datura stramonium.* COMMON NAME: Thornapple, jimsonweed, Jamestownweed, devil's apple, devil's trumpet, datura, mad apple, stinkweed, apple of Peru.

OCCURRENCE: a plant of unknown origin that is currently found throughout the world except in cold or Arctic areas.

PARTS USED: the whole plant has medicinal qualities but it is the leaves and seeds that are most commonly used today. The leaves contain the same alkaloids as belladonna, but in slightly smaller amounts. The alkaloids include lyoscyamine, atropine, lyoscine along with malic acid, volatile oil, gum, resin and starch. The seeds are made up of fixed oil and the same alkaloids as the leaves, but the fixed oil makes the alkaloids difficult to extract so the leaves are the most extensively utilized.

MEDICINAL USES: antispasmodic, anodyne, narcotic. A herb which acts in a very similar manner to belladonna except it does not cause constipation. An extract of the seeds is given in pill form to stop coughing in spasmodic bronchial asthma, to ease whooping cough and spasm of the bladder. It is considered a better cough remedy than opium, but is used with extreme care as it can act as a narcotic poison in overdoses. When smoked with tobacco, alone or with other herbs, e.g. sage and belladonna, stramonium can ease asthma by relaxing spasms of the bronchioles during an attack. Taken in this form, it can also help control the spasms that occur in Parkinson's disease. The herb can relieve the pain of sciatica and rheumatism when used externally in the form of an ointment. Signs of an overdose of stramonium include dryness of the throat and mouth and an overdose can cause double vision, thirst, palpitations, restlessness, confusion and hallucinations. This drug is highly toxic and should only be used under the guidance of a herbal medicine practitioner or doctor. In India, thieves and assassins used to give their victims Stramonium in order to make them insensible while history states that the herb was taken by the priests of Apollo at Delphi, in Ancient Greece, to assist them in their prophecies. Stramonium was considered to be a plant which aided witches in their ill-doing, and during the time of the witch and wizard hunt in England, it was exceedingly dangerous to grow stramonium in your garden as it was said to confirm the supernatural powers of the householder. Many people were sentenced to death purely because stramonium was found in their garden.

ADMINISTERED AS: powdered leaves, powdered seeds, fluid extract, tincture and ointment.

Strawberry *Fragaria vesca.*

OCCURRENCE: found through the whole of the northern hemisphere, excluding the tropics.

PARTS USED: the leaves, which contain cissotanic, malic and citric acids, sugar, mucilage and a volatile aromatic chemical which is, as yet, unidentified.

MEDICINAL USES: laxative, diuretic, astringent. The berries are of great benefit for rheumatic gout while the root is good against diarrhoea. The leaves have similar properties and are used to stop dysentery. Fresh strawberries remove discolouration of the teeth if the juice is left on for about five minutes and then the teeth are cleaned with warm water, to which a pinch of bicarbonate of soda has been added. Sunburn could be relieved by rubbing a cut strawberry over a freshly washed face.

ADMINISTERED AS: infusion, fresh berries.

Sundew *Drosera rotundifolia.* COMMON NAME: Roundleaved sundew, dew plant, red rot, youthwort, rosa solis, herba rosellae ros+e du soleil.

OCCURRENCE: an insectivorous plant found in bogs, wet places and river edges throughout Britain, Europe, India, China, North and South America and Russian Asia.

PARTS USED: the air-dried flowering plant.

MEDICINAL USES: pectoral, expectorant, demulcent, anti-asthmatic. In small doses sundew is a specific in dry, spasmodic tickling coughs and is considered very good in whooping cough for which it may also be used as a prophylactic drug. The fresh juice is used to remove corns and warts. In America, the sundew has been advocated as a cure for old age and has been used with colloidal silicates in cases of thickening of arteries due to old age, or calcium or fat deposition.

ADMINISTERED AS: fluid extract, expressed juice, solid extract.

Sunflower *Helicanthus annuus.* COMMON NAME: Helianthus, marigold of Peru, *Sola indianus*, *Chrysanthemum peruvianum*, *Corona solis.*

OCCURRENCE: native to Peru and Mexico and was introduced into America, Europe and Great Britain as a garden plant.

PARTS USED: the seeds. These contain a vegetable oil, carbonate of potash, tannin and vitamins B1, B3 and B6. The oil is expressed from the crushed seeds and, according to the range of temperature to which the seeds are heated, several grades of oil are obtained.

MEDICINAL USES: diuretic, expectorant. It has been used successfully in treating pulmonary, bronchial and laryngeal afflictions as well as whooping cough, colds and coughs. The leaves are used, in some parts of the world, to treat malaria and the tincture may replace quinine in easing intermittent fevers and the ague. Sunflowers produce the seed cake which is used as cattle food; the fresh leaves are given to poultry; the plants can be used as a vegetable; the stems are used as bedding for ducks; the plant used for silage, fuel, manure, textiles and as a soil improver.

ADMINISTERED AS: sunflower oil, tincture, decoction, poultice.

Tag alder *Alnus semulata*. COMMON NAME: Smooth alder, red alder, common alder, *Alnus rubra*.

OCCURRENCE: a common tree found in Europe, Great Britain and the United States of America.

PARTS USED: the bark and cones.

MEDICINAL USES: tonic, alterative, emetic, astringent. This plant is good for scrofula, diarrhoea, dyspepsia, indigestion, secondary syphilis and debility of the stomach. A decoction of the cones was said to be astringent in effect and of use in all types of haemorrhages. The bark was also of benefit to some cutaneous diseases and intermittent fevers.

ADMINISTERED AS: infusion, decoction, fluid extract.

Tansy *Tanacetum vulgare*. COMMON NAME: Buttons.

OCCURRENCE: a hardy perennial plant, commonly seen in he and on waste ground all over Europe and Great Britain.

PARTS USED: the herb. It contains the chemicals tanacetin, tannic acid, a volatile oil, thujone, sugar and a colouring matter.

MEDICINAL USES: anthelmintic, tonic, emmenagogue, stimulant.

471

Tansy is largely used for expelling worms from children. |t is good in female disorders, like hysteria and nausea and in kidney weakness. The herb is also used for slight fevers, for allaying spasms and as a nervine drug. In large doses, the herb is violently irritant and induces venous congestion of the abdominal organs. In Scotland, an infusion was administered to cure gout. Tansy essential oil, when given in small doses, has helped in epilepsy and has also been used externally to help some eruptive diseases of the skin. Bruised fresh leaves can reduce swelling and relieve sprains, as can a hot infusion used as a poultice.

ADMINISTERED AS: essential oil, infusion, poultice, fresh leaves, solid extract.

Tarragon *Artemisia dracunculus.* COMMON NAME: Mugwort, little dragon.

OCCURRENCE: cultivated in kitchen gardens across Europe and Great Britain. Tarragon originally arose from both Siberia and southern Europe to form the French and Russian tarragon we know today.

PARTS USED: the leaves, which contain an essential volatile oil which is lost on drying.

MEDICINAL USES: today there are few medicinal uses for tarragon but it has been used previously to stimulate the appetite and to cure toothache. Tarragon is mostly used in cooking – particularly on the European continent. It is used for dressings, salads, vinegar and pickles.

ADMINISTERED AS: fresh root, fresh herb.

Tea *Camellia thea.* COMMON NAME: *Camellia theifera, Thea sinensis Thea veridis, Thea bohea, Thea stricta jassamica.*

OCCURRENCE: native to Assam in India, and the plant has spread to Sri Lanka, Java, China and Japan.

PARTS USED: the dried leaves.

MEDICINAL USES: stimulant, astringent. The infusion of the leaves has a stimulating effect on the nervous system, producing a feeling of comfort. It may also act as a nerve sedative where it can relieve headaches. When drunk in excessive quantities, tea can produce unpleasant nervous symptoms, dyspepsia and un-natural wakefulness.

ADMINISTERED AS: infusion.

Thistle, Holy *Carbenia benedicta*. COMMON NAME: Blessed thistle, *Cnicus benedictus, Carduus benedictus*.

OCCURRENCE: a native of southern Europe and has been culti-vated in Britain for hundreds of years.

PARTS USED: the whole herb which contains a volatile oil, a bitter crystalline compound called cnicin which is said to be similar to salicin in its properties.

MEDICINAL USES: tonic, stimulant, diaphoretic, emetic and em-menagogue. Very useful as an infusion to weak and debilitating stomach conditions, creating appetite and preventing sickness. It is said to be good in all fevers, as a purifier of the blood and circulation and its main modern day use is for bringing on a proper supply of milk in nursing mothers. In large doses, how-ever, holy thistle is a strong emetic, producing vomiting. It may be used as a vermifuge.

ADMINISTERED AS: infusion and fluid extract.

Thistle, Scotch *Onopordon acanthium*. COMMON NAME: Woolly thistle, cotton thistle.

OCCURRENCE: a common plant in all of Great Britain, found in waste ground and roadsides.

PARTS USED: the leaves and root.

MEDICINAL USES: ancient herbalists believed that the Scotch thistle was a specific against cancer and even today the ex-pressed juice of the plant has been used to good effect on can-cers and ulcers. A decoction of thistles was thought to restore a healthy, growing head of hair when applied to a bald head, while a root decoction has astringent effects and reduces production from mucous membranes. Thistles were also supposed to be effective against rickets in children, a crick in the neck and nervous complaints.

ADMINISTERED AS: expressed juice, decoction.

Thyme *Thymus vulgaris*. COMMON NAME: Garden or common thyme, tomillo.

OCCURRENCE: cultivated in temperate countries in northern Europe.

PARTS USED: the herb. Thyme gives rise to oil of thyme after distillation of the fresh leaves. This oil contains the phenols, thymol and carvacrol, as well as cymene, pinene and borneol.

MEDICINAL USES: antiseptic, antispasmodic, tonic, carminative. The fresh herb, in syrup, forms a safe cure for whooping cough, as is an infusion of the dried herb. The infusion or tea is beneficial for catarrh, sore throat, wind spasms, colic and in allaying fevers and colds. Thyme is generally used in conjunction with other remedies in herbal medicine.

ADMINISTERED AS: fluid extract, essential oil and infusion.

Tobacco *Nicotiana tabacum, N. acuminata, N. rustica* and other varieties. COMMON NAME: Leaf tobacco, tabacca.

occurrence: native to America and cultivated in many sub-tropical countries including China, Greece, France and Turkey.

parts used: the cured and dried leaves, which contain five alkaloids including nicotine. Upon smoking, nicotine decomposes into various chemicals – the very poisonous carbon monoxide, pyridine and hydrogen cyanide.

medicinal uses: narcotic, sedative, diuretic, expectorant, emetic. Medicinally, tobacco has been used internally for hernias, constipation, tetanus, retention of urine, worms and hysterical convulsions. It is best utilized externally as a plaster or poultice to ease cutaneous diseases, haemorrhoids and facial neuralgia. A combination of tobacco leaves along with the leaves of stramonium or belladonna make a very good treatment for spasmodic afflictions, painful tumours and obstinate ulcers. Tobacco is a local irritant and the nicotine within it is very poisonous, causing heart palpitations and irregularity and disturbing the digestive and circulatory organs. The use of tobacco as a medicine is unusual in today's western herbal medicine, although it is still used in some native societies. The poisonous nature of the alkaloids within the plant have discouraged its use as use of tobacco, even within small doses, can cause depression, convulsions and even death.

administered as: poultice, ointment, suppositories, smoking herb.

Turpentine oil distilled from *Pinus palustris*, *Pinus maritima* and other species.

MEDICINAL USES: rubefacient, irritant, diuretic. When taken internally, turpentine forms a valuable remedy in bladder, kidney, and rheumatic problems and diseases of the mucous membranes. The oil is also used for respiratory complaints and externally as a liniment, an embrocation and an inhalant for rheumatism and chest problems. Turpentine may be combined with other aromatic oils as a remedy.

ADMINISTERED AS: essential oil.

Valerian *Valeriana officinalis*. COMMON NAME: all-heal, great wild valerian, amantilla, setwall, sete-wale, capon's tail.

OCCURRENCE: found throughout Europe and northern Asia. It is common in England in marshy thickets, riverbanks and ditches.

PARTS USED: the root, which contains a volatile oil, two alkaloids called chatarine and valerianine as well as several unidentified compounds.

MEDICINAL USES: powerful nervine, stimulant, carminative anodyne and antispasmodic herb. It may be given in all cases of nervous debility and irritation as it is not narcotic. The expressed juice of the fresh root has been used as a narcotic in insomnia and as an anticonvulsant in epilepsy. The oil of valerian is of use against cholera and in strengthening the eyesight. A herbal compound containing valerian was given to civilians during the Second World War, to reduce the effects of stress caused by repeated air raids and to minimize damage to health.

ADMINISTERED AS: fluid and solid extract, tincture, oil, expressed juice.

Verbena, Lemon *Lippia citriodora*. COMMON NAME: Herb louisa, lemon-scented verbena, *Verveine citronelle* or *odorante*, *Verbena triphylla*, *Lippia triphylla*, *Aloysia citriodora*.

OCCURRENCE: originally from Peru and Chile, it was introduced into England in 1784 and is now a common garden plant.

PARTS USED: the leaves and flowering tops.

MEDICINAL USES: febrifuge, sedative. This herb has similar uses to BALM, PEPPERMINT, ORANGE flowers and SPEARMINT in relieving flatulence, indigestion and dyspepsia through its antispasmodic and stomachic actions. It is commonly made into a refreshing tisane. The leaves of lemon verbena were once used in finger bowls at banquets and the essential oil distilled from the herb was used to impart a strong lemon scent to cosmetics and soaps.

ADMINISTERED AS: tea.

Vervain *Verbena officinalis.* COMMON NAME: Herb of grace, herbe sacré, herba veneris, *Verbena hastrata*.

OCCURRENCE: grows across Europe, China, Japan and Barbary. Also found in England by roadsides and in sunny pastures.

PARTS USED: the herb. Vervain contains a peculiar tannin, which has not yet been fully investigated.

MEDICINAL USES: nervine, tonic, emetic, sudorific, astringent, diaphoretic, antispasmodic. This herb is recommended in many complaints including intermittent fevers, ulcers, pleurisy, oph-thalmic disorders and is said to be a good galactogogue. May also be administered as a poultice to ease headache, ear neu-ralgia, rheumatism and taken as a decoction to ease bowel pain during purging. Vervain is often applied externally for piles.

ADMINISTERED AS: fluid extract, decoction.

Vine *Vitis vinifera.* COMMON NAME: Grape vine.

OCCURRENCE: a very ancient plant, frequently mentioned in the Bible after the Great Flood. It now grows in Asia, central and southern Europe, Africa, Australia, Greece, California and South America.

PARTS USED: the fruit, leaves and juice. The wine sold commer-cially is made from fermented fruit juice. This juice, which is called 'must', contains malic acid, gum, sugar, inorganic salts and potassium bicarbonate. The leaves contain tartaric acid, tannin, malic acid, gum, quercetine, quercitrin, potassium bi-tartrate, cane sugar and glucose.

MEDICINAL USES: the leaves and seeds have an astringent action, with the leaves previously used to stop haemorrhages and bleed-ing. Ripe grapes, when eaten in some quantity, increase the flow of urine and can be of great benefit in exhaustion, anaemia, smallpox, sleeplessness and neuralgia. They are also eaten for poor biliary function and torpid liver. Grape sugar is chemically different to other sugars, as the saliva has no enzymatic effect on it. Thus it acts faster to warm up the body and build tissues, to increase strength and repair the body after illness. Raisins, have demulcent, nutritive and slightly laxative effects on the body.

administered as: fermented fruit juice, fresh or dried leaves, fresh or dried fruits.

Violet *Viola adorata.* COMMON NAME: Blue violet, sweet violet, sweet-scented violet.

occurrence: native to Great Britain and found widely over Europe, northern Asia and North America.

parts used: the dried flowers and leaves and whole plant when fresh.

medicinal uses: antiseptic, expectorant, laxative. The herb is mainly taken as syrup of violets which has been used to cure the ague, epilepsy, eye inflammation, pleurisy, jaundice and sleeplessness which are some of the many other complaints that benefit from treatment with this herb. The flowers possess expectorant properties and have long been used to treat coughs. The flowers may also be crystallized as a sweetmeat or added to salads. The rhizome is strongly emetic and purgative and has violent effects when administered. The seeds also have purgative and diuretic effects and are beneficial in treating urinary complaints and gravel. In the early part of this century, violet preparations were used to great effect against cancer. Fresh violet leaves are made into an infusion which was drunk regularly, and a poultice of the leaves was applied to the affected area. The herb has been used successfully to both allay pain and perhaps cure the cancer. It is said to be particularly good against throat cancer.

administered as: infusion, poultice, injection, ointment, syrup and powdered root.

Walnut *Juglans nigra.* COMMON NAME: Carya, Jupiter's nuts, *Juglans regia.*

OCCURRENCE: cultivated throughout Europe and was probably native to Persia.

PARTS USED: the bark and leaves. The active principle of the walnut tree is nucin or juglon, while the kernels also contain oil, mucilage, albumin, cellulose, mineral matter and water.

MEDICINAL USES: alterative, laxative, detergent, astringent. The bark and leaves are used in skin problems, e.g. scrofulous diseases, herpes, eczema and for healing indolent ulcers. A strong infusion of the powdered bark has purgative effects, while the walnut has various properties dependent upon its stage of ripeness. Green walnuts are anthelminthic and vermifuge in action and are pickled in vinegar, which is then used as a gargle for sore and ulcerated throats. The wood is used for furniture, gun-stocks and for cabinets. Walnut oil expressed from the kernels is used in wood polishing, painting and is used as butter or frying oil.

ADMINISTERED AS: fluid extract, infusion, expressed oil, whole fruit.

Water betony *Scrophularia aquatica*. COMMON NAME: Water figwort, brownwort, bishop's leaves, crowdy kit, fiddlewood, fiddler, *Betonica aquatica*.

OCCURRENCE: found growing wild in damp places, on the banks of rivers and ponds throughout Great Britain and Europe.

PARTS USED: the leaves, fresh and dried.

MEDICINAL USES: detergent, vulnerary. The leaves are used as a poultice, or as an ointment for wounds, sores, haemorrhoids, ulcers and scrofulous glands in the neck. It was also used to expel nightmares, cure toothache and as a cosmetic for blemished or sunburnt skin.

ADMINISTERED AS: decoction, poultice, ointment.

Watercress *Nasturtium officinale*

OCCURRENCE: a perennial creeping plant often growing near springs and running water across Great Britain and Europe.

PARTS USED: the stem and leaves, which contain nicotinamide, volatile oil, a glucoside, gluconasturtin and vitamins A, C and E.

MEDICINAL USES: stimulant, expectorant, nutritive, antiscorbutic, diuretic. Watercress was proposed as a specific in tuberculosis and has a very long history of medical use. It is used to treat bronchitis and coughs as well as boosting digestion, lowering blood sugar and helping the body to remove toxic wastes from the blood and tissues. The herb is of value nutritionally as it contains many vitamins and mineral salts which help during convalescence and general debility. It can be bruised and made into a poultice for arthritis and gout, and is chewed raw to strengthen gums.

ADMINISTERED AS: expressed juice, poultice, dietary item.

Water dock *Rumex aquaticus.* COMMON NAME: Red Dock, bloodwort.

OCCURRENCE: found frequently in fields, meadows, pools and ditches throughout Europe and Great Britain and is particularly common in the northern latitudes.

PARTS USED: the root.

MEDICINAL USES: alterative, deobstruent, detergent. It has a tonic action and is used externally to clean ulcers in afflictions of the mouth. It is applied to eruptive and scorbutic diseases, skin ulcers and sores. As a powder, Water dock has a cleansing and detergent effect upon the teeth.

ADMINISTERED AS: fluid extract and infusion.

Willow, White *Salix alba.* COMMON NAME: European willow.

OCCURRENCE: a large tree growing in moist places and running streams around Great Britain and Europe.

PARTS USED: the bark and leaves. The bark contains tannin and salicin.

MEDICINAL USES: tonic, antiperiodic, astringent. The bark has been used in febrile diseases of rheumatic or gouty origin, diarrhoea and dysentery. It has been used in dyspepsia connected with digestive organ disorders. The bark has also been of benefit in convalescence after acute diseases and against parasitic worms.

ADMINISTERED AS: decoction, powdered root.

Wintergreen *Gaultheria procumbens.* COMMON NAME: Mountain tea, teaberry, boxberry, thé du Canada, aromatic wintergreen, partridge berry, deerberry, checkerberry.

OCCURRENCE: native to the northern United States and Canada from Georgia northwards.

PARTS USED: the leaves, which produce a volatile oil upon distillation. The oil is made up of methyl salicylate, gaultherilene, an aldehyde, a secondary alcohol and an ester. The aromatic odour of the plant is due to the alcohol and the ester.

MEDICINAL USES: aromatic, tonic, stimulant, diuretic, emmenagogue, astringent, galactogogue. The oil is of great benefit in acute rheumatism, but must be given in the form of capsules so stomach inflammation does not occur. The true distilled oil when applied to the skin can give rise to an eruption and so the synthetic oil of wintergreen is recommended for external use as it still contains methyl salicylate, but with no deleterious effects. The synthetic oil is exceedingly valuable for all chronic joint and muscular troubles, lumbago, sciatica and rheumatism. The oil is also used as a flavouring for toothpowders and mouth washes, particularly when combined with menthol and EUCALYPTUS. The berries are a winter food for many animals and also produce a bitter tonic, after being steeped in brandy. The leaves are either used to flavour tea or as a substitute for tea itself.

ADMINISTERED AS: capsules, synthetic oil, infusion, tincture.

Witch hazel *Hamamelis virginiana.* COMMON NAME: Spotted alder, winterbloom, snapping hazelnut.

OCCURRENCE: native to the United States of America and Canada.

PARTS USED: the dried bark, both fresh and dried leaves. The leaves contain tannic and gallic acids, volatile oil and an unknown bitter principle. The bark contains tannin, gallic acid, physterol, resin, fat and other bitter and odorous bodies.

MEDICINAL USES: astringent, tonic, sedative. Valuable in stopping internal and external haemorrhages and in treating piles. Mainly used for bruises, swelling, inflammation and tumours as a poultice. It may also be utilized for diarrhoea, dysentery and mucous discharges. A decoction is used against tuberculosis gonorrhoea, menorrhagia and the debilitated state resulting from abortion. Tea made from the bark or leaves aids bleeding of the stomach, bowel complaints and may be given as an injection for bleeding piles. Witch hazel is used to treat varicose veins as a moist poultice, as an extract to ease burns, scalds and insect and mosquito bites, and to help inflammation of the eyelids.

ADMINISTERED AS: liquid extract, injection, tincture, lotion, ointment, suppositories, poultice, infusion and decoction.

Woodruff *Asperula odorata*. COMMON NAME: Wuderove, wood-rova, sweet woodruff, woodroof, waldmeister tea.

OCCURRENCE: grows in woods or shaded hedges in England.

PARTS USED: the herb, which contains coumarin, a fragrant crystalline chemical, citric, malic and rubichloric acids and tannic acid.

MEDICINAL USES: diuretic, tonic. The fresh leaves, when applied to wounds, were said to have a strong healing effect. A strong decoction of the fresh herb was used as a cordial and stomachic and is said to be useful in removing biliary obstructions of the liver.

ADMINISTERED AS: a poultice and decoction.

Woundwort *Stachys palustris*. COMMON NAME: all-heal, panay, opopanewort, clown's woundwort, rusticum vulna herba, downy woundwort, stinking marsh stachys.

OCCURRENCE: common to marshy meadows, riversides and ditches in most parts of Great Britain.

PARTS USED: the herb.

MEDICINAL USES: antiseptic, antispasmodic. The herb relieves cramp, gout, painful joints and vertigo, while bruised leaves will stop bleeding and encourage healing when applied to a wound. Woundwort had an excellent reputation as a vulnerary among all of the early herbalists. A syrup made of the fresh juice will stop haemorrhages and dysentery when taken internally. The tuberous roots are edible as are the young shoot which resemble ASPARAGUS.

ADMINISTERED AS: poultice or syrup.

Yam, wild *dioscorea villosa*. COMMON NAME: Dioscorea, colic root, rheumatism root, wilde yamwurzel.

OCCURRENCE: native to the southern United States and Canada
PARTS USED: the roots and rhizome, which contain steroidal sa
ponins, phytosterols, tannins, starch and various alkaloids in
cluding dioscorine.
MEDICINAL USES: antispasmodic, diuretic. This plant has a his
tory of traditional use in relieving menstrual cramps and in stop
ping threatened miscarriage. It brings quick relief for biliou
colic and flatulence, particularly in pregnant women. It is pre
scribed for the inflammatory stage of rheumatoid arthritis and
in painful disorders of the urinary tract. Wild Yam is also ben
eficial for poor circulation, spasmodic hiccoughs, neuralgi
complaints and spasmodic asthma. Prior to 1970, the wild yam
was the only source of diosgenin, one of the starting material
used in commercial manufacturing of steroid hormones for the
contraceptive pill.
ADMINISTERED AS: fluid extract, powdered bark, infusion.

Yew *Taxus baccata.*

OCCURRENCE: found in Europe, North Africa and Western Asia
The tree has been closely associated with the history and leg
ends of Europe.
PARTS USED: the leaves, seeds and fruit. The seeds and fruit ar
the most poisonous parts of the plant and contain an alkaloi
toxine and another principle milrossin.
MEDICINAL USES: it has few medicinal uses due to its poisonou
nature but the leaves were once used effectively in treating epi
lepsy. The wood was used for making longbows.
ADMINISTERED AS: powdered leaves.

Forms of Herbal Preparations

capsule this is a gelatine container for swallowing and holdin
oils or balsams that would otherwise be difficult to administe
due to their unpleasant taste or smell. It is used for cod liver o
and castor oil.

decoction this is prepared using cut, bruised or ground bar
and roots placed into a stainless steel or enamel pan (not alu

minium) with cold water poured on. The mixture is boiled for 20–30 minutes, cooled and strained. It is best drunk when warm.

herbal dressing this may be a compress or poultice. A compress is made of cloth or cotton wool soaked in cold or warm herbal decoctions or infusions while a poultice can be made with fresh or dried herbs. Bruised fresh herbs are applied directly to the affected area and dried herbs are made into a paste with water and placed on gauze on the required area. Both dressings are very effective in easing pain, swelling and inflammation of the skin and tissues.

infusion this liquid is made from ground or bruised roots, bark, herbs or seeds, by pouring boiling water onto the herb and leaving it to stand for 10-30 minutes, possibly stirring the mixture occasionally. The resultant liquid is strained and used. Cold infusions may be made if the active principles are yielded from the herb without heat. Today, infusions may be packaged into teabags for convenience.

liquid extract this preparation, if correctly made, is the most concentrated fluid form in which herbal drugs may be obtained and, as such, is very popular and convenient. Each herb is treated by various means dependent upon the individual properties of the herb, e.g. cold percolation, high pressure, evaporation by heat in a vacuum. These extracts are commonly held in a household stock of domestic remedies.

pessary similar to suppositories, but it is used in female complaints to apply a preparation to the walls of the vagina and cervix.

pill probably the best known and most widely used herbal preparation. It is normally composed of concentrated extracts and alkaloids, in combination with active crude drugs. The pill may be coated with sugar or another pleasant-tasting substance that is readily soluble in the stomach.

solid extract this type of preparation is prepared by evaporating the fresh juices or strong infusions of herbal drugs to the consistency of honey. It may also be prepared from an alcoholic tincture base. It is used mainly to produce pills, plasters, ointments and compressed tablets.

Homeopathy

Introduction

The aim of homeopathy is to cure an illness or disorder by treating the whole person rather than merely concentrating on a set of symptoms. Hence, in homeopathy the approach is holistic, and the overall state of health of the patient, especially his or her emotional and psychological wellbeing, is regarded as being significant. A homeopath notes the symptoms that the person wishes to have cured but also takes time to discover other signs or indications of disorder that the patient may regard as being less important. The reasoning behind this is that illness is a sign of disorder or imbalance within the body. It is believed that the whole 'make-up' of a person determines, to a great extent, the type of disorders to which that individual is prone and the symptoms likely to occur. A homeopathic remedy must be suitable both for the symptoms and the characteristics and temperament of the patient. Hence, two patients with the same illness may be offered different remedies according to their individual natures. One remedy may also be used to treat different groups of symptoms or ailments.

Like cures like

Homeopathic remedies are based on the concept that 'like cures like', an ancient philosophy that can be traced back to the 5th century BC, when it was formulated by Hippocrates. In the early 1800s, this idea awakened the interest of a German doctor, Samuel Hahnemann, who believed that the medical practices at the time were too harsh and tended to hinder rather than aid healing. Hahnemann observed that a treatment for malaria, based on an extract of cinchona bark (quinine), actually produced symptoms of this disease when taken in a small dose by a healthy person. Further extensive studies convinced him that the production of symptoms was the body's way of combating illness. Hence, to give a minute dose of a substance that stimulated the symptoms of an illness in a healthy person could be used to fight that illness in someone who was sick. Hahnemann conducted numerous trials (called 'provings'), giving minute doses of substances to healthy people and recording the symptoms produced. Eventually, these very dilute remedies were given to people with illnesses, often with encouraging results.

Modern homeopathy is based on the work of Hahnemann, and the medicines derived from plant, mineral and animal sources are used in extremely dilute amounts. Indeed, it is believed that the curative properties are enhanced by each dilution because impurities that might cause unwanted side effects are lost. Substances used in homeopathy are first soaked in alcohol to extract their essential ingredients. This initial solution, called the 'mother tincture', is diluted successively either by factors of ten (called the 'decimal scale' and designated X) or 100 (the 'centesimal scale' and designated C). Each dilution is shaken vigorously before further ones are made, and this is thought to make the properties more powerful by adding energy at each stage while impurities are removed. The thorough shakings of each dilution are said to energize, or 'potentiate', the medicine. The remedies are made into tablets or may be used in the form of ointment, solutions, powders, suppositories, etc. High potency (i.e. more dilute) remedies are used for severe symptoms and lower potency (less dilute) for milder ones.

The homeopathic view is that during the process of healing symptoms are redirected from more important to less important body systems. It is also held that healing is from innermost to outermost parts of the body and that more recent symptoms disappear first, this being known as the 'law of direction of cure'

Occasionally, symptoms may worsen initially when a homeopathic remedy is taken, but this is usually short-lived and is known as a 'healing crisis'. It is taken to indicate a change and that improvement is likely to follow. Usually, with a homeopathic remedy, an improvement is noticed fairly quickly although this depends upon the nature of the ailment, health, age and wellbeing of the patient and potency of the remedy.

A first homeopathic consultation is likely to last about one hour so that the specialist can obtain a full picture of the patient's medical history and personal circumstances. On the basis of this information, the homeopathic doctor decides on an appropriate remedy and potency (which is usually 6C). Subsequent consultations are generally shorter, and full advice is given on how to store and take the medicine. It is widely accepted that homeopathic remedies are safe and non-addictive, but they are covered by the legal requirements governing all medicines and should be obtained from a recognized source.

Potency table for homeopathic medicines
The centesimal scale

1C =	1/100	$(1/100^1)$	of mother tincture
2C =	1/10 000	$(1/100^2)$	of mother tincture
3C =	1/1 000 000	$(1/100^3)$	of mother tincture
6C =	1/1 000 000 000 000	$(1/100^6)$	of mother tincture

The decimal scale

1X =	1/10	$(1/10^1)$	of mother tincture
2X =	1/100	$(1/10^2)$	of mother tincture
6X =	1/1 000 000	$(1/10^6)$	of mother tincture

The development of homeopathy

The Greek physician Hippocrates, who lived several hundred years before the birth of Christ (460–370 BC), is regarded as the founding father of all medicine. The Hippocratic Oath taken by newly qualified doctors in orthodox medicine binds them to an ethical code of medical practice in honour of Hippocrates. Hippocrates believed that disease resulted from natural elements in the world in which people lived. This contrasted with the view that held sway for centuries that disease was some form of punishment from the gods or God. He believed that it was essential to observe and take account of the course and progress of a disease in each individual, and that any cure should encourage that person's own innate healing power. Hippocrates embraced the idea of 'like being able to cure like' and had many remedies that were based on this principle. Hence, in his practice and study of medicine he laid the foundations of the homeopathic approach although this was not to be appreciated and developed for many centuries.

During the period of Roman civilization a greater knowledge and insight into the nature of the human body was developed. Many herbs and plants were used for healing by people throughout the world, and much knowledge was gained and handed down from generation to generation. The belief persisted, however, that diseases were caused by supernatural or divine forces. It was not until the early 1500s that a Swiss doctor, Paracelsus (1493–1541), put forward the view that disease resulted from external environmental forces. He also believed that plants and natural substances held the key to healing and embraced the 'like can cure like' principle. One of his ideas, known as the 'doctrine of signatures', was that the appearance of a plant, or the substances it contained, gave an idea of the disorders it could cure.

In the succeeding centuries, increased knowledge was gained about the healing properties of plants and the way the human body worked. In spite of this, the methods of medical practice were extremely harsh, and there is no doubt that many people suffered needlessly and died because of the treatment they received. It was against this background that Samuel Hahnemann (1755–1843), the founding father of modern homeopathy, began his work as a doctor in the late 1700s. In his early writings, Hahnemann criticized the severe practices of medicine and advocated a healthy diet, clean living conditions and high standards of hygiene as a means of improving health and warding off disease. In 1790, he became interested in quinine, extracted from the bark of the cinchona tree, which was known to be an effective treatment for malaria. He tested the substance first on himself, and later on friends and close family members, and recorded the results. These 'provings' led him to conduct many further investigations and provings of other natural substances, during the course of which he rediscovered and established the principle of like being able to cure like.

By 1812, the principle and practice of homeopathy had become established, and many other doctors adopted the homeopathic approach. Hahnemann himself became a teacher in homeopathy at the University of Leipzig and published many important writings – the results of his years of research. He continued to practise, teach and conduct research throughout his life, especially in producing more dilute remedies that were succussed, or shaken, at each stage and were found to be more potent. Although his work was not without its detractors, Hahnemann had attracted a considerable following by the 1830s. In 1831 there was a widespread cholera epidemic in central Europe for which Hahnemann recommended treatment with camphor. Many people were cured, including Dr Frederick Quin (1799–1878), a medical practitioner at that time. He went on to establish the first homeopathic hospital in London in 1849. A later resurgence of cholera in Britain enabled the effectiveness of camphor to be established beyond doubt, as the numbers of people cured at the homeopathic hospital were far greater than those treated at other hospitals.

In the United States of America, homeopathy became firmly established in the early part of the 19th century, and there were several eminent practitioners who further enhanced knowledge and practice. These included Dr Constantine Hering (1800–80), who formulated the 'laws of cure', explaining how symptoms affect organ systems and move from one part of the body to another as a cure occurs. Dr James Tyler Kent (1849–1916) introduced the idea of constitutional types, which is now the basis of classical homeopathy , and advocated the use of high potency remedies.

In the later years of the 19th century, a fundamental split

occurred in the practice of homeopathy, which was brought about by Dr Richard Hughes (1836-1902), who worked in London and Brighton. He insisted that physical symptoms and the nature of the disease itself was the important factor rather than the holistic approach based on the make-up of the whole individual person. Hughes rejected the concept of constitutional types and advocated the use of low potency remedies. Although he worked as a homeopath, his approach was to attempt to make homeopathy more scientific and to bring it closer to the practices of conventional medicine. Some other homeopathic doctors followed the approach of Hughes, and the split led to a collapse in faith in the whole practice of homeopathy during the earlier part of the 20th century. As the 20th century advanced, however, homeopathy regained its following and respect. Conventional medicine and homeopathy have continued to advance, and there is now a greater sympathy and understanding between the practitioners in both these important disciplines.

Homeopathic Remedies in Common Use

Aconitum napellus

Aconite, monkshood, wolfsbane, friar's cap, mousebane

Aconitum is a native plant of Switzerland and other mountainous regions of Europe, where it grows in the damp conditions of alpine meadows. Attractive purple/dark blue flowers are borne on tall, upright stems produced from tubers developed from the root system. Aconite is highly poisonous, and its sap was used by ancient hunters on the ends of their arrows. 'Wolfsbane' refers to this use, and *Aconitum* is derived from the Latin word *acon*, meaning 'dart'. This was one of the homeopathic remedies extensively tested and proved by Hahnemann. He used it for the acute infections and fevers, accompanied by severe pain, that were usually treated by blood-letting by the physicians of his day. This remains its main use in modern homeopathy , and the whole plant is used to produce the remedy.

Aconite is a valuable treatment for acute illnesses of rapid onset in people who have previously been healthy and well. These often occur after the person has been out in cold wet weather. It is used especially at the start of feverish respiratory infections, such as colds and influenza and those affecting the eyes and ears. The person usually experiences restlessness, a hot, flushed face and pains and disturbed sleep but may be pale when first getting up. It is also used to treat the menopausal symptoms of hot flushes. It is an effective remedy for some mental symptoms, including extreme anxiety and fear, palpitations and attacks of panic, especially the belief that death is imminent during illness. The remedy encourages sweating and is sometimes used in conjunction with BELLADONNA.

Symptoms are made worse by cold, draughts, tobacco smoke, stuffy, airless, warm rooms, listening to music, at midnight and by lying on the painful part. They improve out in the fresh air and with warmth. The people who benefit from Aconite are typically strong, solid or well-built, high-coloured and usually enjoy good health but have a poor opinion of themselves. Because of this, they tend to have a constant need to prove their own worth, to the point of insensitivity or unkindness to others. When in good health, Aconite people have a need for the company of others. However, they also have fears that they keep concealed and may be frightened of going out or of being in a crowd. When ill, they are inclined to be morbid and to believe that death is imminent, and they cope badly with any kind of shock.

Allium

Allium cepa; Spanish onion

The onion has been cultivated and used for many centuries, both for culinary and medicinal purposes, and was important in the ancient Egyptian civilization. The volatile oil released when an onion is sliced stimulates the tear glands of the eyes and mucous membranes of the nose, throat and air passages. Hence, in homeopathy the onion is used to treat ailments with symptoms of a streaming nose and watering eyes. The red Spanish onion, which is cultivated throughout the world, is used to make the homeopathic remedy. It is used to treat allergic conditions, such as hay fever, colds and pains or symptoms that go from one side to the other. It is useful for shooting, stabbing or burning pains associated with neuralgia, which may alternate from side to side, frontal headaches, painful molar teeth and earache in children. The symptoms are made worse by cold, damp conditions and improve in fresh air and cool, dry surroundings.

Apis mellifica

Apis; *Apis mellifera*, the honey bee

The source of the medicine is the entire body of the honey bee which is crushed or ground to prepare the remedy. It is used particularly to treat inflammation, redness, swelling and itching of the skin, which is sensitive to touch, and with stinging hot pains. There is usually feverishness and thirst and the pains are worsened by heat and relieved by cold. The remedy is used for insect stings, nettle rash, allergic conditions, blisters, whitlow (an abscess on the fingertip) and infections of the urinary tract, including cystitis, with stabbing hot pains. Also for urinary incontinence in elderly persons, fluid retention causing swelling of the eyelids or other areas, allergic conditions that cause sore throat and swallowing difficulty, and tonsillitis. The person often experiences hot, stabbing headaches and has dry skin. Apis is additionally valued as a remedy for swollen, painful inflammation of the joints as in arthritic conditions and for peritonitis and pleurisy. The symptoms are made worse by heat and touch, stuffy airless rooms following sleep and in the early evening. They improve in the fresh, cool open air, after taking a cold bath, or any cold application. A person suitable for the Apis remedy tends to expect high standards and may be rather irritable and hard to please. He (or she) likes to organize others and is jealous of his own domain, tending to be resentful of anyone new. Apis types may seem to be rushing around and working hard but may achieve very little as a result.

Argenticum nitricum

Argent. nit; silver nitrate, devil's stone, lunar caustic, hellstone
Silver nitrate is obtained from the mineral acanthite, which is a natural ore of silver. White silver nitrate crystals are derived from a chemical solution of the mineral ore and these are used to make the homeopathic remedy. Silver nitrate is poisonous in large doses and has antiseptic and caustic properties. In the past it was used to clean out wounds and prevent infection. In homeopathy , it is used to treat states of great anxiety, panic, fear or apprehension about a forthcoming event, e.g. taking an examination, having to perform a public role (speech-making, chairing a public meeting, acting, singing), going for an interview, or any activity involving scrutiny and criticism by others. It was also used as a remedy for digestive complaints including

indigestion, abdominal pain, wind, nausea and headache. Often, there is a longing for sweet 'comfort' or other types of food. Argent. nit. may be given for laryngitis, sore throat and hoarseness, eye inflammation such as conjunctivitis, and period pains. Other types of pain, asthma and warts may benefit from Argent. nit.

Often, a person experiences symptoms mainly on the left side, and these are worse with heat and at night. Also, they are made worse by anxiety and overwork, emotional tension and resting on the left side. Pains are made worse with talking and movement. Symptoms improve in cold or cool fresh air and are relieved by belching. Pains are helped by applying pressure to the painful part. People suitable for Argent nit. are quick-witted and rapid in thought and action. They may appear outgoing and happy but are prey to worry, anxiety and ungrounded fears that make them tense. All the emotions are quick to surface, and Argent nit. people are able to put on an impressive performance. They enjoy a wide variety of foods, particularly salty and sweet things although these may upset the digestion. They have a fear of heights, crowds, of being burgled and of failure and arriving late for an appointment. Also, of serious illness, dying and madness. Argent. nit. people are generally slim and full of restless energy and tension. They may have deeply etched features and lines on the skin that make them appear older than their real age.

Arnica montana

Arnica; leopard's bane, sneezewort, mountain tobacco

Arnica is a native plant of woodland and mountainous regions of central Europe and Siberia. It has a dark brown root system from which a central stem arises, producing pairs of elongated green leaves and bright yellow flowers. If the flowers are crushed or bruised and a person then inhales the scent, this cause sneezing. All the fresh parts of the flowering plant are used to prepare the homeopathic remedy. It is a commonly used first aid remedy for symptoms relating to injury or trauma of any kind, e.g. bruising, swelling, pain and bleeding. It is also used

494

to treat physical and mental shock. It is helpful following surgery, childbirth or tooth extraction, promoting healing, and also for gout, rheumatic joints with pain, heat and inflammation, sore sprained or strained muscles, concussion, and osteoarthritis. Taken internally, it is a remedy for black eyes, eye strain, skin conditions such as eczema and boils. Arnica is helpful in the treatment of whooping cough in children and also wetting the bed when the cause is nightmares. Symptoms are made worse with heat, touch and continued movement, and also with heat and resting for a long period. The symptoms improve when the person first begins to move and with lying down with the head at a lower level than the feet. A person suitable for this remedy tends to be solemn, fatalistic and subject to morbid fears. Arnica types usually deny the existence of any illness, even when obviously not well, and do not seek medical help, preferring to manage on their own.

Arsenicum album

Arsen. alb.; white arsenic trioxide

This is a widely used homeopathic remedy, the source being white arsenic trioxide derived from arsenopyrite, a metallic mineral ore of arsenic. Arsenic has been known for centuries as a poison and was once used as a treatment for syphilis. White arsenic trioxide used to be given to improve muscles and skin in animals such as horses. It is used to treat acute conditions of the digestive system and chest and mental symptoms of anxiety and fear. Hence it is a remedy for diarrhoea and vomiting caused by eating the wrong kinds of food, or food poisoning or overindulgence in alcohol. Also, for dehydration in children following gastroenteritis or feverish illness. It is a remedy for asthma and breathing difficulty, mouth ulcers, carbuncle (a collection of boils), dry, cracked lips, burning skin, inflamed, watering stinging eyes and psoriasis. Also, for sciatica, shingles, sore throat and painful swallowing, candidiasis (fungal infection) of the mouth and motion sickness. There may be oedema (retention of fluid) showing as a puffiness around the ankles.

An ill person who benefits from Arsen. alb. experiences

burning pains but also feels cold. The skin may be either hot or cold to the touch. The symptoms are worse with cold in any form, including cold food and drink, and between midnight and 3 a.m. They are worse on the right side and if the person is near the coast. Symptoms improve with warmth, including warm drinks, gentle movement and lying down with the head raised. People suitable for Arsen. alb. are precise, meticulous and ambitious and loathe any form of disorder. They are always immaculately dressed and everything in their life is neat and tidy. However, they tend to have great worries, especially about their financial security and their own health and that of their family. They fear illness and dying, loss of financial and personal status, being burgled, darkness and the supernatural. Arsen. alb. people have strongly held views and do not readily tolerate contrary opinions or those with a more relaxed or disordered lifestyle. They enjoy a variety of different foods, coffee and alcoholic drinks. They are usually thin, with delicate, fine features and pale skin that may show worry lines. Their movements tend to be rapid and their manner serious and somewhat restless, although always polite.

Atropa belladonna

Belladonna, deadly nightshade, black cherry, devil's cherries, naughty man's cherries, devil's herb

Belladonna is a native plant of most of Europe although it is uncommon in Scotland. The plant is extremely poisonous, and many children have died as a result of being tempted to eat the shiny black berries of deadly nightshade. It is a stout, stocky plant with light brown roots, growing to about four feet high with green oval leaves and pale purple, bell-shaped flowers. In medieval times, the plant had its place in the potions of witchcraft. Italian women used extracts of the plant as eye drops to widen the pupils of the eye and make them more beautiful (hence *bella donna*, which means 'beautiful woman'). The plant contains atropine, an alkaloid substance that induces paralysis of nerves and is used in orthodox medicine to relieve painful spasms and in ophthalmic (eye) procedures.

In homeopathy, the remedy is obtained from the pulped leaves and flowers. It was investigated and proved by Hahnemann as a treatment for scarlet fever. Belladonna is used to treat acute conditions that arise suddenly in which there is a throbbing, pulsing headache and red, flushed skin, high fever and staring wide eyes. The skin around the mouth and lips may be pale, but the tongue is a fiery red and the hands and feet are cold. It is used as a remedy for infectious diseases such as influenza, scarlet fever, measles, whooping cough, chicken pox, mumps and the early stages of pneumonia. Also for boils, earache (particularly on the right side and worse when the head is cold or wet), cystitis, boils, conjunctivitis, tonsillitis, inflammation of the kidneys, neuralgia (sharp pain along the course of a nerve) and sore throat. Other conditions that benefit from this remedy include labour pains, soreness of the breasts in breast-feeding, fever and teething in children, with broken sleep and whitlow (an infection of a fingernail). The symptoms are worse at night and with lying down, and occur more intensely on the right side. Also, they are exacerbated by loud noises, bright lights, jarring of the body, touch or pressure and with cool surroundings.

They improve with sitting upright or standing and keeping warm or warm applications to the painful area. People suitable for belladonna usually enjoy good health, being fit, energetic and ready to tackle any task. They are amusing, sociable and popular when in good health. However, if they become ill the reverse is often true and they may be restless, irritable and possibly even violent.

Aurum metallicum

Aurum met.; gold

Gold was highly prized by Arabian physicians in the early Middle Ages who used it to treat heart disorders. In the early part of this century, it was used in the treatment of tuberculosis. Gold is now used in conventional medicine for some cancer treatments and for rheumatic and arthritic complaints. In homeopathy, pure gold is ground down to produce a fine powder, and it is used to treat both physical and mental symptoms. It is used as a remedy for congestive circulatory disorders and heart diseases including angina pectoris. The symptoms include a throbbing, pulsing headache, chest pain, breathlessness and palpitations. It is also used to treat liver disorders with symptoms of jaundice, painful conditions of bones and joints (especially the hip and knee), inflammation of the testes and an undescended testicle in small boys (especially if the right side is affected). It is a remedy for sinusitis and severe mental symptoms of despair, depression and thoughts of suicide. The person who is suitable for this remedy tends to drive himself very hard to the point of being a workaholic. He (or she) is excessively conscientious but usually feels that he has not done enough and is oversensitive to the criticism of other people. The person may come to regard himself as a failure and become severely clinically depressed or even suicidal. Symptoms are made worse by mental effort and concentration, or physical exercise, especially in the evening or night and by emotional upheaval. They improve with cold bathing, walking in the fresh air and with rest and quiet.

Calcarea carbonica

Calc. carb.; calcium carbonate

This important homeopathic remedy is made from powdered mother-of-pearl, the beautiful, translucent inner layer of oyster shells. Calcium is an essential mineral in the body, being especially important for the healthy development of bones and teeth. The Calc. carb. remedy is used to treat a number of different disorders, especially those relating to bones and teeth and also certain skin conditions and symptoms relating to the female reproductive system. It is a remedy for weak or slow growth of bones and teeth and fractures that take a long time to heal. Also, for teething problems in children, pains in bones, teeth and joints, headaches and eye inflammations affecting the right side, and ear infections with an unpleasant-smelling discharge. Premenstrual syndrome, heavy periods and menopausal disorders are helped by Calc. carb., and also chapped skin and eczema.

Calc. carb. may be used as a remedy for verruca (a type of wart) and thrush infections. People who benefit from Calc. carb. are very sensitive to the cold, particularly in the hands and feet and tend to sweat profusely. They suffer from fatigue and anxiety, and body secretions (sweat and urine) smell unpleasant. Children who benefit from Calc. carb. have recurrent ear, nose and throat infections, especially tonsillitis and glue ear. Symptoms are made worse by draughts and cold, damp weather and also at night. They are worse when the person first wakens up in the morning and for physical exercise and sweating. In women, symptoms are worse premenstrually. They improve in warm, dry weather and are better later on in the morning and after the person has eaten breakfast. People suitable for Calc. carb. are often overweight or even obese with a pale complexion. They are shy and very sensitive, quiet in company and always worried about what other people think of them. Calc. carb. people are hard-working, conscientious and reliable and easily upset by the suffering of others. They need constant reassurance from friends and family and tend to feel that they are a failure. Usually, Calc. carb. people enjoy good health but have a tendency for skeletal weakness. They enjoy a wide variety of different foods and tend to overeat, but are upset by coffee and milk. They are afraid of dying and serious illness, the supernatural, madness, being a failure and becoming poor, and they tend to be claustrophobic.

Calcarea fluorica

Calc. fluor.; fluorite, calcium fluoride, fluoride of lime

This homeopathic remedy is one of the Schussler tissue salts. Calcium fluoride occurs naturally in the body in the enamel of the teeth, bones, skin and connective tissue. It is used to treat disorders of these body tissues or to maintain their elasticity. It is used to treat chronic lumbago, scars, and to prevent the formation of adhesions after operations, gout and arthritic nodules. Also, for rickets, slow growth of bones in children, enlarged adenoids that become stony because of persistent, recurrent respiratory tract infections and cataracts. It is used to strengthen weak tooth enamel and strained and stretched ligaments and muscles, e.g. around a joint. People suitable for Calc. fluor. are intelligent and punctual but tend to make mistakes through lack of planning. They benefit from the guidance of others to work efficiently and fear poverty and illness. They are often prone to piles, varicose veins, swollen glands and muscle and ligament strain. The manner of walking may be rapid with jerking of the limbs. Symptoms are made worse on beginning movement and in cold, damp, draughty conditions. They improve with warmth and heat and for continual gentle movement.

Calcarea phosphorica

Calc. phos., phosphate of lime, calcium phosphate

This homeopathic remedy is a Schussler tissue salt and calcium phosphate is the mineral that gives hardness to bones and teeth. It is obtained by a chemical reaction between dilute phosphoric acid and calcium hydroxide, when a white precipitate of calcium phosphate is formed. Since calcium phosphate is an essential mineral in the normal, healthy development of bones and teeth, it is used to treat disorders in these tissues. It is particularly helpful as a remedy for painful bones, difficult fractures that are slow to heal, teeth prone to decay, problems of bone growth and teething in children and 'growing pains'. Also, it is beneficial during convalescence when a person is weakened and tired after an illness, and for digestive problems including diarrhoea, stomach pains and indigestion. It may be used as a remedy for tonsillitis, sore throats and swollen glands. Children who benefit from this remedy tend to be thin, pale, miserable and fail to thrive, and are prone to sickness and headaches. They are often fretful and demanding. Adults are also unhappy and discontented with their circumstances, although endeavour to be friendly towards others. They are restless and need plenty of different activities and stimulation, hating routine and needing a good reason to get out of bed in the morning. Symptoms are made worse by any change in the weather and in cold, wet conditions, e.g. thawing snow. Also for worry or grief and too much physical activity. Symptoms improve when the weather is warm and dry, in summer, and from taking a hot bath.

Calendula officinalis

Calendula, marigold, garden marigold, marygold

This is a familiar garden plant that grows well in all parts of the United Kingdom, having light green leaves and bright orange flowers. The plant has been known for centuries for its healing properties and was used in the treatment of various ailments. The parts used in homeopathy are the leaves and flowers, and the remedy is of value in first aid for its antiseptic and anti-inflammatory activity. It is used in the treatment of boils, stings, cuts and wounds, and to stem bleeding, often in the form of an ointment that can be applied to broken skin. It is helpful when applied to skin tears following childbirth. It is used in the form of an antiseptic tincture as a mouth wash and gargle after tooth extraction, for mouth ulcers or a septic sore throat. When taken internally it prevents suppuration (pus formation) and may be used for persistent chronic ulcers and varicose ulcers, fever and jaundice. It is a useful remedy in the treatment of children's ailments. The symptoms are made worse in damp, draughty conditions and cloudy weather and after eating. They improve with walking about and lying absolutely still.

Cantharis vesicatoria

Cantharis, Spanish fly

This remedy is derived from the body and wings of a bright green iridescent beetle that is found mainly in the southern parts of Spain and France. The beetle, *Cantharis vesicatoria*, secretes a substance called canthardin, which has irritant prop-erties, is also poisonous and is an ancient remedy to cure warts. It was also used as an aphrodisiac, reputedly by the notorious Maquis de Sade. The beetles are dried and ground to produce a powder that is then used in homeopathy . It is an irritant, blistering agent acting externally on the part of the body to which it is applied and internally on the bladder, urinary tract and genital organs. Hence it is used to treat conditions in which there are stinging and burning pains. An accompanying symptom is often a great thirst but a reluctance to drink. It is used to treat cystitis with cutting hot pains on passing urine, urinary frequency with pain and other urinary infections. Also, certain inflammations of the digestive system in which there is abdominal distension and burning pains and diarrhoea. In general it is used as a remedy for conditions that worsen rapidly. It is a remedy for burns and scalds of the skin, including sunburn, insect stings, and rashes with spots that contain pus. Some mental symptoms are eased by Cantharis, including angry and irritable or violent behaviour, extreme anxiety and excessive sexual appetite. Symptoms are made worse with movement, touch and after drinking coffee or chilled water. They improve when gastro-intestinal wind is eliminated and with warmth, at night time and with very light massage.

Carbo vegetabilis

Carbo veg., vegetable charcoal

The homeopathic remedy Carbo veg. is made from charcoal, which itself is obtained from heating or partially burning wood without oxygen. The charcoal is hard and black or dark grey, and is a form of carbon that is present in all living things. Charcoal has been made for centuries, and usually silver birch, beech or poplar trees are the source of wood that is used. The homeopathic remedy is used to treat a person who is run down, weak or exhausted, especially after a debilitating illness or operation. It is also used for postoperative shock, when there is a clammy, cold, pale skin but the person feels a sensation of heat or burning inside. It is helpful as a remedy for ailments of poor circulation such as varicose veins. Again, the skin tends to be pale, clammy and chilly with a bluish colour and the extremities feel cold. The legs may be puffy, and additional symptoms include hoarseness and laryngitis and lack of energy. Carbo veg is a useful remedy for digestive problems, and carbon is also used for this purpose in orthodox medicine. Symptoms are those of indigestion, heartburn and flatulence with a sour taste in the mouth. Morning headaches with accompanying symptoms of nausea and giddiness or fainting may be relieved by Carbo veg., particularly if the cause is a large, heavy meal the night before. People suitable for this remedy often complain of a lack of energy and may indeed be physically and mentally exhausted, with poor powers of concentration and lapses of memory. They usually have fixed attitudes, with a lack of interest in news of the wider world. They do not like the night and are fearful of the supernatural. Symptoms are made worse by warm, moist weather, in the evening and night, and with lying down. They are also exacerbated after eating meals of fatty foods, coffee and milk and drinks of wine. They improve with burping and with circulating cool, fresh air.

Chamomilla

Camomile, chamomile, common camomile, double camomile

A creeping and trailing plant that produces daisy-like flowers in summer and prefers dry, sandy soils. Chamomiles are native to Britain and others part of northern Europe and have been used in medicine since ancient times, being described by Hippocrates. When walked on, it gives off an aromatic perfume and was gathered and strewn on the floor in medieval dwellings to counter unpleasant odours. It is prized for its many medicinal uses, the flowers and leaves both being used for a number of different ailments. Herbalists use chamomile to treat skin conditions such as eczema, and for asthma and disturbed sleep. In homeopathy , it is used for its soothing and sedative effect on all conditions producing restlessness, irritability and pains. It is a useful remedy for children's complaints such as teething where the child is fretful and cries if put down, colicky pains and disturbed sleep. Also, for toothache, when one cheek is red and the other white, that is exacerbated by heat and relieved by cold. It is used to treat a blocked ear and earache, painful, heavy periods and soreness and inflammation associated with breast-feeding. People suitable for this remedy are very sensitive to pain, which causes sweating or fainting, especially in children and women. They are irritable and fretful when ill. Symptoms are made worse if the person becomes angry or in cold winds and the open air. They improve if the person fasts for a time and if the weather is wet and warm. People who are suitable for chamomile are noisy sleepers, in that they frequently cry out or talk while dreaming. If woken suddenly from sleep they are extremely irritable and they like to poke their feet out from the bed covers to keep them cool.

Chincona officinalis

Cinchona succirubra; china, Peruvian bark, Jesuit's bark

This homeopathic remedy, known as china, is obtained from the dried bark of the cinchona tree and contains quinine. The attractive evergreen cinchona, with its red bark, is a native of the hot tropical forests of South America, but it is also cultivated in India, Sri Lanka and southeast Asia. A preparation of powdered bark was used to treat a feverish illness suffered by the Countess of Cinchon, wife of the viceroy of Peru in 1638. After her recovery she publicized the remedy, and the tree was called cinchona from this time. The value of the bark as a cure for malaria had long been known and used by Jesuit priests. This was the first homeopathic substance tested and proved by Hahnemann on himself.

In modern homeopathy it is used mainly as a remedy for nervous and physical exhaustion resulting from chronic debilitating illnesses. It is used for weakness because of dehydration, sweating, chills and fever, and headaches that are relieved if firm pressure is applied. The person wants drinks during periods of chills and shivering rather than when feverish and hot. He or she usually has a washed-out unhealthy complexion with very sensitive skin. China is also used as a remedy for neuralgia, muscles that twitch because of extreme fatigue, bleeding, including nosebleeds, and tinnitus (noises in the ears). It has a helpful effect on the digestion and is used to treat gastrointestinal wind, gall bladder disorders and digestive upset. Some mental symptoms are helped by this remedy, including irritability and tetchy behaviour that is out of character, apathy and loss of concentration and sleeplessness.

People who are suitable for this remedy tend to be artistic, imaginative and highly strung. They find it easier to empathize with the natural world rather than with the people around them. They are intense and dislike trivial conversation and fatty foods such as butter, but have a liking for alcoholic drinks. Their nature makes them prone to irritability and depression, and they tend to draw up grand schemes at night that are later abandoned. Symptoms are made better by warmth and plenty of sleep and by the application of steady continuous pressure to a painful area. They are made worse by cold, draughty weather, particularly in the autumn, and in the evening and night.

Cuprum metallicum

Cuprum met.; copper

Copper ore, which is found in rocks in many parts of the world, has been mined and used for many centuries in the manufacture of weapons, utensils and jewellery, etc. In earlier times, physicians made an ointment from the ground metal and this was applied to raw wounds to aid healing. Copper is poisonous in large doses affecting the nervous system and causing convulsions, paralysis and possibly death because of its effects upon respiratory muscles. Toxic effects were recognized in those who worked with the metal and who developed wasting because of poor absorption of food, coughs and respiratory symptoms, and colicky pains. The ruddy, gold-coloured metal is ground to produce a fine red powder that is used in homeopathy to treat cramping, colicky pains in the abdomen, and muscular spasms in the calves of the legs, feet and ankles. It is also used as a remedy for epilepsy and problems of breathing and respiration such as asthma, croup and whooping cough in which there are spasms. The person may turn blue because of the effort of breathing.

The symptoms are made worse by touch, hot, sunny weather and for keeping emotions bottled up. They improve with sweating and drinking cold fluids. People who benefit from Cuprum met. have mood swings that alternate from stubbornness to passivity, weepiness and depression. They tend to be serious people who judge themselves severely and keep their emotions very much suppressed. As babies or toddlers, they may be breath-holders who turn blue with anger or as a result of a tantrum. As children, some are destructive and others are loners who dislike the company of others.

Drosera rotundifolia

Drosera, sundew, youthwort, red rot, moor grass

This small, carnivorous (insect-eating) plant is found widely throughout Europe and in Britain, where it grows in the poor, acidic soils of bogs, damp uplands, moorlands and woodlands. It is a small plant growing close to the ground, and needs to trap insects for extra nutrients as the soil in which it grows is so poor. It is remarkable for its leaves, which are covered with long red hairs, each with a small, fluid-containing gland at the top. When the sun shines on the leaves it resembles dew, hence the name sundew. An insect landing on the leaf is trapped because this curls over and inwards, and the sticky fluid secreted by the hairs holds it fast. The secretion contains enzymes that digest the body and the nutrients are absorbed by the plant. The small, white flowers of sundew are fully open in the early morning but close up when the sun is shining strongly. In medieval times, the plant was used to treat tuberculosis and the plague, and it was employed as a remedy for skin disorders in early Asian medicine. It was noticed that sheep who inadvertently cropped sundew developed a paroxysmal type of cough like whooping cough. It was investigated and proved as a remedy for this illness in homeopathy , and the whole plant is used to prepare the medicine. Any condition in which there is a violent, dry, persistent barking cough of a spasmodic nature, as in whooping cough, benefits from the use of sundew, which has a particular action on the upper respiratory tract. Accompanying symptoms are gagging, sickness, sweating and nosebleeds. It is also used to treat bronchitis, asthma, corns and warts, growing pains and pains in the bones.

People who benefit from this remedy are restless and fearful of being alone when they are ill, and they tend to be stubborn and lack concentration. They are suspicious and may feel that others are talking about them or concealing bad news. They are sensitive to the supernatural and are afraid of ghosts. The symptoms are worse for being too warm in bed, after midnight, with crying, lying down, laughing, singing and talking. Also, for meals of cold food and drinks. Symptoms improve out in the fresh air, with walking or gentle exercise, sitting propped up in bed, with pressure applied to the painful part and in quiet surroundings.

Euphrasia officinalis

Euphrasia, eyebright

Eyebright is an attractive wild flower that is variable in size and grows widely throughout Europe, including Britain, and in North America. It has been known since medieval times as a remedy for inflammation of the eyes, and this remains its main use in homeopathy . The plant flourishes on well-drained, chalky soils and may be between two and eight inches in height, depending upon conditions. It is partly parasitic, deriving some nourishment from the roots of grass, and produces pretty white, purple-veined flowers with yellow centres. The whole plant and flowers are used in homeopathy , and the remedy is used to treat eye disorders characterized by redness, inflammation, watering, burning, stinging or itching. These include conjunctivitis, blepharitis (inflammation of eyelids), injuries to the eye and dry eyes. It is also used as a remedy for allergic conditions such as hay fever, in which the eyes are very much affected, and colds producing eye symptoms. It is a remedy for the early stages of measles, headaches, some menstrual problems and inflammation of the prostate gland in men. Symptoms are worse in the evening, in windy and warm weather and for being inside. They improve in subdued light, with drinking a cup of coffee and with cold applications.

Ferrum phosphoricum

Ferrum phos.; ferric phosphate of iron, iron phosphate

Ferrum phos. is one of the Schussler tissue salts, and the iron phosphate powder is obtained by chemical reaction between sodium phosphate, sodium acetate and iron sulphate. Iron is a

very important substance in the body, being found in the hae-
moglobin pigment of red blood cells that transports oxygen to
all the tissues and organs. The homeopathic remedy is used to
treat the early stages of infections, inflammations and feverish
conditions, before any other particular symptoms occur. It is
used to treat colds and coughs in which there may be a slowly
developing fever, headache, nosebleeds, bronchitis, hoarseness
and loss of the voice, earache and rheumatic pains. Digestive
symptoms such as sour indigestion, inflammation of the stomach (gastritis), and vomiting and some disorders of menstruation are helped by this remedy. It is also used to treat the early
symptoms of dysentery. The person tends to be pale but is prone
to flushing, and feels cold in the early afternoon. There may be
a rapid weak pulse. Symptoms are worse at night and in the
early morning between 4 a.m. and 6 a.m. Also, they are worse
for heat and hot sun, movement and jarring of the body, pressure and touch and resting on the right side and suppressing
sweating by the use of deodorants, etc. Symptoms improve for
cold applications and with gentle movements. People who are
suitable for Ferrum phos. tend to be thin and pale but may be
liable to flush easily. They are intelligent and quick to absorb
new concepts, having plenty of original ideas of their own. They
may be prone to digestive and respiratory complaints, stomach
upsets and coughs and colds.

Gelsemium sempervirens

Gelsemium, yellow jasmine, false jasmine, Carolina jasmine, wild
  woodbine

This attractive climbing plant is a native of the southern United
States and parts of Mexico. It has a woody stem that twists
around any available tree trunk, and grows on stream banks
and on the sea coast. It produces attractive, large, bell-shaped,
perfumed yellow flowers in the early spring, which belie the
poisonous nature of the plant. It has an underground stem, or
rhizome, from which arise a tangle of yellow roots that have an
aromatic smell. The root is the part used in homeopathy and,
if eaten in significant amounts, it affects the central nervous

system, causing paralysis and possible death through failure of the nerves and muscles of the respiratory system. In homeopathy it is used to treat both physical and mental symptoms. The physical ailments treated mainly involve the nervous and respiratory systems. These include headaches that are worsened with bright light and movement, multiple sclerosis, eye pain, especially on the right side, sore throat and influenza-like symptoms, earache and feverish muscular pains. Accompanying symptoms include chills and shivering, flushed face and malaise. It is used to treat some menstrual problems including pain. Mental symptoms that are helped by Gelsemium include fears and phobias with symptoms of fatigue, weakness, trembling and apprehension. These fears may arise before an examination, interview or public performance (stage fright). Excitement or fear that causes the heart to skip a beat and extreme anxiety causing sleeplessness are helped by Gelsemium. Symptoms are made worse in the sun and in warm, moist, humid weather or damp and fog. They are also worse with smoking and for excitement, anticipation, stress or bad news. Symptoms improve with movement in the fresh air and after sweating and drinking alcohol or a stimulant drink. They improve after urinating – a large quantity of pale urine is usually passed. People suitable for Gelsemium tend to be well-built with a blue-tinged skin and often complain of feeling weak and tired. They are beset by fears, and may be cowardly and too fearful to lead or enjoy a normal active life.

Graphites

Graphite; black pencil lead

Graphite is a form of carbon that is the basis of all life. It is found in older igneous or metamorphic rocks, such as granite and marble, and is mined for its industrial uses, e.g. in batteries, motors, pencil leads, cleaning and lubricating fluids. It was investigated and proved by Hahnemann after he learned that it was being used by some factory workers to heal cold sores. The powder used in homeopathy is ground graphite, and it is mainly used for skin disorders that may be caused by metabolic imbalances and stomach ulcers. It is a remedy for eczema, psoriasis, acne, rough, dry skin conditions with pustules or blisters, scarring and thickened cracked nails and cold sores. Also for stomach ulcers caused by a thinning or weakness in the lining of the stomach wall, problems caused by excessive catarrh, loss of hair, and cramping pains or numbing of the feet and hands. In women it is used to treat some menstrual problems. The symptoms are worse in draughty, cold and damp conditions and for eating sweet meals or sea foods. Also, the use of steroids for skin complaints and, in women, during menstruation. Symptoms are often worse on the left side. They improve with warmth as long as the air is fresh and it is not stuffy, when it is dark and for eating and sleep. People suitable for Graphites are usually well-built and may be overweight, often having dark hair. They like to eat well but lack physical fitness, and sweat or flush with slight exertion. They are prone to dry, flaky skin conditions that may affect the scalp. Graphites people are usually lethargic and may be irritable, lacking in concentration for intellectual activities. They are prone to mood swings and subject to bouts of weeping, especially when listening to music. A Graphites person feels that he or she is unlucky and is inclined to self-pity, often feeling fearful and timid.

Hamamelis virginiana

Hamamelis, witch hazel, spotted alder, snapping hazelnut, winterbloom

This plant is a native of the eastern United States and Canada but it is also grown in Europe. It is a shrub with grey-green leaves and yellow flowers that appear in the autumn. The part used in homeopathy is the bark of stems and twigs and the outer part of the fresh root. This has the effect of causing body tissues, especially blood vessels, to contract, and it is used to arrest bleeding. Its curative properties were known to the native North American Indians, and it was first investigated and proved in homeopathy by Dr Hering. Its main effect is on the blood circulation of the veins, particularly when the walls of the vessels are inflamed and weakened, and bleeding does no stop easily. It is used as a remedy for haemorrhoids, or piles with bleeding, varicose veins and ulcers, phlebitis (inflamed veins), nosebleeds, heavy periods, internal bleeding and pain associated with bruising or bleeding. Some headaches are helped by Hamamelis and, also, mental symptoms of depression, irritability and impatience. The symptoms are made worse by warmth and moisture and with physical activity. They improve out in the fresh air and for concentrating on a particular task or event and for conversation, thinking and reading.

Hypericum perforatum
Hypericum, St John's wort

A perennial herbaceous plant that is a native of Britain, Europe and Asia, but is cultivated throughout the world. It grows between one and three feet in height, producing elongated, oval dark green leaves that appear to be covered in minute spots or holes (hence *perforatum*, or perforate). In fact, these are minute oil-secreting glands that secrete a bright red solution. The large, bright yellow flowers appear in June, July and August and have small black dots around the edges of the petals. The crushed flowers produce a blood-coloured juice that was used, in early times, to treat raw wounds. It was also believed that the plant could be hung up to ward off evil spirits (the name *Hypericum* being derived from the Greek, meaning 'over an apparition'). There are two traditions associated with the common name, St John's wort. One links the plant with 29 August, believed to be the anniversary of the execution of St John the Baptist. The other is that the plant is named after an ancient order of knights going back to the time of the Crusades, the knights of St John of Jerusalem.

The whole fresh green plant and flowers are used in homeopathy to produce the mother tincture. It is mainly used to treat damage to nerves and nerve pain following accidental injury. Typically, there are shooting, stabbing pains that radiate upwards, and it is indicated especially where there are many nerve endings concentrated in a particular part of the body, e.g. the fingers and toes. It is very effective in pains associated

with the spinal nerves and spinal cord, concussion, head or eye
injuries. It is also a remedy for wounds and lacerations producing stabbing pains indicating nerve damage, and accidental
crushing injuries. It is useful for bites, stings, splinters and
puncture wounds, toothache and pain following dental extrac-
tions. In addition, it is a treatment for asthma and some digestive complaints of indigestion, sickness and diarrhoea. It is
sometimes helpful in the treatment of piles, or haemorrhoids,
and some menstrual problems with accompanying headache.
The symptoms are made worse by cold, damp or foggy weather,
before a storm and getting chilled when undressing. Also for
touch and for a close, stuffy atmosphere. Symptoms improve
when the person remains still and tilts the head backwards.

Ignatia amara

Agnate; *Strychnos ignatii*, St Ignatius' bean

Ignatia amara is a large tree that is native to the Philippine
Islands, China and the East Indies. The tree has many branches
and twining stems and produces stalked white flowers. Later
seed pods are produced, each containing ten to twenty large
oval seeds, that are about one inch long and are embedded in
pulp. The seeds are highly poisonous and contain strychnine,
which affects the central nervous system. Similar active constituents and properties are found in nux vomica. The tree is
named after the founder of the Jesuits, Ignatius Loyola
(1491-1556), and Spanish priests belonging to this order
brought the seeds to Europe during the 1600s. The homeopathic remedy is made from the powdered seeds and is used
especially for emotional symptoms. It is used for grief, bereavement, shock and loss, particularly when a person is having difficulty coming to terms with his or her feelings and is inclined
to suppress the natural responses. Accompanying symptoms
include sleeplessness, anger and hysteria. Similar emotional
and psychological problems are helped by this remedy, including anxiety and fear, especially of appearing too forward to others, a tendency to burst into fits of crying, self-doubt, pity and
blame, and depression. Nervous tension headaches and

digestive upsets, feverish symptoms, chills and pains in the abdomen may be helped by Ignatia. Some problems associated with menstruation, especially sharp pains or absence of periods are relieved by this remedy, as are conditions with changeable symptoms. These are worse in cold weather or conditions, with emotional trauma, being touched, for smoking and drinking coffee. They improve with warmth, moving about, eating, lying on the side or area that is painful and after passing urine.

The person for whom Ignatia is suitable is usually female and with a tendency towards harsh, self criticism and blame; she is usually a creative artistic person, highly sensitive but with a tendency to suppress the emotions. She is perceptive and intelligent but inclined to be hysterical and subject to erratic swings of mood. Typically, the person expects a high standard in those she loves. The person enjoys dairy products, bread and sour foods but sweets, alcoholic drinks and fruit upset her system. She is afraid of crowds, tends to be claustrophobic, and fears being burgled. Also, she is afraid of being hurt emotionally, and is very sensitive to pain. The person is usually dark-haired and of slim build with a worried expression and prone to sighing, yawning and excessive blinking.

pecacuanha

pecac.; *Cephaelis ipecacuanha, Psychotria ipecacuanha*, the ipecac plant

This plant is a native of South America, particularly Brazil, Bolivia and New Grenada. The plant contains the alkaloids emetine and cephaeline, and different varieties contain differing proportions of these alkaloids. The root is the part used in homeopathy , and the preparations may be in a number of different forms. It is used to treat conditions where the main symptoms are nausea and vomiting, which are intractable and persistent, e.g. motion sickness and morning sickness. It is also used as a remedy for bronchitis, breathlessness because of the presence of fluid in the lung, whooping cough and heart failure. The symptoms are made worse by cold weather and lying down, and after a meal of pork or veal. They improve in the fresh open air and while resting with the eyes shut.

Kalium bichromicum

Kali bich.; potassium dichromate, potassium bichromate

This substance has several uses in industry (e.g. in the prepa rations of dyes and in batteries) as well as its medicinal pur poses. The crystals of potassium dichromate are bright orang and are prepared from a chemical reaction involving the addi tion of a solution of potassium chromate to an acid. It is use for discharges of mucus and disorders of the mucous mem branes, particularly involving the vagina and genital and uri nary tracts, throat, nose and stomach. The remedy is useful fo catarrhal colds and sinusitis, feelings of fullness and pressure headache, migraine and glue ear. Also, for joint and rheumati disorders with pains that may move about or even disappea People who benefit from this remedy are highly sensitive to col and chills when ill, but also experience a worsening of symp toms in hot, sunny conditions. They tend to be people wh adhere very closely to a regular routine and may be somewha rigid and inflexible. They like everything to be done properl down to the smallest detail and are law-abiding, moral and con formist. Symptoms are worse during the summer and also i wet and chilly conditions. They are at their height in the earl hours of the morning between 3 and 5 a.m., and also on firs waking up. Drinking alcohol and becoming chilled while tak ing off clothes exacerbates the symptoms. They improve wit moving around and after eating a meal. Also, symptoms improv with warmth and heat (but not hot sun) and after vomiting.

Kalium iodatum

Kali iod.; *Kali hydriodicum*, potassium iodide

This is prepared by chemical reaction from potassium hydrox ide and iodine and is an old remedy for syphilis. It is recom mended that potassium iodide should be added to animal fee concentrates and table salt to prevent deficiency in iodine. Th homeopathic remedy is used to relieve catarrh in those who ar prone to chesty conditions. It is also used to treat swollen gland sore throats, sinusitis, hay fever and influenza-type infection It is used to treat male prostate gland disorders. The symp toms tend to improve with movement and from being out in the fresh air. They are made worse by heat and touch and are at their most severe between two and five in the early morning. People who suit this remedy tend to be dogmatic, knowing exactly what they think about a particular subject. They may be irritable or bad-tempered and not easy to get along with. They have a preference for cool rather than warm or hot weather.

Kalium phosphoricum

Kali phos.; potassium phosphate, phosphate of potash

This remedy is one of the Schussler tissue salts, and it is obtained from a chemical reaction between dilute phosphoric acid and solution of potassium carbonate. Potassium carbonate is derived from potash, the white powder that is left when wood is burnt completely. Potassium is an essential element in the body, vital for the healthy functioning of nerve tissue. Kali phos. is used to treat mental and physical exhaustion and depression, particularly in young persons in whom it may have been caused by too much work or studying. Accompanying symptoms include jumping at noise or interruption and a desire to be alone. Also, there may be a pus-containing discharge from the bladder, vagina, bowels or lungs and extreme muscular fatigue. They may suffer from gnawing hunger pains, anxiety, insomnia, tremor and have a tendency to perspire on the face when excited or after a meal. People who are suitable for Kali phos. are usually extrovert, hold clearly formed ideas and are easily exhausted. They become distressed by bad news, including that which does not affect them directly, such as a disaster in another country. They tend to crave sweet foods and dislike bread. Symptoms are made worse by any anxiety, in cold, dry weather and in winter and on drinking cold drinks. Also, they are exacerbated by noise, conversation, touch and physical activity. Symptoms improve with heat, gentle exercise, in cloudy conditions and after eating.

Lachesis

Trigonocephalus lachesis, *Lachesis muta*, venom of the bushmaster or surukuku snake

This South African snake produces a deadly venom that may prove instantly fatal because of its effects upon the heart. The venom causes the blood to thin and flow more freely, hence increasing the likelihood of haemorrhage. Even a slight bite bleeds copiously with a risk of blood poisoning or septicaemia. The snake is a ferocious hunter, and its African name, surukuku, describes the sound it makes while in pursuit of prey. The properties of the venom were investigated by the eminent American homeopathic doctor Constantine Hering during the 1800s. He tested and proved the remedy on himself. It is effective in treating a variety of disorders, particularly those relating to the blood circulation and where there is a risk of blood poisoning or septicaemia. It is used to treat varicose veins and problems of the circulation indicated by a bluish tinge to the skin. The remedy is useful for those suffering from a weak heart or angina, palpitations and an irregular, fast or weak pulse. There may be symptoms of chest pain and breathing difficulty. It is of great benefit in treating uterine problems, particularly premenstrual congestion and pain that is relieved once the period starts. It is also an excellent remedy for menopausal symptoms, especially hot flushes, and for infections of the bladder and rectum. It is used to treat conditions and infections where symptoms are mainly on the left side, such as headache or stroke. Also, as a treatment for sore throats and throat infections, tonsillitis, lung abscess, boils, ulcers, wounds that heal slowly, vomiting because of appendicitis and digestive disorders, fevers with chills and shivering, nosebleeds and bleeding piles.

It is used to treat severe symptoms of measles and serious infections including scarlet fever and smallpox. Symptoms are made worse by touch and after sleep and by tight clothing. They are worse for hot drinks and baths, exposure to hot sun or direct heat in any form. For women, symptoms are worse during the menopause. They improve for being out in the fresh air and drinking cold drinks and for release of normal bodily discharges. People suitable for Lachesis tend to be intelligent, creative, intense and ambitious. They have strong views abou

516

politics and world affairs and may be impatient of the views of others. They may be somewhat self-centred, possessive and jealous, which can cause problems in close relationships with others. They dislike being tied down and so may be reluctant to commit themselves to a relationship. Lachesis people have a liking for sour pickled foods, bread, rice and oysters and alcoholic drinks. They like coffee, but hot drinks and wheat-based food tends to upset them. They have a fear of water, people they do not know, being burgled and of dying or being suffocated. Lachesis people may be somewhat overweight and are sometimes red-haired and freckled. Alternatively, they may be thin and dark-haired, pale and with a lot of energy. Children tend to be somewhat jealous of others and possessive of their friends, which can lead to naughty or trying behaviour.

Ledum palustre

Ledum; marsh tea, wild rosemary

Wild rosemary is an evergreen shrub that grows in the bogs and cold upland conditions of the northern United States, Canada and northern Europe, especially Scandinavia, Ireland and parts of Asia. The bush produces elongated, dark green leaves, about one or two inches long, that are smooth and shiny on the upper surface but underneath are covered with brown woolly hairs. ('Ledum' is derived from the Greek word *ledos*, meaning 'woolly robe'). The leaves contain a volatile, aromatic oil like camphor, and the plant has been used for centuries by Scandinavian people to repel insects, moths and mice. The plant produces attractive white flowers and is valued for its antiseptic properties. The fresh parts of the plant are gathered, dried and ground to make a powder used in homeopathy , and it is a valuable first aid remedy. It is taken internally for animal bites, insect stings, lacerations and wounds in which there is bruising and sharp stabbing pains. There is usually inflammation, redness, swelling and throbbing accompanied by feverish symptoms of chills and shivering. It is additionally used as a remedy for gout in the big toe, rheumatic pains in the feet that radiate upwards, hot, painful, stiff joints and tendons but with

suppository this preparation is a small cone of a convenient and easily soluble base with herbal extracts added, which is used to apply medicines to the rectum. It is very effective in the treatment of piles, cancers, etc.

tablet this is made by compressing drugs into a small compass. It is more easily administered and has a quicker action as it dissolves more rapidly in the stomach.

tincture this is the most prescribed form of herbal medicine. It is based on alcohol and, as such, removes certain active principles from herbs that will not dissolve in water, or in the presence of heat. The tincture produced is long-lasting, highly concentrated and only needs to be taken in small doses for beneficial effects. The ground or chopped dried herb is placed in a container with 40 per cent alcohol such as gin or vodka and left for two weeks. The tincture is then decanted into a dark bottle and sealed before use.

cold skin. People who benefit from this remedy tend to get hot and sweaty at night when ill, and usually throw off the bed coverings. They often have itchy skin on the feet and ankles and have a tendency to sprain their ankles. When ill, they are irritable and hard to please or may be withdrawn, and do not want the company of others. The symptoms are made worse by warmth or heat, touch and at night. They improve with cold applications to the painful part and for cool conditions.

Lycopodium clavatum

Lycopodium; club moss, wolf's claw, vegetable sulphur, stag's-horn moss, running pine

This plant is found throughout the northern hemisphere, in high moorlands, forests and mountains. The plant produces spore cases on the end of upright forked stalks, which contain the spores. These produce yellow dust or powder that is resistant to water and was once used as a coating on pills and tablets to keep them separate from one another. The powder was also used as a constituent of fireworks. It has been used medicinally for many centuries, as a remedy for digestive disorders and kidney stones in Arabian countries and in the treatment of gout. The powder and spores are collected by shaking the fresh, flowering stalks of the plant, and its main use in homeopathy is for digestive and kidney disorders. It is used to treat indigestion, heartburn, the effects of eating a large meal late at night, sickness, nausea, wind, bloatedness and constipation. Also, in men, for kidney stones, with the production of a red-coloured urine containing a sand-like sediment and enlarged prostate gland. It is used in the treatment of some problems of male impotence and bleeding haemorrhoids, or piles. Symptoms that occur on the right side are helped by Lycopodium, and the patient additionally tends to crave sweet, comfort foods. Nettle rash, psoriasis affecting the hands, fatigue because of illness and ME (myalgic encephalomyelitis), some types of headache, cough and sore throat are relieved by this remedy. It is used to relieve emotional states of anxiety, fear and apprehension caused by chronic insecurity or relating to forthcoming events, such as taking an examination or appearing in public (stage fright). Also, night terrors, sleeplessness, shouting or talking in the sleep and being frightened on first waking up can all benefit from this treatment.

The symptoms are worse between 4 p.m. and 8 p.m. and in warm, stuffy rooms and with wearing clothes that are too tight. They are also worse in the early morning between 4 a.m. and 8 a.m., for eating too much and during the spring. They improve outside in cool fresh air, after a hot meal or drink and with loosening tight clothing, with light exercise and at night. People suitable for Lycopodium tend to be serious, hard-working and intelligent, often in professional positions. They seem to be self-possessed and confident but are in reality rather insecure with a low self-opinion. They are impatient of what they perceive as being weakness and are not tolerant or sympathetic of illness. Lycopodium people are sociable but may keep their distance and not get involved; they may be sexually promiscuous. They have a great liking for sweet foods of all kinds and enjoy hot meals and drinks. They are easily filled but may carry on eating regardless of this and usually complain of symptoms on the right side. Lycopodium people are afraid of being left on their own, of failure in life, of crowds, darkness and the supernatural, and tend to be claustrophobic. They are often tall, thin and pale with receding hair or hair that turns grey early in life. They may be bald, with a forehead lined with worry lines and a serious appearance. They tend to have weak muscles and are easily tired after physical exercise. They may have a tendency to unconsciously twitch the muscles of the face and to flare the nostrils.

Mercurius solubilis

Merc. sol.; quicksilver

The mineral cinnabar, which is found in volcanic crystalline rocks, is an important ore of mercury and is extracted for a variety of uses, including dental fillings and in thermometers. Mercury is toxic in large doses, and an affected person produces great quantities of saliva and suffers repeated bouts of vomiting. Mercury has been used since ancient times and was once given as a remedy for syphilis. A powder of precipitate of mercury is obtained from dissolving liquid mercury in a dilute solution of nitric acid, and this is the source of the remedy used in homeopathy . It is used as a remedy for conditions that produce copious bodily secretions that often smell unpleasant, with accompanying symptoms of heat or burning and a great sensitivity to temperature. It is used as a remedy for fevers with profuse, unpleasant sweating, bad breath, inflammation of the gums, mouth ulcers, candidiasis (fungal infection) of the mouth, infected painful teeth and gums, and excessive production of saliva. Also, for a sore infected throat, tonsillitis, mumps, discharging infected ear, and a congested severe headache and pains in the joints. It is good for eye complaints, including severe conjunctivitis, allergic conditions with a running nose, skin complaints that produce pus-filled pustules, spots, and ulcers, including varicose ulcers. The symptoms are made worse by extremes of heat and cold and also by wet and rapidly changing weather. They are worse at night and for sweating and being too hot in bed.

Symptoms improve with rest and in comfortable temperatures where the person is neither too hot nor too cold. People suitable for Merc. sol. tend to be very insecure although they have an outwardly calm appearance. They are cautious and reserved with other people and consider what they are about to say before speaking so that conversation may seem laboured. Merc. sol. types do not like criticism of any kind and may suddenly become angry if someone disagrees with their point of view. They tend to be introverted, but their innermost thoughts may be in turmoil. They tend to be hungry and enjoy bread and butter, milk and other cold drinks but dislike alcohol with the exception of beer. They usually do not eat meat and do not have a sweet tooth. They dislike coffee and salt. Merc. sol. people often have fair hair with fine, unlined skin and an air of detachment. They are afraid of dying and of mental illness leading to insanity, and worry about the wellbeing of their family. They fear being burgled and are afraid or fearful during a thunder-storm.

Natrum muriaticum

Natrum mur.; common salt, sodium chloride

Salt has long been prized for its seasoning and preservative qualities, and Roman soldiers were once paid in salt, such was its value (the word 'salary' comes from the Latin word *salarium*, which refers to this practice). Sodium and chlorine are essential chemicals in the body, being needed for many metabolic processes, particularly the functioning of nerve tissue. In fact, there is seldom a need to add salt to food as usually enough is present naturally in a healthy, well-balanced diet. (An exception is when people are working very hard physically in a hot climate and losing a lot of salt in sweat). However, people and many other mammals frequently have a great liking for salt. If the salt/water balance in the body is disturbed, a person soon becomes very ill and may even die.

In ancient times, salt was usually obtained by boiling sea water, but natural evaporation around the shallow edges of salt lakes results in deposits of rock salt being formed. Rock salt is the usual source of table salt and also of the remedy used in homeopathy . This remedy has an effect on the functioning of the kidneys and the salt/water balance of body fluids, and is used to treat both mental and physical symptoms. Emotional symptoms that benefit from Natrum mur. include sensitivity and irritability, tearfulness and depression, suppressed grief and premenstrual tension. Physical ailments that respond to this remedy are often those in which there is a thin, watery discharge of mucus and in which symptoms are made worse by heat. Hence Natrum mur. is used in the treatment of colds with a runny nose or other catarrhal problems. Also, for some menstrual and vaginal problems, headaches and migraines, cold sores, candidiasis (fungal infection) of the mouth, mouth ulcers, inflamed and infected gums and bad breath. Some skin disorders are helped by Natrum mur., including verruca (a wart on the foot), warts, spots and boils, and cracked, dry lips. It may be used in the treatment of fluid retention with puffiness around the face, eyelids and abdomen, etc, urine retention, constipation, anal fissure, indigestion, anaemia and thyroid disorders (goitre). When ill, people who benefit from this remedy feel cold and shivery, but their symptoms are made worse, or even brought on, by heat. Heat, whether from hot sun and fire or a warm, stuffy room, exacerbate the symptoms, which also are made worse by cold and thundery weather. They are worse on the coast from the sea breeze, and in the morning between 9 and 11 o'clock. Too much physical activity and the sympathy of others exacerbate the symptoms. They improve in the fresh, open air and for cold applications or a cold bath or swim. Also, sleeping on a hard bed and sweating and fasting make the symptoms better. People suitable for Natrum mur. are often women who are highly sensitive, serious-minded, intelligent and reliable. They have high ideals and feel things very deeply, being easily hurt and stung by slights and criticism. They need the company of other people but, being so sensitive, can actually shun them for fear of being hurt. They are afraid of mental illness leading to loss of self-control and insanity, and of dying. Also, they fear the dark, failure in work, crowds, being burgled and have a tendency to be claustrophobic. They worry about being late and are fearful during a thunderstorm. Merc. sol. people tend to become introverted and react badly to the criticism of others. They are highly sensitive to the influence of music, which easily moves them to tears. Natrum mur. people are usually of squat or solid build with dark or fairish hair. They are prone to reddened, watery eyes as though they have been crying, and a cracked lower lip. The face may appear puffy and shiny with an air of stoicism.

Nux vomica

Strychnos nux vomica; poison nut, Quaker buttons

The *Strychnos nux vomica* tree is a native of India but also grows in Burma, Thailand, China and Australia. It produces small, greenish-white flowers and, later, apple-sized fruits, containing small, flat, circular pale seeds covered in fine hair. The seeds, bark and leaves are highly poisonous, containing strychnine, and have been used in medicine for many centuries. In medieval times, the seeds were used as a treatment for the plague. Strychnine has severe effects upon the nervous system but in minute amounts can help increase urination and aid digestion. The seeds are cleaned and dried and used to produce the homeopathic remedy. Nux vomica is used in the treatment of a variety of digestive complaints, including cramping, colicky abdominal pains, indigestion, nausea and vomiting, diarrhoea and constipation. Also, indigestion or stomach upset caused by overindulgence in alcohol or rich food and piles, which cause painful contractions of the rectum. Sometimes these complaints are brought on by a tendency to keep emotions, particularly anger, suppressed and not allowing it to show or be expressed outwardly. Nux vomica is a remedy for irritability, headache and migraine, colds, coughs and influenza-like symptoms of fever, aching bones and muscles and chills and shivering. It is a useful remedy for women who experience heavy, painful periods that may cause fainting, morning sickness during pregnancy and pain in labour. It is also used to treat urinary frequency and cystitis.

The type of person who benefits from this remedy is frequently under stress and experiences a periodic flare-up of symptoms. The person may be prone to indigestion and heartburn, gastritis and stomach ulcer, and piles, or haemorrhoids. The person usually has a tendency to keep everything bottled up but has a passionate nature and is liable to outbursts of anger. Nux vomica people are very ambitious and competitive, demanding a high standard of themselves and others and intolerant of anything less than perfection. They enjoy challenges and using their wits to keep one step ahead. Often they are to be found as managers, company directors, scientists, etc, at the cutting edge of their particular occupation. They are ungracious and irritable when ill and cannot abide the criticism of others. This type of person is afraid of being a failure at work and fears or dislikes crowded public places. He or she is afraid of dying. The person enjoys rich, fattening foods containing cholesterol and spicy meals, alcohol and coffee, although these upset the digestive system. Symptoms are worse in cold, windy, dry weather and in winter and in the early morning between 3 and 4 a.m. They are aggravated by certain noises, music, bright lights and touch, eating (especially spicy meals) and overwork of mental faculties. Nux vomica people usually look serious, tense and are thin with a worried expression. They have sallow skin and tend to have dark shadows beneath the eyes.

Phosphorus

Phos; white phosphorus

Phosphorus is an essential mineral in the body found in the genetic material (DNA), bones and teeth. White phosphorus is extremely flammable and poisonous and was once used in the manufacture of matches and fireworks. As it tends to catch fire spontaneously when exposed to air, it is stored under water. In the past it has been used to treat a number of disorders and infectious diseases such as measles. In homeopathy , the remedy is used to treat nervous tension caused by stress and worry, with symptoms of sleeplessness, exhaustion and digestive upset. Often there are pains of a burning nature in the chest or abdomen. It is a remedy for vomiting and nausea, heartburn, acid indigestion, stomach ulcer and gastroenteritis. It is also used to treat bleeding, e.g. from minor wounds, the gums, nosebleeds, gastric and profuse menstrual bleeding.

Severe coughs, which may be accompanied by retching, vomiting and production of a blood-tinged phlegm, are treated with Phos. as well as some other severe respiratory complaints. These include pneumonia, bronchitis, asthma and laryngitis. Styes that tend to recur and poor circulation may be helped by Phos. Symptoms are worse in the evening and morning and before or during a thunderstorm. They are also made worse for too much physical activity, hot food and drink and lying on the left side. Symptoms improve in the fresh open air and with lying on the back or right side. They are better after sleep or when the person is touched or stroked. People who need Phos. do not like to be alone when ill and improve with the sympathy and attention of others. They are warm, kind, affectionate people who are highly creative, imaginative and artistic. They enjoy the company of other people and need stimulation to give impetus to their ideas. Phos. people have an optimistic outlook, are full of enthusiasm but sometimes promise much and deliver little. They are very tactile and like to be touched or stroked and offered sympathy when unhappy or unwell. They enjoy a variety of different foods but tend to suffer from digestive upsets. Phos. people are usually tall, slim and may be dark or fair-haired, with an attractive, open appearance. They like to wear brightly coloured clothes and are usually popular. They have a fear of illness, especially cancer, and of dying and also of the dark and supernatural forces. They are apprehensive of water and fear being a failure in their work. Thunderstorms make them nervous.

Pulsatilla nigricans

Pulsatilla, *Anemone pratensis*, meadow anemone

This attractive plant closely resembles *Anemone pulsatilla*, the pasqueflower, which is used in herbal medicine but has smaller flowers. *Anemone pratensis* is a native of Germany, Denmark and Scandinavia and has been used medicinally for hundreds of years. The plant produces beautiful deep purple flowers with orange centres and both leaves and flowers are covered with fine, silky hairs. The whole fresh plant is gathered and made into a pulp, and liquid is extracted to make the homeopathic remedy. It is used to treat a wide variety of disorders with both physical and mental symptoms. It is useful for ailments in which there is a greenish, yellowish discharge. Hence it is used for colds and coughs and sinusitis with the production of profuse catarrh or phlegm. Also, eye infections with discharge such as styes and conjunctivitis. Digestive disorders are helped by it, particularly indigestion, heartburn, nausea and sickness caused by eating too much fatty or rich food. The remedy is helpful for female disorders in which there are a variety of physical and emotional symptoms. These include premenstrual tension, menstrual problems, menopausal symptoms and cystitis, with accompanying symptoms of mood swings, depression and tearfulness. It is a remedy for headaches and migraine, swollen glands, inflammation and pain in the bones and joints as in rheumatic and arthritic disorders, nosebleeds, varicose veins, mumps, measles, toothache, acne, frequent urination and incontinence.

Symptoms are worse at night or when it is hot, and after eating heavy, rich food. Symptoms improve out in the cool fresh air and for gentle exercise such as walking. The person feels better after crying and being treated sympathetically by others. Pulsatilla people are usually women who have a mild, passive nature and are kind, gentle and loving. They are easily moved to tears by the plight of others and love animals and people alike. The person yields easily to the requests and demands of others and is a peacemaker who likes to avoid a scene. An outburst of anger is very much out of character, and a Pulsatilla person usually has many friends. The person likes rich and sweet foods, although these may upset the digestion, and dislikes spicy meals. Pulsatilla people may fear darkness, being left alone, dying and any illness leading to insanity. They are fearful of crowds, the supernatural and tend to be claustrophobic. Usually, they are fair and blue-eyed with clear, delicate skin that blushes readily. They are attractive and slightly overweight or plump.

Rhus toxicodendron

Rhus tox.; *Rhus radicaris*, American poison ivy, poison oak, poison vine.

This large bush or small tree is a native species of the United States and Canada. Its leaves are extremely irritant to the touch causing an inflamed and painful rash, swelling and ulceration Often the person experiences malaise, swollen glands headache, feverishness and a lack of appetite. The plant produces white flowers with a green or yellow tinge in June, followed later by clusters of berries. The fresh leaves are gathered and pulped to make the remedy used in homeopathy . It is used especially as a treatment for skin rashes and lesions with hot, burning sensations and also for inflammation of muscles and joints. Hence it is used to treat eczema, chilblains, cold sores, shingles, nappy rash and other conditions in which there is a dry, scaling or blistered skin. Also, for rheumatism, sciatica, lumbago, gout, synovitis (inflammation of the synovial membranes surrounding joints), osteoarthritis, ligament and tendon strains. Feverish symptoms caused by viral infections, such as high temperature, chills and shivering, swollen, watering eyes, aching joints, nausea and vomiting, may be helped by Rhus tox. Some menstrual problems, including heavy bleeding and abdominal pains that are relieved by lying down, benefit from this remedy. People who are helped by Rhus tox tend to be depressed and miserable when ill, with a tendency to burst into tears, and are highly susceptible to cold, damp weather. Usually they have a dry, irritating cough and thirst and are irritable, anxious and restless. The symptoms are made worse in stormy, wet, windy weather and at night, and when the person moves after a period of rest. Also, for becoming chilled when undressing. Warm, dry conditions and gentle exercise improve and lessen the symptoms. Rhus tox people may be initially shy in company, but when they lose this are charming, entertaining and lively and make friends easily. They are usually conscientious and highly motivated and serious about their work to the extent of being somewhat workaholic. Rhus tox people often have an inner restlessness and become depressed and moody when affected by illness. They may be prone to carry out small compulsive rituals in order to function.

Ruta graveolens

Ruta grav.; rue, garden rue, herbygrass, ave-grace, herb-of-grace, bitter herb

This hardy, evergreen plant is a native of southern Europe but has been cultivated in Britain for centuries, having been first brought here by the Romans. It thrives in poor soil in a dry and partially shaded situation, producing yellow-green flowers. The whole plant has a distinctive, pungent, unpleasant smell and was once used to repel insects, pestilence and infections. It has been used medicinally throughout history to treat ailments in both animals and people, and was used to guard against the plague. It was believed to be effective in guarding against witchcraft, and Hippocrates recommended it as an antidote to poisoning. Rue was believed to have beneficial effects on sight and was used by the great artists, such as Michelangelo, to keep vision sharp. In the Catholic High Mass, brushes made from rue were once used to sprinkle the holy water, hence the name herb-of-grace. Taken internally in large doses, rue has toxic effects causing vomiting, a swollen tongue, fits and delirium.

The homeopathic remedy is prepared from the sap of the green parts of the plant before the flowers open. It is indicated especially for bone and joint injuries and disorders, and those affecting tendons, ligaments and muscles where there is severe, deep, tearing pain. Hence it is used for synovitis (inflammation of the synovial membranes lining joints), rheumatism, sprains, strains, bruising, fractures and dislocations and also sciatica. Also, it is a useful remedy for eyestrain with tired, aching eyes, redness and inflammation and headache. Chest problems may be relieved by Ruta grav., particularly painful deep coughs, and some problems affecting the rectum, such as prolapse. Pain and infection in the socket of a tooth after dental extraction may be helped by this remedy. A person who is ill and who benefits from Ruta grav. tends to feel low, anxious, depressed and dissatisfied both with himself (or herself) and others. The symptoms are usually worse in cold, damp weather, for resting and lying down and for exercise out of doors. They improve with heat and gentle movement indoors.

Sepia officinalis

Sepia; ink of the cuttlefish

Cuttlefish ink has been used since ancient times, both for medicinal purposes and as a colour in artists' paint. The cuttlefish has the ability to change colour to blend in with its surroundings and squirts out the dark brown-black ink when threatened by predators. Sepia was known to Roman physicians who used it as a cure for baldness. In homeopathy it is mainly used as an excellent remedy for women experiencing menstrual and menopausal problems. It was investigated and proved by Hahnemann in 1834. It is used to treat premenstrual tension, menstrual pain and heavy bleeding, infrequent or suppressed periods, menopausal symptoms such as hot flushes, and post-natal depression. Physical and emotional symptoms caused by an imbalance of hormones are helped by Sepia. Also, conditions in which there is extreme fatigue or exhaustion with muscular aches and pains. Digestive complaints, including nausea and sickness, abdominal pain and wind, caused by eating dairy products, and headaches with giddiness and nausea are relieved by Sepia. Also, it is a remedy for incontinence, hot, sweaty feet and verruca (a wart on the foot). A woman often experiences pelvic, dragging pains frequently associated with prolapse of the womb. Disorders of the circulation, especially varicose veins and cold extremities, benefit from sepia.

Symptoms are worse in cold weather and before a thunderstorm, and in the late afternoon, evening and early in the morning. Also, before a period in women and if the person receives sympathy from others. The symptoms are better with heat and warmth, quick vigorous movements, having plenty to do and out in the fresh open air. People suitable for Sepia are usually, but not exclusively, women. They tend to be tall, thin and with a yellowish complexion, and are rather self-contained and indifferent to others. Sepia people may become easily cross, especially with family and close friends, and harbour resentment. In company, they make a great effort to appear outgoing and love to dance. A woman may be either an externally hard, successful career person or someone who constantly feels unable to cope, especially with looking after the home and family. Sepia people have strongly held beliefs and cannot stand others taking a contrary opinion. When ill, they hate to be fussed over or have the sympathy of others. They like both sour and sweet foods and alcoholic drinks but are upset by milk products and fatty meals. They harbour deep insecurity and fear being left alone, illness resulting in madness, and loss of their material possessions and wealth. One physical attribute is that they often have a brown mark in the shape of a saddle across the bridge of the nose.

Silicea terra

Silicea; silica

Silica is one of the main rock-forming minerals and is also found in living things, where its main function is to confer strength and resilience. In homeopathy , it is used to treat disorders of the skin, nails and bones and recurring inflammations and infections, especially those that occur because the person is somewhat rundown or has an inadequate diet. Also, some disorders of the nervous system are relieved by Silicea. The homeopathic remedy used to be derived from ground flint or quartz but is now prepared by chemical reaction. The remedy is used for catarrhal infections such as colds, influenza, sinusitis, eye infections including glue ear. Also, for inflammations producing pus, such as a boil, carbuncle, abscess, stye, whitlow (infection of the fingernail) and peritonsillar abscess. It is beneficial in helping the natural expulsion of a foreign body, such as a splinter in the skin. It is a remedy for a headache beginning at the back of the head and radiating forwards over the right eye, and for stress-related conditions of overwork and sleeplessness.

Symptoms are worse for cold, wet weather, especially when clothing is inadequate, draughts, swimming and bathing, becoming chilled after removing clothes and in the morning. They are better for warmth and heat, summer weather, warm clothing, particularly a hat or head covering, and not lying on the left side. People who are suitable for Silicea tend to be thin with a fine build and pale skin. They often have thin straight hair. They are prone to dry, cracked skin and nails and may suffer from skin infections. Silicea people are usually unassuming and lacking in confidence and physical stamina. They are conscientious and hard-working to the point of working too hard once a task has been undertaken. However, they may hesitate to commit themselves through lack of confidence and fear of responsibility. Silicea people are tidy and obsessive about small details. They may feel 'put upon' but lack the courage to speak out, and may take this out on others who are not responsible for the situation. They fear failure and dislike exercise because of physical weakness, often feeling mentally and physically exhausted. They enjoy cold foods and drinks.

Sulphur

Sulphur, flowers of sulphur, brimstone

Sulphur has a long history of use in medicine going back to very ancient times. Sulphur gives off sulphur dioxide when burnt, which smells unpleasant ('rotten eggs' odour) but acts as a disinfectant. This was used in mediaeval times to limit the spread of infectious diseases. Sulphur is deposited around the edges of hot springs and geysers and where there is volcanic activity. Flowers of sulphur, which is a bright yellow powder, is obtained from the natural mineral deposit and is used to make the homeopathic remedy. Sulphur is found naturally in all body tissues, and in both orthodox medicine and homeopathy is used to treat skin disorders. It is a useful remedy for dermatitis, eczema, psoriasis and a dry, flaky, itchy skin or scalp. Some digestive disorders benefit from it, especially a tendency for food to rise back up to the mouth and indigestion caused by drinking milk. Sulphur is helpful in the treatment of haemorrhoids, or piles, premenstrual and menopausal symptoms, eye inflamma-tions such as conjunctivitis, pain in the lower part of the back, catarrhal colds and coughs, migraine headaches and feverish symptoms. Some mental symptoms are helped by this remedy, particularly those brought about by stress or worry, including depression, irritability, insomnia and lethargy. When ill, people who benefit from sulphur feel thirsty rather than hungry and are upset by unpleasant smells. The person soon becomes exhausted and usually sleeps poorly at night and is tired through the day. The symptoms are worse in cold, damp conditions, in the middle of the morning around 11 a.m., and in stuffy, hot, airless rooms. Also, for becoming too hot at night in bed and for wearing too many layers of clothes. Long periods of standing and sitting aggravate the symptoms, and they are worse if the person drinks alcohol or has a wash. Symptoms improve in dry, clear, warm weather and for taking exercise. They are better if the person lies on the right side.

Sulphur people tend to look rather untidy and have dry, flaky skin and coarse, rough hair. They may be thin, round-shouldered and inclined to slouch or be overweight, round and red-faced. Sulphur people have lively, intelligent minds full of schemes and inventions, but are often useless on a practical level. They may be somewhat self-centred with a need to be praised, and fussy over small unimportant details. They enjoy intellectual discussion on subjects that they find interesting and may become quite heated although the anger soon subsides. Sulphur people are often warm and generous with their time and money. They enjoy a wide range of foods but are upset by milk and eggs. They have a fear of being a failure in their work, of heights and the supernatural.

Tarentula cubensis

Tarentula cub.; Cuban tarantula

The bite of the Cuban tarantula spider produces a delayed response in the victim. About 24 hours after a bite, the site becomes inflamed and red, and swelling, fever and abscess follow. The homeopathic remedy, made from the poison of the spider, is used to treat similar septic conditions, such as an abscess, boil, carbuncle or whitlow (an infection of the fingernail) and genital itching. Also, it is a remedy for anthrax and shock, and is of value as a last-resort treatment in severe conditions. The infected areas are often tinged blue, and there may be burning sensations of pain that are especially severe at night. It is of particular value in the treatment of recurring boils or carbuncles. The symptoms tend to improve with smoking and are made worse by physical activity and consuming cold drinks.

Thuja occidentalis

Thuja; tree of life, yellow cedar, arbor vitae, false white cedar

This coniferous, evergreen tree is a native species of the

northern United States and Canada and grows to a height of about 30 feet. It has feathery green leaves with a strong, aromatic smell resembling that of camphor. The leaves and twigs were used by the Indian peoples to treat a variety of infections and disorders, and the plant has long been used in herbal medicine. It is an important remedy in aromatherapy. The fresh green leaves and twigs are used to prepare the homeopathic remedy, which is especially valuable in the treatment of warts and wartlike tumours on any part of the body. It is a useful remedy for shingles and also has an effect on the genital and urinary tracts. Hence it is used to treat inflammations and infections such as cystitis and urethritis and also pain on ovulation. It may be given as a remedy for infections of the mouth, teeth and gums, catarrh and for tension headaches.

People who benefit from Thuja tend to sweat profusely, and it helps to alleviate this symptom. They tend to suffer from insomnia and when they do manage to sleep, may talk or cry out. They are prone to severe left-sided frontal headaches that may be present on waking in the morning. Symptoms are worse at night, from being too hot in bed and after breakfast. Also, at 3 a.m. and 3 p.m. and in weather that is cold and wet. Symptoms are felt more severely on the left side. Symptoms improve for movement and stretching of the limbs, massage and after sweating. People suitable for Thuja tend to be insecure and unsure about themselves. They try hard to please others but are very sensitive to criticism and soon become depressed. This may lead them to neglect their appearance. Thuja people are often thin and pale and tend to have greasy skin and perspire easily.

Urtica urens

Urtica; stinging nettle

One of the few plants that is familiar to all and that, for hundreds of years, has been valued for its medicinal and culinary uses. Nettles have always been used as a source of food both for people and animals, the young leaves being a nutritious vegetable with a high content of vitamin C. Nettles were thought to purify the blood, and an ancient cure for rheumatism and muscular weakness was the practice of 'urtication', or lashing the body with stinging nettles. The hairs covering the leaves of the nettle release a volatile liquid when touched, which causes the familiar skin reaction of painful, white bumps to appear. The fresh, green parts of the plant are used to prepare the homeopathic remedy, which is used as a treatment for burning and stinging of the skin. Hence it is used to treat allergic reactions of the skin, urticaria, or nettle rash, insect bites and stings and skin lesions caused by burns and scalds. Also, for eczema, chicken pox, nerve inflammation and pain (neuritis and neuralgia), shingles, rheumatism, gout and cystitis in which there are burning, stinging pains. The person who benefits from this remedy is prone to inflamed, itching and irritated skin complaints and may be fretful, impatient and restless. Symptoms are made worse by touch and in cold, wet weather, snow and for contact with water. Allergic skin reactions may occur if the person eats shellfish such as prawns. The symptoms improve if the affected skin is rubbed and also if the person rests and lies down.

Index

543